PRINCIPLES *of* VASCULAR *and* INTRAVASCULAR ULTRASOUND

PRINCIPLES *of* VASCULAR *and* INTRAVASCULAR ULTRASOUND

STUART J. HUTCHISON, MD, FRCPC, FACC, FAHA

Clinical Professor of Medicine
University of Calgary
Departments of Cardiac Sciences, Medicine, and Radiology
Director of Echocardiography
Foothills Medical Center
Calgary, Ontario
Canada

KATHERINE C. HOLMES, RVT, RT(R)

Team Leader, Vascular Ultrasound Laboratory
Division of Cardiology
St. Michael's Hospital
Toronto, Ontario
Canada

ELSEVIER
SAUNDERS

1600 John F. Kennedy Blvd.
Ste 1800
Philadelphia, PA 19103-2899

PRINCIPLES OF VASCULAR AND INTRAVASCULAR ULTRASOUND   ISBN 978-1-4377-0404-4
Copyright © 2012 by Saunders, an imprint of Elsevier Inc.

Notice

Knowledge and best practice in this field are constantly changing. As new research and experience broaden our understanding, changes in research methods, professional practices, or medical treatment may become necessary.

Practitioners and researchers must always rely on their own experience and knowledge in evaluating and using any information, methods, compounds, or experiments described herein. In using such information or methods, they should be mindful of their own safety and the safety of others, including parties for whom they have a professional responsibility.

With respect to any drug or pharmaceutical products identified, readers are advised to check the most current information provided (i) on procedures featured or (ii) by the manufacturer of each product to be administered, to verify the recommended dose or formula, the method and duration of administration, and contraindications. It is the responsibility of practitioners, relying on their own experience and knowledge of their patients, to make diagnoses, to determine dosages and the best treatment for each individual patient, and to take all appropriate safety precautions.

To the fullest extent of the law, neither the Publisher nor the authors, contributors, or editors, assume any liability for any injury and/or damage to persons or property as a matter of products liability, negligence or otherwise, or from any use or operation of any methods, products, instructions, or ideas contained in the material herein.

ISBN 978-1-4377-0404-4

Acquisitions Editor: Natasha Andjelkovic
Developmental Editor: Bradley McIlwain
Publishing Services Manager: Pat Joiner-Myers
Project Manager: Marlene Weeks
Designer: Steven Stave

Printed in China.
Last digit is the print number: 9 8 7 6 5 4 3 2 1

To my Cindy, Noel Keith, and Liam James. Your gifts of love, time, and belief can only ever be repaid in kind.

SJH

To Miles Cramer, RVT, for incredible teaching, encouragement, example, collegiality and friendship.

SJH and KCH

My deep appreciation goes to Stuart Hutchison for giving me the opportunity to participate in this adventure.

I dedicate this book to Maggie, whose love and support have enabled me to realize a dream.

KCH

CONTRIBUTORS

Junya Ako, MD
Center for Research in Cardiovascular
   Interventions
Stanford University Medical Center
Stanford, California

Joe Chauvapun, MD
Department of Surgery
Harbor-UCLA Medical Center
Torrance, California

Katherine C. Holmes, RVT, RT(R)
Team Leader, Vascular Ultrasound Laboratory
Division of Cardiology
St. Michael's Hospital
Toronto, Ontario
Canada

Stuart J. Hutchison, MD, FRCPC, FACC, FAHA
Clinical Professor of Medicine
University of Calgary
Departments of Cardiac Sciences, Medicine,
   and Radiology
Director of Echocardiography
Foothills Medical Center
Calgary, Ontario
Canada

George E. Kopchok, BS
Los Angeles Biomedical Research Institute
Harbor-UCLA Medical Center
Torrance, California

Katsuhisa Waseda, MD
Center for Research in Cardiovascular
   Interventions
Stanford University Medical Center
Stanford, California

Rodney A. White, MD
Vascular Surgery Division Chief
Vascular Surgery Fellowship Program Director
Vice Chairman of Research
Harbor-UCLA Medical Center
David Geffen School of Medicine
University of California, Los Angeles
Torrance, California

PREFACE

Vascular ultrasound represents one of the first successful applications of Doppler ultrasound to clinical medicine, and it has evolved to be a versatile diagnostic test for the assessment of both arterial and venous disease. Given the anatomic extent and potential complexities of arterial and venous trees and the inherent requirements of ultrasound imaging, vascular ultrasound has its limitations, but when approached properly and formally (with thorough and structured protocols), it is a very useful diagnostic tool. Attention to technique and to detail and an attempt to have the greatest knowledge possible of native anatomy and its variants, vascular diseases and their permutations, and interventional and surgical techniques maximize the yield of vascular ultrasound.

The historic standard of comparison of vascular ultrasound has been conventional angiography/venography. With the progress and developments of computed tomography (CT) angiography and magnetic resonance (MR) angiography, both of which also have as their basis of comparison conventional angiography, the respective roles of vascular ultrasound, CT angiography, and MR angiography are evolving and are slowly being defined. Each modality has its strengths and weaknesses. CT and MR angiography are anatomic tests; vascular ultrasound is both a physiologic and an anatomic test. Vascular ultrasound is still currently the pre-eminent noninvasive test of venous disease; CT venography is less competitive. CT angiography is certainly a rising contributor to the assessment of arterial disease, but vascular ultrasound remains a radiation-free means to initially assess arterial disease.

This book is our attempt to summarize and provide our experience, principles, and approach to the application of vascular ultrasound to the arterial and venous vascular fields, and also a platform from which to stalwartly encourage structured and thorough technique and protocol, as well as awareness of disease permutations.

It is our hope that this book will prove useful to those who are dedicated to providing care to patients through the clinical application of vascular ultrasound.

Acknowledgments. We acknowledge with appreciation Adrien Boutin, Vern M. Campbell, Tony M. Chou, Melma J. Evangelista, Allan J. Lossing, Krishnankutty Sudhir, Inga Tomas, William S. Tucker, and contributors Junya Ako, Joe Chauvapun, George E. Kopchok, Katsuhisa Waseda, and Rodney A. White.

Stuart J. Hutchison
Katherine C. Holmes

CONTENTS

Technical Issues in Vascular Ultrasound

1

Key Points

- Maximizing and easing optimal image acquisition is achieved by:
  - Integration of knowledge of anatomy, disease, machine factors, and scanning technique
  - Effort and persistence

BASIC GUIDELINES

Optimizing Settings: Beyond Factory Presets

Although providing a useful starting point, factory settings and algorithms are designed for optimal scanning of patients of average body habitus, without consideration of precisely what is to be depicted or measured. Further optimization and enhancement of the image and color or spectral Doppler for a particular study/zone can be achieved by directed empiric manual adjustment of machine settings. Knowledge and confidence with machine settings provides incremental diagnostic yield and avoidance of many artifacts.

Knowledge of Anatomic Variants: As Important As Knowledge of Normal Anatomy

Arterial, and especially venous, anatomy is subject to a considerable range of variation. Failing to consider anatomic variation in the evaluation of a suspected disease may preclude its recognition. For example, normally, the superficial femoral vein lies posterior to the superficial femoral artery. However, in as many as 30% of cases, the superficial femoral vein/popliteal venous anatomy is that of a bifid, and occasionally trifid, variant. Thrombosis of such an anatomic variant system commonly involves only one of its limbs. If the thrombosed limb of a bifid system is situated posterior to the artery, then only the anterior venous limb is seen at first glance. Failure to search for the presence of a diseased posterior limb may miss the presence of thrombosis. Failure to search the entire field may lead to failure to detect thrombosis of an anomalous vein.

Flow Direction: Should Be Determined Rather Than Assumed

The direction of flow within a vessel should never be assumed. In several pathologies (those that involve upstream tight stenosis or occlusion with large downstream collaterals or complex recanalization), flow within an artery may be reversed in direction, which would therefore clearly establish the presence of significant pathology. Examples, such as subtotal or complete occlusion of the common carotid artery where collaterals from the external carotid artery reconstitute flow at the bifurcation to maintain patency of the internal carotid artery, abound.

Encountering Technical Difficulties

If part of a scan is technically difficult, try the following maneuvers: (1) change the patient/body part position, (2) change the scanning angle of approach, (3) change the transducer frequency, or (4) call in a colleague—sometimes a different hand or eye can help. If these do not yield improved image quality, proceed to scan another vessel or segment and return to the difficult section later.

Optimal Sonographer Positioning for Carotid Scanning

For all scanning, when possible, use the elbow of the scanning arm and part of the scanning hand (such as a finger) as a fulcrum to maximize manual stability and to minimize muscle and joint strain. Perform hand and arm stretches and exercises before scanning every day to minimize repetitive strain injury. Consider scanning with both left and right hands and learn to scan with the ultrasound machine at both the foot and the head of the patient. This is useful on the ward, where monitoring equipment is inevitably in the way.

Scanning with the Nondominant Hand

Scanning with the nondominant arm and hand is easier than it first appears and can be learned quickly (often within a week). Distribution of the repetitive strain of scanning between the upper extremities may help stave off wear-and-tear injuries to the upper extremities and spine. Developing some versatility of scanning with both hands is particularly useful when having to perform portable scans at the bedside, such as in the intensive care unit, where there is medical equipment around the bed, rendering it impossible for the sonographer to stand in the ideal/usual position for scanning. In such a case, lack of access to positioning oneself above the head of the patient for carotid scanning results in the need to scan facing the patient and use of the hands in the reverse position from usual. Use of a triangle-wedge sponge pad or towel to support the scanning limb may also avoid excess strain.

Optimal Patient Position for Scanning

Patient comfort during scanning is important, and the patients' position should be such that they are comfortable throughout. Patients who are uncomfortable may: (1) adjust their body position to alleviate the discomfort and move during scanning, (2) often tense their limb muscles, and (3) be unable to undergo a complete scan. Neck stretches for carotid scanning are not necessary and may be counterproductive because they provoke discomfort in many patients. Similarly, leg abduction (to scan the popliteal fossa) in elderly or orthopedic patients with hip or other leg problems is often uncomfortable for patients and unnecessary because the distal superficial femoral and popliteal vessels can be scanned from the posterolateral side.

Internal Consistency of Testing

Retain an understanding of the "big picture"—how all the pieces may (or may not) fit together. If, for instance, a lower extremity study consists of both ankle-brachial index recordings and an arterial lower extremity duplex scan, and the results from the two components do not lead to the same conclusion, consider: (1) repeating one or part of one of the tests, (2) disease-based reasons that may explain the observations, and (3) the role of further testing.

Standardization of Laboratory Algorithms and Criteria

A standard diagnostic algorithm, per pathology, should be established and adhered to in the laboratory. Just as importantly, diagnostic criteria should be standardized. Standard, but adaptable, diagnostic algorithms and diagnostic criteria keep results consistent from one patient visit to the next, from one patient to another, and from one sonographer to another.

Clinical Context and Complementary Data

Review available notes and compile an appropriate medical history to establish and understand the clinical profile of the case. Whenever possible, seek the results of subsequent follow-up testing.

Scanning the Anatomic Length of the Vessel

To maximize the recognition of disease within an artery or vein, scan along the complete length of the vessel from its ostium to terminus when possible. Although the more proximal and distal aspects of vessels are regularly more difficult to image, they are particularly important to scan. For example, atherosclerosis occasionally occurs at the origin of the common carotid artery, as it may at the ostia of the vertebral and innominate arteries. Ostial lesions are often, but not necessarily, suggested by the detection of turbulent flow encountered further downstream in the more readily imaged portions of vessels, and there is no plausible explanation of the origin of the turbulence, other than downstream transmission from an upstream lesion. Ostial lesions that send elevated velocities downstream render assessment of more distal stenoses difficult, unless there has been recovery of flow velocity to normal levels before such downstream lesions.

Avoiding Singularization of Focus and Findings

Beware of focusing on one lesion to the exclusion of others that are present. This can readily occur, particularly when the scan is difficult. Common examples include (1) finding one endoleak but missing others, (2) finding an iatrogenically created pseudoaneurysm but missing an arteriovenous fistula, and (3) finding an extensive deep venous thrombosis but missing concomitant superficial venous thrombosis.

Localizing Lesions by Anatomic Reference Points

Using landmarks to localize the position is helpful when comparing findings with radiographic studies. For example, lesional position in the superficial femoral artery measured with respect to inguinal ligament/groin crease, with respect to the lower border of the patellar (knee joint), or of the internal carotid artery with respect to the angle of mandible may facilitate comparison with findings from angiographic, computed tomography, or magnetic resonance angiography studies. The referencing of lesions by superficial or deep anatomy facilitates intertest comparisons, such as preintervention and postintervention.

Avoiding Mistaken Identity: Differentiation of Collateral from Native Vessels

When interrogating peripheral arteries, beware of mistaking a stem vessel (the collateral or efferent artery that is the first part of the bypass system around a significant occlusion) for a stenosis. Typically, flow at the point where the stem vessel branches out exhibits a high velocity profile (because flow in the branch is being sampled off-axis with angle possibly unknown and flow velocity will be higher as compensation for the stenosis/occlusion downstream) and turbulent (because flow in the branch vessel is not being sampled necessarily in midstream, because most are small arteries).

Similarly, when scanning the superficial femoral artery, it is possible to mistake a straight segment of bridging collaterals as the anticipated/intended native vessel, particularly if the course of the collateral vessels is near to and parallel with the occluded vessel, facilitating "mistaken identity." A midzone collateral network may be distinguished from a diseased, stringy, but patent native lumen by use of a lower frequency transducer that enables a wider field of view and often allows visualization of both collateral and patent native vessel segments in the same planes. Identification of the vein that accompanies the artery and knowledge of the vessels' usual alignment may assist with distinguishing parallel collaterals from an occluded main artery, because a collateral vessel most likely runs quite separately from the vein.

Always try to follow a vessel from its origin to be certain of its source. This lessens potential confusion in the case of complex, and often very important, lesions. For example, in the presence of distal aortic occlusion, it is common for the inferior mesenteric to enlarge, supply collaterals around the blockage, and, as it invariably runs parallel, take on the appearance of a patent iliac artery.

GRAYSCALE IMAGING ISSUES

Grayscale Settings
To optimize grayscale images, in addition to gain controls, consider adjusting the following settings/parameters to enhance detail:
1. Persistence. Optimization of persistence smoothes the appearance of the image and reduces speckle artifact.
2. Harmonics. Optimization of harmonic frequency enhances the depiction of deep structures as well as improving grayscale contrast (although increasing the selected harmonic frequency reduces the frame rate and can be attempted, for example, when trying to image a poorly depicted distal internal carotid artery, before resorting to a deeper penetrating transducer.
3. Tissue colorization (allows the eye to see detail that was not readily apparent in the plain grayscale image)
4. Scanning initially without color Doppler flow mapping to pick up nuances in grayscale findings, because such fine detail may be washed over by color (as a general rule, only apply color Doppler flow mapping after the grayscale image has been optimized and acquired).

Grayscale imaging issues are illustrated in Figures 1-1 to 1-5.

Recognition of Artifacts
With grayscale imaging, to differentiate between a genuine intraluminal lesion and an artifact, observe carefully to see if the suspected artifact moves with the vessel's movement and whether it extends outside of the lumen of the vessel, which would generally be implausible for an intraluminal lesion such as thrombus or atherosclerosis.

COLOR DOPPLER ISSUES: COLOR DOPPLER SETTINGS

To optimize color Doppler flow mapping, adjustment of the following settings may improve saturation:
1. Color write. When grayscale bleeds through the color Doppler flow mapping, this function assigns more color pixels to the color Doppler map in proportion to the background grayscale.
2. Color maps
3. Selection of a different color Doppler map. This, a change for the eyes, may assist with recognition of detail (e.g., use of color tagging, often called variance [green], in an area of stenosis, illuminates the high-velocity stenotic jet without having to rely on aliasing for localization).

Where significant occlusive disease or venous thrombosis is present, the potential for complicated flow patterns and altered flow directions in both main and branch vessels is high. To minimize the likelihood of reaching an erroneous conclusion, it is essential to understand clearly at the outset how use of color box steering represents flow colorization and direction representation.

Color Doppler imaging issues are illustrated in Figures 1-6 to 1-14.

SPECTRAL DOPPLER SAMPLING AND DISPLAY ISSUES

Spectral Doppler Settings
Spectral maps may help delineate an unclear waveform peak by adding detail and increasing the spectral gain without adding unwanted noise in the form of either background "snow"-type noise or envelope noise, leading to overestimation of measurements. In addition, there is subjective difference in the representation of spectral profiles according to different color displays. Whatever display provides the optimal sense of ease in visual assessment and appears to avoid visual harshness or glare is desirable.

Although color Doppler is, among other things, useful as a guide for spectral Doppler placement, it has the potential to impair visualization of the Doppler cursor and the location of the sampling. Sampling of slightly different areas of a lesion on repeat scans may engender misinterpretation of lesional severity difference. Color Doppler flow mapping should be used to set up sampling. However, a grayscale image following the color Doppler set-up image that precisely establishes the site of sampling and the orientation of the sampling alignment as perpendicular to the vessel wall is useful and a measure of quality assurance.

Although considerable controversy has always existed regarding optimal Doppler cursor angulation (alignment parallel to the walls or to the flow), it is most reasonable to say that whichever method is used, reproducibility can only be achieved if the same method is used throughout a study and for every case. For example, establishing the internal carotid artery–to–common carotid artery peak systolic velocity (PSV) ratio requires recording velocities using the same method of angle correction and at the exact same angle of incidence in both the common carotid and internal carotid arteries.

Effect of Slice Thickness on Spectral Sampling

Slice thickness can contribute more to the spectral Doppler display than is evident. For example, when the internal carotid artery is occluded and the sample volume is placed within the internal carotid artery (occluded) lumen, it is often possible to pick up a strong signal from the adjacent internal jugular vein. Slight movement of the intended sampling away from the intended site may contribute to "sampling error." To further complicate matters, in some instances, flow in the internal jugular vein may be misleading and misinterpreted. For example, flow in the internal jugular vein may be pulsatile and with elements above and below the baseline, such as occurs in cases of severe tricuspid regurgitation. To maintain sampling at the intended site, Doppler acquisition with simultaneous real-time grayscale scanning assists in stabilizing acquisition from within the intended sampling site, although with reduction of the color Doppler frame rate, and rougher/less refined grayscale. Recruitment maneuvers that cause variation in venous flow patterns such as having the patient take a deep breath (which leads initially to flow acceleration followed by brief flow cessation) reveal that the sampled flow is venous rather than arterial.

Spectral Doppler sampling issues are illustrated in Figures 1-15 to 1-33.

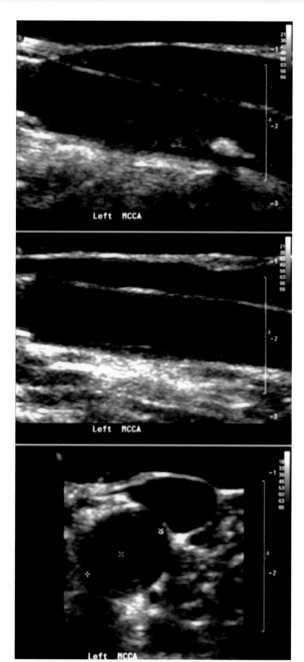

Figure 1-1. The effect of approach angle (of insonation) on grayscale imaging. *Top,* A significant plaque is seen in the common carotid artery. *Middle,* The plaque is not evident, although the image was obtained on nearly the same level. *Bottom,* A short-axis image (SAX) reveals the eccentric plaque in the common carotid artery that is responsible for the depiction of plaque in the middle image and shows the utility of SAX scanning.

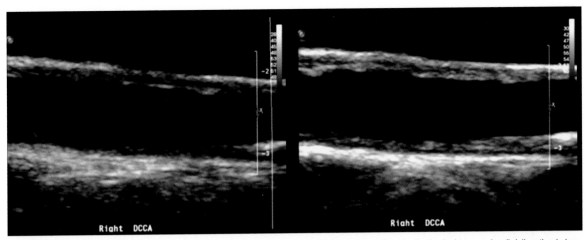

Figure 1-2. The effect of grayscale setting on vessel and lumen depiction. *Left,* With lower grayscale gain, the luminal-to-vessel wall delineation is less. *Right,* With optimal grayscale gain, there is near-continuous delineation of the boundary and a better impression of the intimal topography and the luminal characteristics.

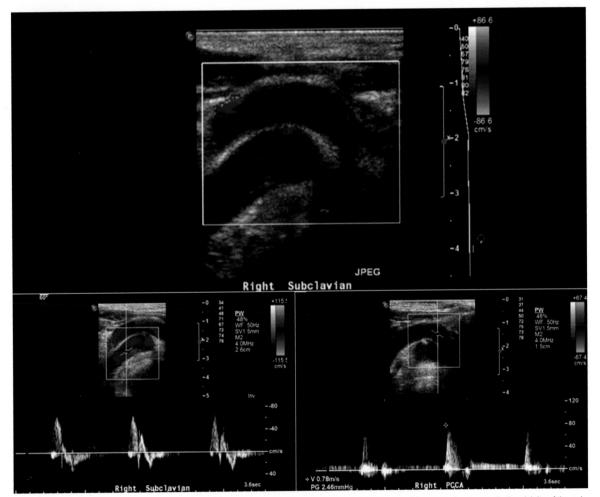

Figure 1-3. Nonphantom image. *Top,* This grayscale image suggests that there might be a phantom vessel image, as is common in the vicinity of the sub-clavian artery, due to reflection of the ultrasound beam from more superficial structures (e.g., clavicle). *Bottom,* The images reveal the different flow patterns in the vessels, which are actually real and the common carotid artery and right subclavian artery.

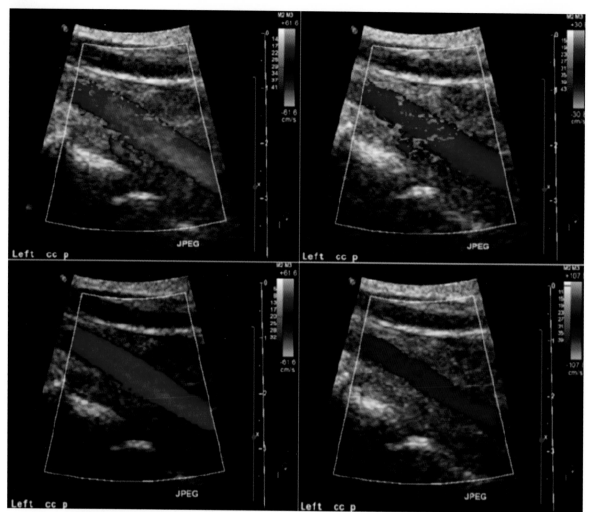

Figure 1-4. The effect of color Doppler gain, pulse repetition frequency (PRF), grayscale gain, and color write settings on optimizing hybrid grayscale and color Doppler flow mapping images. *Top left,* Color Doppler and grayscale gain settings are both too high, resulting in color bleeding onto nearby tissue and grayscale bleeding onto the color flow map. *Top right,* Attempting to optimize the color flow mapping and lessen the grayscale gain artifact by reducing color Doppler PRF, the image quality is still suboptimal with compromise of the quality of the flow mapping, and with more color bleeding onto nearby tissue. *Bottom left,* With grayscale gain optimized (reduced), the grayscale bleeding onto the flow mapping has been successfully eliminated. Also, the color bleeding has also been largely corrected, without adjusting PRF or color Doppler gain. The saturation of the color Doppler mapping is also improved, if not exquisite. *Bottom right,* Original grayscale and color gain settings with adjustment of the color write/PRF. Color Doppler flow mapping gives a good impression of homogeneous flow and a different impression of the intimal surface. Which of the two bottom images gives the truer impression of the intimal surfaces is ambiguous, but they do offer a congruent impression of the flow.

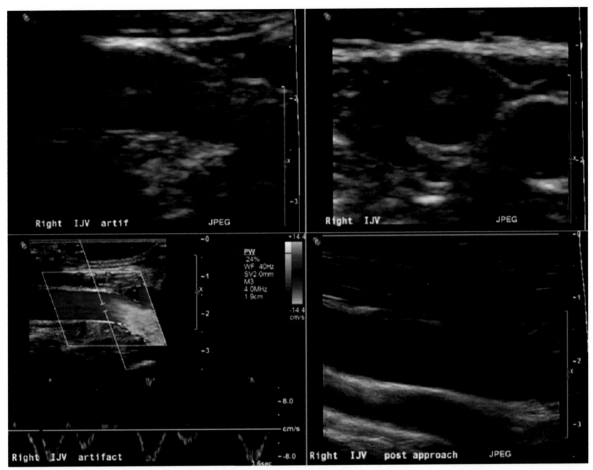

Figure 1-5. Grayscale artifacts suggesting intraluminal material. *Top left and right,* These images represent an artifact of soft tissue within the lumen of the internal jugular vein. *Bottom left,* Color Doppler depiction and spectral flow display discounted the presence of intraluminal material. *Bottom right,* Image taken from a more posterior approach eliminates the artifact.

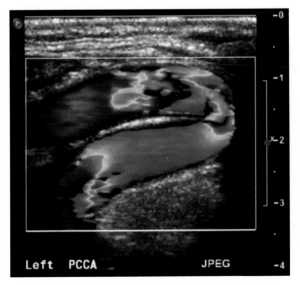

Figure 1-6. The effect of tortuosity and varying angle of incidence on color Doppler flow-mapping. At the site of curvature of the right side of the image, flow mapping depicts convergence (isovelocity zones). This may result from near-perfect alignment of sampling that depicts the highest frequency shift or from folding and actual narrowing. The complex flow in the upper segment may similarly be due to either downstream turbulence to slight narrowing at the fold or to alignment so near to 90 degrees that small directional variation is depicted as flow in different directions. Pulsed-wave Doppler sampling at the site of the fold would be a technical challenge to maintain angle correction of 60 degrees and parallelism with the vessels walls. Most carotid atherosclerotic disease is situated within the first 1 to 3 cm of the internal carotid artery, and tortuosity is generally proximal or distal to that.

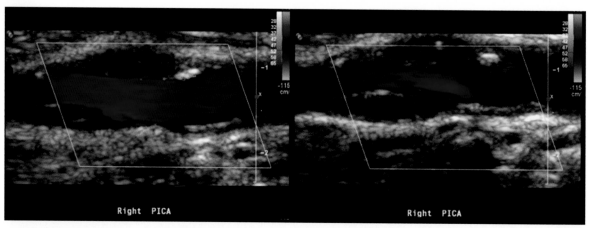

Figure 1-7. In these images of the internal carotid artery, the influence of color Doppler gain is exemplified. *Left,* The gain is too high, and the color representation of flow exceeds the actual lumen and extends over the plaque, over-representing the luminal width. *Right,* The color Doppler gain has been adjusted to map the true lumen.

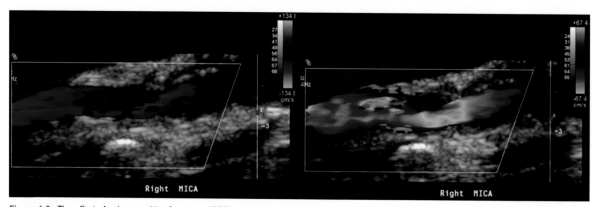

Figure 1-8. The effect of pulse repetition frequency (PRF) settings on flow mapping, lumen depiction, and the impression of stenosis severity. *Left,* The image is fairly successful in flow-mapping the vessel without bleeding artifact, but there are color voids within the vessel. Some grayscale bleeding onto the flow voids in the center affords confusion about whether there is a bulk of hypoechoic material. *Right,* The PRF has been reduced to capture flow in low velocity/low Doppler shift pixels. The lower PRF has enabled depiction of the nearfield jugular venous flow and also resulted in some color Doppler bleeding onto structures away from the lumen.

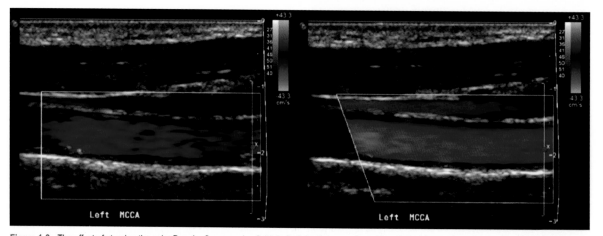

Figure 1-9. The effect of steering the color Doppler flow mapping field. *Left,* Color flow mapping without left–right steering of the profile. *Right,* Steering the field into the flow has optimized the flow mapping.

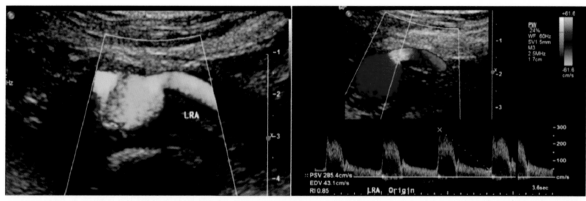

Figure 1-10. The effect of power Doppler flow-mapping on flow mapping depiction and on flow convergence. *Left,* Power Doppler flow mapping clearly delineates the left renal artery ostium and proximal segment. *Right,* The standard color Doppler flow mapping depicts isovelocity flow convergence consistent with stenosis, which is confirmed by pulsed Doppler sampling/spectral display of elevated velocities. Both modes of color Doppler imaging are useful and complement each other. (Courtesy of Miles Cramer, RVT, Bellingham, WA.)

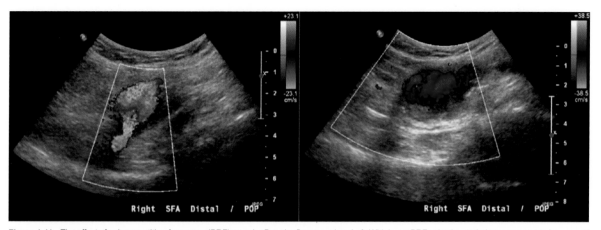

Figure 1-11. The effect of pulse repetition frequency (PRF) on color Doppler flow mapping. *Left,* With lower PRF selection, turbulence appears to be present within an aneurysm. *Right,* With an increase in PRF, flow within the aneurysm appears to be normal.

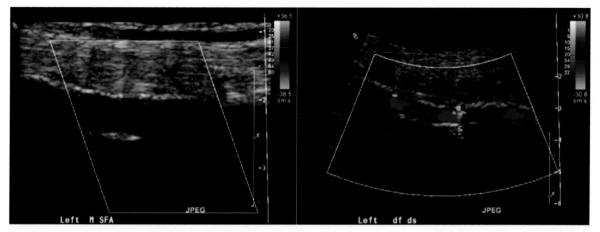

Figure 1-12. The effect of medial calcinosis shadowing on flow and of transducer selection on flow imaging. *Left,* Linear transducer selection and steerage of the color flow mapping field into the flow. No flow is detected, due to shadowing from the medial calcinosis. *Right,* Imaging via a more posterior site, enabled by use of a curved linear transducer, depicts flow within the lumen, although with apparent flow voids that may be due to near-wall shadowing artifact.

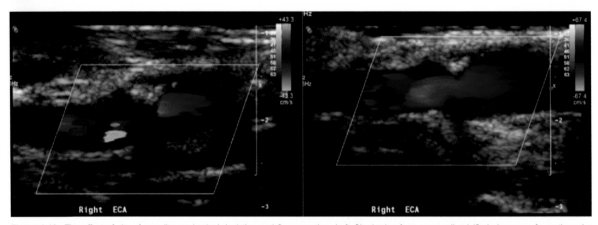

Figure 1-13. The effect of site of sampling on luminal depiction and flow mapping. *Left,* Shadowing from near wall calcified plaque confuses the color Doppler depiction of flow and the lumen. *Right,* In an image obtained from a different orientation, the calcium shadowing artifact is avoided by sampling through another plane of the eccentrically calcified lesion, enabling depiction of the lumen by grayscale and of the flow by color Doppler flow mapping.

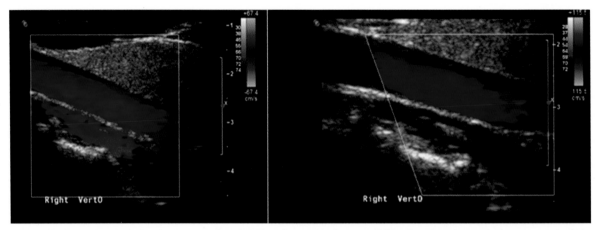

Figure 1-14. Grayscale and color Doppler phantom artifacts. *Left,* The pulse repetition frequency (PRF), color gain, and steer selections generate the depiction of a deeper vessel with flow in it, parallel to the vertebral artery. However, there are no vessels beside the vertebral artery with similarly aligned flow. *Right,* With an increase in the PRF and color field steer selection toward the flow, the apparent deeper field vessel, a phantom, has disappeared.

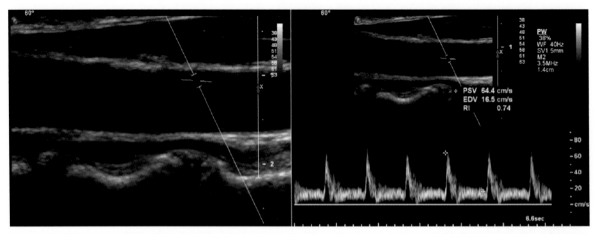

Figure 1-15. Optimizing pulsed-wave Doppler sampling. The angle correction wings of the sample volume (set to 60 degrees) should be parallel to both the vessel wall and the flow. To set up the sampling ideally, the cursor is positioned initially near to a wall to verify the parallelism before shifting the sample volume, now ideally aligned, into the midstream. When the flow vector and the wall are not parallel, alignment of sampling with the flow vector is preferred.

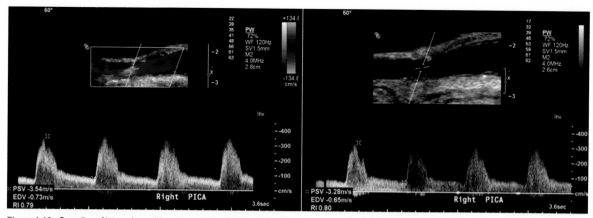

Figure 1-16. Sampling of internal carotid anatomy with and without color Doppler. Localizing the site of sampling, so that the lesion can be directly compared on a follow-up study, is best guided by grayscale imaging. The spectral display on the left was recorded from a color Doppler flow-mapped grayscale image. The detail, and site, of the plaque are largely obscured by the flow mapping. The spectral display on the right was recorded from grayscale image, where the location and detail of the plaque are seen.

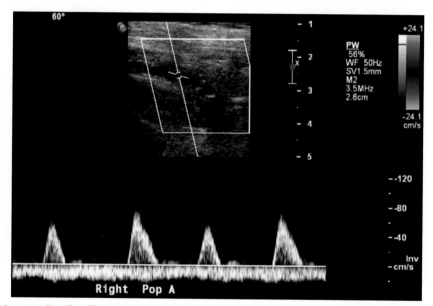

Figure 1-17. The volume sampling effect. The sample volume appears to be within the popliteal artery (as intended), but the spectral display reveals that flow from the adjacent popliteal vein has also been sampled. Pulsed-wave Doppler may sample more than the reference image may suggest because the volume of sampling may exceed the depicted plane in a Z-axis and sample flow deep to or superficial to what is imaged.

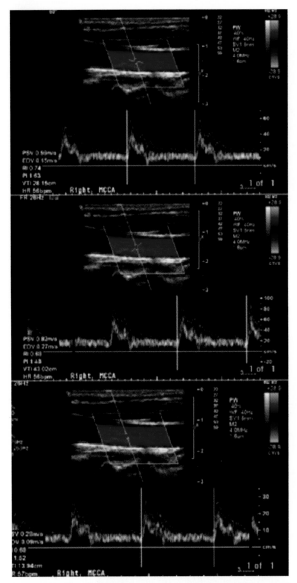

Figure 1-18. The effect of angle correction and alignment with the vessel wall, on recording of flow velocities. *Top,* 60 degrees. *Middle,* 70 degrees. *Bottom,* 0 degrees. By convention, sampling should be between 45 degrees and 60 degrees.

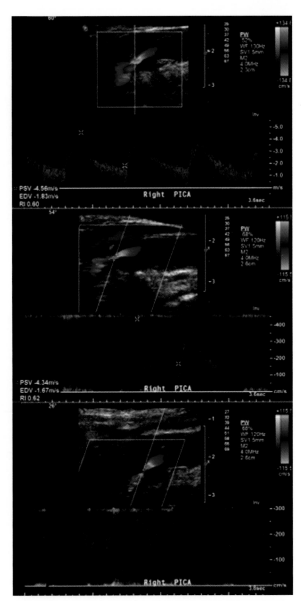

Figure 1-19. The effect of angle correction on depicted flow velocities. *Top,* The sampling of flow is with alignment to the vessel wall and flow and at 60 degrees of angle correction. *Middle,* The angle correction has been changed to 54 degrees, and the depicted velocity, as well as the display scale, has also been changed. *Bottom,* The angle correction has been further reduced to 26 degrees, resulting in a different velocity scale.

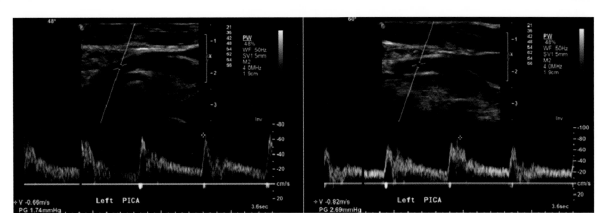

Figure 1-20. The need for manipulation of the transducer to maintain accuracy and uphold convention. Each image uses a different Doppler angle of insonation, and although they are all acceptable according to convention, they produce different velocity values.

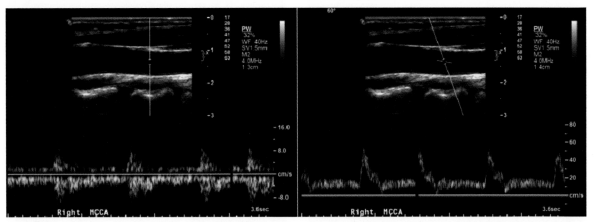

Figure 1-21. The incident angle and angle correction have a prominent effect on spectral Doppler display. *Left,* The image involves an incident angle of about 90 degrees, sampling perpendicular to the vessel walls, and no angle correction. The spectral display infers turbulence and even reversed flow. *Right,* With sampling parallel to the vessel walls and an angle correction of 60 degrees, the image yields a more plausible depiction of laminar and biphasic (physiologic) flow.

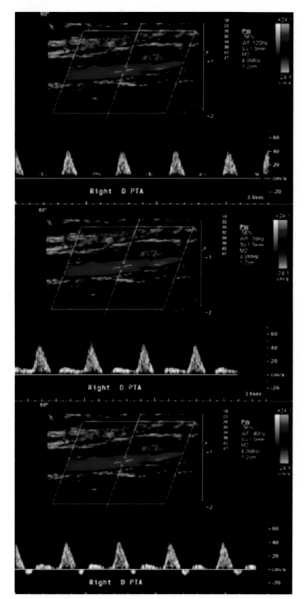

Figure 1-22. The effect of optimizing the Doppler filter setting on the depiction of spectral waveforms on a lower extremity arterial study. *Top,* The filter setting is too high, with the effect of representing flow as monophasic. *Middle,* The filter setting is still too high, with the effect of representing flow as biphasic. *Bottom,* The filter setting is optimal, revealing the true flow pattern as triphasic.

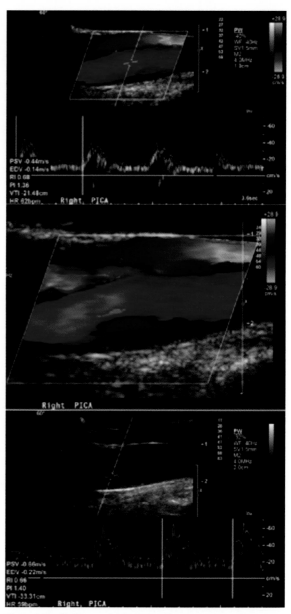

Figure 1-23. Challenges of pulsed-wave Doppler sampling of flow in the proximal bulb portion of the internal carotid artery (ICA). The "bulb" of the proximal ICA (distal common carotid artery) generates eddy currents and challenges flow sampling. *Top,* The site of pulsed-wave flow sampling appears optimal, but the spectral display depicts lower-than-normal velocities. *Middle,* Image of flow mapping in the bulb portion of the ICA reveals a lateral wall eddy current and how nonoptimal location of pulsed-wave sampling may capture different flow streams in the bulb portion of the ICA. In the bottom image, flow is sampled distal to the bulb portion, away from the bulb and its lateral wall eddy currents. *Bottom,* The spectral display yields higher velocities than the sampling of the more proximal bulb site, and a less turbulent, more laminar pattern, as the site of sampling is away from the bulb eddy currents.

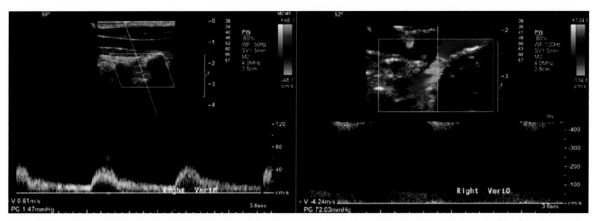

Figure 1-24. *Left,* The vertebral artery is usually sampled in its mid-portion, because that is the easiest site within which to sample flow. Current transducer technology allows the characterization of flow at the origin of the vertebral artery—a previously unlikely depiction. *Right,* The spectral display of the flow at the ostium depicts very elevated velocities consistent with ostial stenosis. Hence, despite significant ostial stenosis, flow in the mid-vertebral artery is unremarkable. Whether the mid-vertebral artery flow has a tardus profile is debatable.

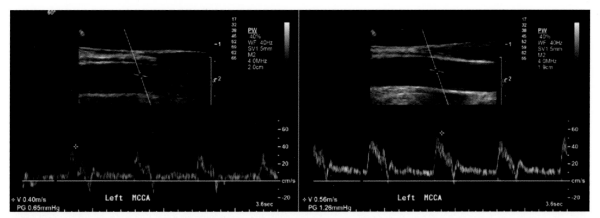

Figure 1-25. The effect of off-axis sampling on spectral flow recording. *Left,* Flow velocity is sampled from where the grayscale image depicts that the plane of imaging exits tangentially from the vessel, yielding lower-than-average velocities and cyclical flow reversal. *Right,* Image of flow sampled from what is more convincingly the center of the lumen yields higher velocities, lesser depiction of turbulence, and lesser depiction of flow reversal.

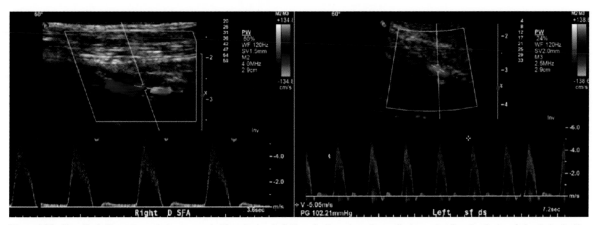

Figure 1-26. The effect of transducer choice on spectral flow display. *Left,* Use of a linear transducer affords spectral Doppler display of elevated velocities that achieve the limit of the display scale. *Right,* Use of a curved linear transducer affords a higher velocity scale and more confident determination of the peak velocity.

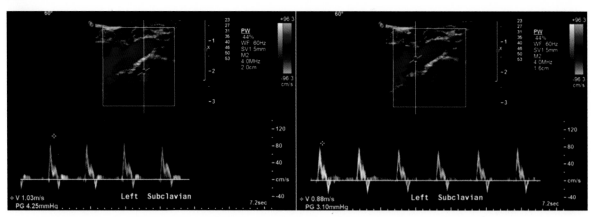

Figure 1-27. Spectral Doppler phantom artifacts. *Left,* The pulse repetition frequency (PRF), color gain, and steer selections generate the depiction of a deeper vessel with flow in it, parallel to the subclavian artery. There are no vessels beside the subclavian artery with similarly aligned flow and yet the Doppler spectral display appears convincing. *Right,* With an increase in the PRF and color field steer selection toward the flow, the apparent deeper field vessel, a phantom, has disappeared.

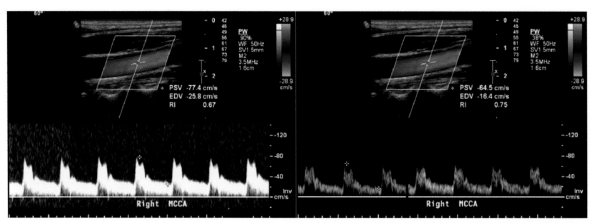

Figure 1-28. The effect of overgain on spectral display. *Left,* Image shows excessive gain. *Right,* The gain is optimal. There is a 20% difference in peak systolic velocity according to gain output.

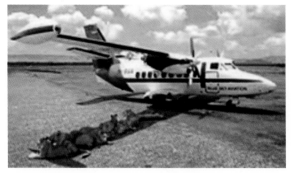

Figure 1-29. Shadowing, of lions.

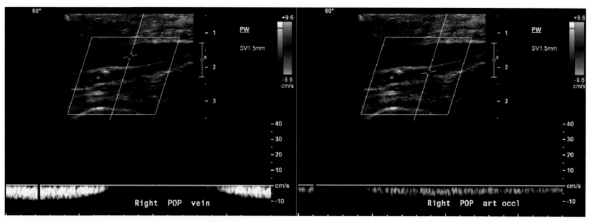

Figure 1-30. The volume sampling effect. The sample volume appears to be within the popliteal artery (*left*), but the spectral display reveals that flow from the adjacent popliteal vein has also been sampled and that the popliteal artery is occluded (*right*). Pulsed-wave Doppler may sample more than the reference image would suggest, due to the fact that the volume of sampling may exceed the depicted plane in a Z-axis and sample flow deep to or superficial to what is actually imaged.

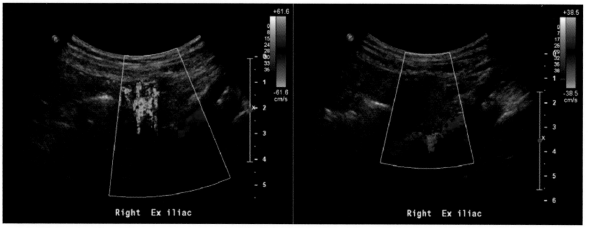

Figure 1-31. *Left,* The image shows a twinkle artifact and inadequate color filling of the external iliac artery. *Right,* The solution to the problem was to use a combination of pulse repetition frequency reduction, to better delineate the course of the artery, as well as adjustment of the color write setting (thin green line) downward, to enhance the grayscale detail.

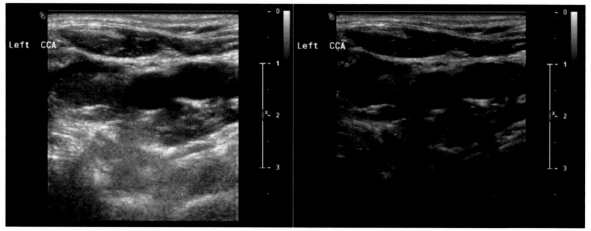

Figure 1-32. Grayscale detail can be enhanced by selection of the single button gain control available on most duplex machines today. This can then serve as a baseline from which refinements are made. *Left,* An example of the limited detail of a "raw" unadjusted image. *Right,* View after the application of the single gain setting.

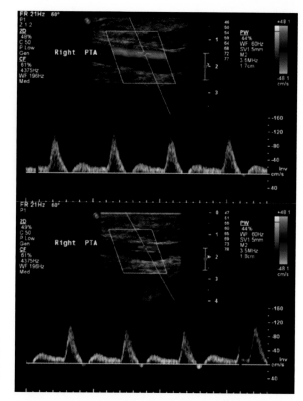

Figure 1-33. Minuscule transducer angle changes can affect the accuracy of the Doppler waveform, shown by the appearance of the normal reversal of flow in early diastole (*bottom*). This reversal was absent in the other image (*top*), which was taken first and before optimal transducer manipulation had been sought.

2

Carotid Artery Disease and Extracranial Cerebrovascular Disease

CAROTID ARTERY AND VARIANT ANATOMY

Anatomic variants of the aortic arch occur in about one third of cases.[1] The innominate artery branch of the aorta gives rise first to the right common carotid artery (CCA) and subsequently the right vertebral artery, beyond which it becomes the subclavian artery. On the distal aortic arch, the left CCA and further distally the left subclavian artery normally arise from the aortic arch with independent ostia. Anomalously, they may arise from a common ostium, and rarely they may arise from a common brachiocephalic artery. The left vertebral artery normally arises from the left subclavian artery.

Normally, the CCAs, which have no branches, divide into the internal and external carotid artery at approximately the level of the upper border of the thyroid cartilage. The main branches of the external carotid artery (ECA), in order of ascension, include the superior thyroid artery, ascending pharyngeal artery, lingual artery, occipital artery, facial artery, posterior auricular artery, maxillary artery, transverse facial artery, and superficial temporal artery.

The first three ECA branch vessels (superior thyroid artery, ascending pharyngeal artery, and lingual artery) are often seen on duplex scanning, and they are visualized more frequently in the presence of an ICA occlusion because they commonly enlarge to become important collateral vessels interconnecting the vertebral artery and ICA via the ophthalmic artery. The facial and superficial temporal arteries are the principal vessels that supply collateral flow around an occlusion of the ICA. The facial artery runs along the lateral border of the mandible and along the cheek to eventually join the ophthalmic artery via the nasal artery. The superficial temporal artery, which runs in front of the tragus of the ear, divides into two vessels, runs across the forehead, and communicates with branches of the terminal ophthalmic artery.

Because the ECA and ICA may be anatomically indistinguishable on grayscale scanning and their flow patterns may be rendered similar by disease, the superficial temporal artery branch of the ECA is sometimes used to attempt to distinguish the ECA from the ICA. The temporal tap technique, which is widely used, has the sonographer simultaneously recoding the spectral flow pattern of the ECA while tapping the superficial temporal artery and observing for waveform artifacts of the same frequency of the tapping. These artifacts are most easily recognized in the diastolic component of flow. However, this technique may fail to depict artifacts of sufficient clarity to avoid confusion of the ECA and ICA. Thus, the temporal tap technique is not adequately reliable to distinguish the ECA from the ICA (see Common Technical Problems).

The ICA has no branches along its extracranial portion and is arbitrarily divided into four segments. The extracranial/cervical segment runs between the carotid bifurcation and the carotid canal, where it becomes the petrous segment. From here, the artery passes through the petrous bone to the cavernous sinus, where it becomes the cavernous segment. After penetration through the dura, it becomes the supraclinoid segment and extends to the bifurcation into the anterior and middle cerebral arteries. There are three branches of the supraclinoid segment (ophthalmic artery, posterior communicating artery, and anterior choroidal artery). In some case, the ophthalmic artery may provide an important collateral of distal (to the ophthalmic artery) occlusion of the ICA.

The vertebral artery extends from the subclavian artery on the left and from the innominate on the right, through the atlanto-occipital membrane and dura mater to join the contralateral vertebral artery and become the basilar artery. There are numerous branches throughout its course.

Common anatomic variants include (1) adjoining or common origin of the innominate artery and the left CCA (16%)[2]; (2) left CCA originating from the innominate artery (13%); (3) left vertebral artery arising from the aortic arch between the left CCA and left subclavian artery (6%); (4) unilateral or bilateral congenital absence of the CCA, which is very rare, with only 25 recorded cases (when the right CCA is absent, the ICA arises from the subclavian artery and the ECA from the innominate artery; when the left CCA is absent, both the ICA and ECA arise from the aortic arch)[3]; and (5) absence of the ICA, which is also very rare, supposedly occurring in less than 0.01% of the population. Collateral flow in this case may occur from the circle of Willis, persistent embryonic branches, or through transcranial vessels interconnected to branches of the ECA (Fig. 2-1).[4]

CAROTID ARTERY DISEASE

Carotid artery disease accounts for approximately 25% of all cases of stroke and is the second largest cause of ischemic stroke (Fig. 2-2). Despite the landmark gains in stroke reduction (>40%) in the past four decades, the total number of strokes per year is increasing due to the aging of the population.

The detection of carotid stenosis by physical diagnosis is relatively poor. Occlusions, lesser severity disease, and inexperience give false-negative results in the detection of carotid disease. Venous hums, ECA stenoses, and tortuosity and "kinking" of the ICA, as well as transmitted aortic stenosis murmurs, give false-positive results in the detection of ICA stenosis. Physical diagnosis sensitivities of 36% to 79% and specificities of 61% to 98% have been reported, establishing the need for more accurate imaging assessment.[5–8] Duplex ultrasound is the usual screening test, although its yield and benefit is significantly determined by the clinical context in which carotid disease is being sought.[9]

Pathology and Pathogenesis

It is recognized that carotid artery disease that results in stroke does so by embolization of atherothrombosis into the intracranial circulation or retina. Occlusion of a carotid artery by itself does not result in stroke if the circle of Willis is complete and has adequate inflow. A complete carotid occlusion may result in propagating distal thrombosis that may yield emboli and result in stroke, although the lesion may also be stable and clinically bland.

The usual location of an atherosclerotic carotid lesion is in the proximal ICA, typically arising off the posterior wall. However, considerable variability of plaque location and length does occur. Stenosis and occlusion of the larger CCA may also occur, as may disease of the intracranial portion of the ICA. ICA stenosis may extend a variable distance up the extracranial carotid artery. In addition to describing the severity of carotid stenosis, detailed description of the morphology of carotid stenosis is important, because successful endarterectomy requires that the entire plaque can be removed. If significant plaque extends further than can be accessed surgically, a shelf is left facing the bloodstream, which may result in dissection.

Treatment

The medical treatment of carotid disease, particularly of symptomatic carotid disease, confers limited benefit (Table 2-1 and Table A-2).[10–17] Medical treatment provides 15% to 20% relative risk reduction of stroke in a secondary prophylaxis with the use of acetylsalicylic acid (50 to 650 mg) or acetylsalicylic acid (50 mg) and dipyridamole (400 mg). It provides little or no proven benefit for primary prevention with acetylsalicylic acid (325 mg/day).[18,19] Recommendations for antithrombotic therapy in patients with extracranial carotid atherosclerotic disease not undergoing revascularization are given in Box 2-1, and guidelines for level of evidence are given in Table A-1 (appendix tables begin on page 277).

TABLE 2-1 Medical Treatment of Carotid Artery Disease

STUDY	SAMPLE SIZE (N)	TREATMENT	OUTCOME	RISK REDUCTION
Meta-analysis[10]	73,247	Antiplatelet therapy	Stroke, death, nonfatal stroke	27% 25% from ASA
Meta-analysis[11]		ASA	Stroke	−16%
CATS,[12] Hass trial[13]		Ticlopidine	Stroke	−23%
CAPRIE[14]		ASA/ticlopidine vs. no treatment	Stroke, MI, vascular death	−9%
ESPS-1[15]		ASA/dipyridamole	Stroke	−33%
ESPS-2[16]	6,602	ASA/dipyridamole	Stroke	−21%
PRoFESS[17]	20,332	Dipyridamole vs. clopidogrel	Stroke, MI, death from vascular causes	—

ASA, acetylsalicylic acid; CAPRIE, Clopidogrel versus Aspirin in Patients at Risk of Ischaemic Events; CATS, Canadian American Ticlopidine Study; ESPS, European Stroke Prevention Study; MI, myocardial infarction; PRoFESS, Preventive Regimen for Effectively Avoiding Second Strokes.

Although the potential revascularization benefit for carotid artery disease is prominent, several factors contribute to achieving, or not achieving, a net benefit, and all have to be carefully considered: (1) symptom status; (2) stenosis severity; (3) patient's comorbidities, operative stroke, and cardiac risk; and (4) the surgeon's operative morbidity and mortality rate.[20,27]

The understanding of the relative merits of surgical endarterectomy and carotid stenting is evolving. By limited trials, they appear similar in overall benefit, with some age influence (Fig. 2-3), and with more myocardial infarction associated with surgical endarterectomy and more stroke associated with stenting.

The optimal combination of nondisabling symptoms, severe stenosis but no occlusion, low comorbidity/patient risk, and low surgeon morbidity/mortality yields an impressive 70% to 85% relative risk reduction of subsequent stroke and mortality from carotid endarterectomy (CEA).[20,21] Following CEA performed in optimal circumstances, survival free of ipsilateral stroke is excellent; it is 97% at 2 years, 93% at 5 years, and 92% at 10 years.[28] Surgical endarterectomy of in cases of greater than 60% stenosis of asymptomatic patients, although validated,[25] remains controversial. The lower (10%) relative risk reduction of endarterectomy for asymptomatic disease renders the outcome critically dependent on patient risk and surgeon risk. Optimally, the stroke and mortality risk for CEA should be less than 6% for symptomatic individuals and less than 3% for asymptomatic individuals.[29] For every 2% complication rate greater than 6% to 7%, the 5-year benefit of CEA falls by 20%. If the complication rate exceeds 6% to 7%, then only severe and symptomatic lesions may have net benefit from CEA (Fig. 2-4).[30,31]

Results of the comparative utility of CEA and modes of therapy are presented in Table A-3.

Results of trials comparing CEA and carotid artery stenting are presented in Tables A-4, A-5, and A-6.

A summary of ASA/ACCF/AHA/AANN/AANS/ACR/ASNR/CNS/SAIP/SCAI/SIR/SNIS/SVM/SVS guideline recommendations regarding the selection of revascularization techniques for patients with carotid artery stenosis is given in Table A-7.

Recommendations for diagnostic testing in patients with symptoms or signs of extracranial carotid artery disease are given in Box 2-2.

Recommendations for carotid artery evaluation and revascularization before cardiac surgery are given in Box 2-3.

Recommendations for selection of patients for carotid revascularization are given in Box 2-4.

Scanning Protocol

Both carotid arteries, as well as the subclavian, vertebral, and brachiocephalic arteries, are scanned. Flow findings in one carotid artery may be influenced by lesions in the contralateral artery; flow patterns (and direction) in the vertebral arteries may be influenced by subclavian artery lesions (Figs. 2-5 to 2-9). The

---

Carotid Scanning Pearls

- Using a curved linear probe for the scanning of the most distal and deep extracranial portion of the internal carotid artery (ICA) not only will achieve better acoustic penetration but will also give (because of its wider field of view) the "big picture" more clearly than a linear probe, especially when the vessel is tortuous.
- Beware of the possibility that the external carotid artery (ECA), depending on the configuration and ostial position of the branches, can and often does have a less resistive waveform shape than the classic pattern. Those branches might not always be in evidence, if imaging is suboptimal. This can sometimes cloud distinction between the ECA and the ICA. (This also applies to the proximal profunda femoris artery.)
- The most comfortable scanning position is from above the head of the patient's bed, using the right hand for the right carotid, and the left hand for the left carotid, supporting the scanning hand as described in Chapter 1 by using the elbow and part of the scanning hand as support.
- When using different angles of approach around the circumference of the neck, it may be necessary to angle steeply to insonate the carotids (e.g., if scanning from a posterior direction angle anteriorly and vice versa).
- With a variation in the angle of approach, the ICA and ECA will change position with respect to one another (e.g., if the ECA was anterior to the ICA with an anterior/mid approach, it will be posterior to the ICA with a posterior approach).
- In the presence of eccentric calcified plaque, first analyzing the artery in short axis to determine the best angle of approach, around the plaque, and then seeking those clear windows in long axis, will provide better color filling and better defined spectral Doppler envelope.
- To facilitate visualization of the vertebral artery, first find the common carotid artery (CCA) in long axis and then either slide the transducer laterally without changing its angle or angle laterally without shifting to left or right and look for segments of the artery lying between the vertebral processes.
- Be aware that as the ICA extends distally in the neck, the caliber will decrease and in a normal vessel flow velocity will consequently rise slightly.
- In addition, in performing spectral Doppler sampling in the distal extracranial ICA, there will be a greater sample volume-to-vessel size ratio, possibly resulting in apparent flow turbulence because a greater cross-section of flow speeds will be included.

---

scanning protocol is summarized in Table 2-2. Scanning pearls are presented in the accompanying box.

Scanning of the Common Carotid Artery

The CCA is scanned as it may harbor significant pathology (e.g., stenosis, dissection), and its flow velocity is used to establish a reference to the ICA flow velocity (peak systolic velocity [PSV] ICA/CCA). Usual (velocity) criteria for ICA stenosis assessment assume nondisturbed prestenotic flow (no CCA stenosis jet contamination of ICA flow characteristics).

BOX 2-1 Recommendations for Antithrombotic Therapy in Patients with Extracranial Carotid Atherosclerotic Disease Not Undergoing Revascularization

Class I

1. Antiplatelet therapy with aspirin, 75 to 325 mg daily, is recommended for patients with obstructive or nonobstructive atherosclerosis that involves the extracranial carotid and/or vertebral arteries for prevention of MI and other ischemic cardiovascular events, although the benefit has not been established for prevention of stroke in asymptomatic patients. (*Level of Evidence: A*)

2. In patients with obstructive or nonobstructive extracranial carotid or vertebral atherosclerosis who have sustained ischemic stroke or TIA, antiplatelet therapy with aspirin alone (75 to 325 mg daily), clopidogrel alone (75 mg daily), or the combination of aspirin plus extended-release dipyridamole (25 and 200 mg twice daily, respectively) is recommended (*Level of Evidence: B*) and preferred over the combination of aspirin with clopidogrel. (*Level of Evidence: B*). Selection of an antiplatelet regimen should be individualized on the basis of patient risk factor profiles, cost, tolerance, and other clinical characteristics, as well as guidance from regulatory agencies.

3. Antiplatelet agents are recommended rather than oral anticoagulation for patients with atherosclerosis of the extracranial carotid or vertebral arteries with (*Level of Evidence: B*) or without (*Level of Evidence: C*) ischemic symptoms. (For patients with allergy or other contraindications to aspirin, see Class IIa recommendation #2.)

Class IIa

1. In patients with extracranial cerebrovascular atherosclerosis who have an indication for anticoagulation, such as atrial fibrillation or a mechanical prosthetic heart valve, it can be beneficial to administer a vitamin K antagonist (such as warfarin, dose-adjusted to achieve a target international normalized ratio [INR] of 2.5 [range 2.0 to 3.0]) for prevention of thromboembolic ischemic events. (*Level of Evidence: C*)

2. For patients with atherosclerosis of the extracranial carotid or vertebral arteries in whom aspirin is contraindicated by factors other than active bleeding, including allergy, either clopidogrel (75 mg daily) or ticlopidine (250 mg twice daily) is a reasonable alternative. (*Level of Evidence: C*)

Class III: No Benefit

1. Full-intensity parenteral anticoagulation with unfractionated heparin or low-molecular-weight heparinoids is not recommended for patients with extracranial cerebrovascular atherosclerosis who develop transient cerebral ischemia or acute ischemic stroke. (*Level of Evidence: B*)

2. Administration of clopidogrel in combination with aspirin is not recommended within 3 months after stroke or TIA. (*Level of Evidence: B*)

From 2011 ASA/ACCF/AHA/AANN/AANS/ACR/ASNR/CNS/SAIP/SCAI/SIR/SNIS/SVM/SVS guideline on the management of patients with extracranial carotid and vertebral artery disease. *J Am Coll Cardiol.* 2011;57:16-94.

A significant CCA stenosis is evident as a greater than 50% narrowing seen on grayscale imaging and a 50% or 100% focal increase in the PSV of the CCA. Advanced congestive heart failure lowers the PSV of the CCA, and it also lowers the PSV of the ICA. Aortic stenosis jets commonly radiate into the CCA, where they are often auscultated. High-grade obstruction of the ICA may increase the pulsatility of the CCA (due to pulse wave reflection) and render the CCA flow profile high resistance, with diminished diastolic velocity or postsystolic flow reversal.

Recommendations for duplex ultrasonography to evaluate asymptomatic patients with known or suspected carotid stenosis are given in Box 2-5.

The CCA sweep is performed to overview the CCA anatomy from the ostium (right CCA: brachiocephalic; left CCA: aorta) to the bifurcation. The distribution and extent of intima-media thickness (IMT), plaque, or other pathology is noted. The CCA sweep is repeated with color Doppler flow mapping to associate anatomic and flow findings. The sweep is performed in both short-axis and long-axis orientations. The intention is to both localize and establish the severity of luminal narrowing by grayscale imaging to provide corroboration with Doppler findings. As well, long-axis grayscale imaging is recorded. In the proximal, middle, and distal CCAs, color Doppler and pulsed-wave

recordings of flow are recorded. Stenosis may occur in any portion of the CCA, particularly the ostium—hence the need to assess for pathology at any level and to endeavor to characterize the grayscale and Doppler findings of the CCAs at all levels.

Scanning of the Brachiocephalic Artery

The brachiocephalic artery is scanned to assess for the presence of significant lesions (e.g., dissection, stenosis) within it. Brachiocephalic lesions influence the flow patterns within the right CCA; hence, interpretation of the right CCA velocity pattern can only be performed with knowledge of the inflow characteristics. In some patients, there are bilateral brachiocephalic arteries (Fig. 2-10).

Scanning of the Internal Carotid Artery

The short-axis and long-axis scanning of the CCA gives a preview of the proximal ICA. As with the CCA, the ICA is scanned with grayscale, color Doppler, and pulsed-wave Doppler recording of its proximal, middle, and distal portions. Although the large majority of atherosclerotic stenoses involve the proximal ICA, some stenoses extend well up into the ICA and are more difficult to remove at endarterectomy. Some lesions, such as spontaneous dissection, are typically present above/beyond the proximal ICA, which is a region commonly difficult to image. The anatomy

BOX 2-2   Recommendations for Diagnostic Testing in Patients with Symptoms or Signs of Extracranial Carotid Artery Disease

Class I

1. The initial evaluation of patients with transient retinal or hemispheric neurological symptoms of possible ischemic origin should include noninvasive imaging for the detection of ECVD. (*Level of Evidence: C*)
2. Duplex ultrasonography is recommended to detect carotid stenosis in patients who develop focal neurological symptoms corresponding to the territory supplied by the left or right internal carotid artery. (*Level of Evidence: C*)
3. In patients with acute, focal ischemic neurological symptoms corresponding to the territory supplied by the left or right internal carotid artery, magnetic resonance angiography (MRA) or computed tomography angiography (CTA) is indicated to detect carotid stenosis when sonography either cannot be obtained or yields equivocal or otherwise nondiagnostic results. (*Level of Evidence: C*)
4. When extracranial or intracranial cerebrovascular disease is not severe enough to account for neurological symptoms of suspected ischemic origin, echocardiography should be performed to search for a source of cardiogenic embolism. (*Level of Evidence: C*)
5. Correlation of findings obtained by several carotid imaging modalities should be part of a program of quality assurance in each laboratory that performs such diagnostic testing. (*Level of Evidence: C*)

Class IIa

1. When an extracranial source of ischemia is not identified in patients with transient retinal or hemispheric neurological symptoms of suspected ischemic origin, CTA, MRA, or selective cerebral angiography can be useful to search for intracranial vascular disease. (*Level of Evidence: C*)
2. When the results of initial noninvasive imaging are inconclusive, additional examination by use of another imaging method is reasonable. In candidates for revascularization, MRA or CTA can be useful when results of carotid duplex ultrasonography are equivocal or indeterminate. (*Level of Evidence: C*)
3. When intervention for significant carotid stenosis detected by carotid duplex ultrasonography is planned, MRA, CTA, or catheter-based contrast angiography can

be useful to evaluate the severity of stenosis and to identify intrathoracic or intracranial vascular lesions that are not adequately assessed by duplex ultrasonography. (*Level of Evidence: C*)
4. When noninvasive imaging is inconclusive or not feasible because of technical limitations or contraindications in patients with transient retinal or hemispheric neurological symptoms of suspected ischemic origin, or when noninvasive imaging studies yield discordant results, it is reasonable to perform catheter-based contrast angiography to detect and characterize extracranial and/or intracranial cerebrovascular disease. (*Level of Evidence: C*)
5. MRA without contrast is reasonable to assess the extent of disease in patients with symptomatic carotid atherosclerosis and renal insufficiency or extensive vascular calcification. (*Level of Evidence: C*)
6. It is reasonable to use MRI systems capable of consistently generating high-quality images while avoiding low-field systems that do not yield diagnostically accurate results. (*Level of Evidence: C*)
7. CTA is reasonable for evaluation of patients with clinically suspected significant carotid atherosclerosis who are not suitable candidates for MRA because of claustrophobia, implanted pacemakers, or other incompatible devices. (*Level of Evidence: C*)

Class IIb

1. Duplex carotid ultrasonography might be considered for patients with nonspecific neurological symptoms when cerebral ischemia is a plausible cause. (*Level of Evidence: C*)
2. When complete carotid arterial occlusion is suggested by duplex ultrasonography, MRA, or CTA in patients with retinal or hemispheric neurological symptoms of suspected ischemic origin, catheter-based contrast angiography may be considered to determine whether the arterial lumen is sufficiently patent to permit carotid revascularization. (*Level of Evidence: C*)
3. Catheter-based angiography may be reasonable in patients with renal dysfunction to limit the amount of radiographic contrast material required for definitive imaging for evaluation of a single vascular territory. (*Level of Evidence: C*)

From 2011 ASA/ACCF/AHA/AANN/AANS/ACR/ASNR/CNS/SAIP/SCAI/SIR/SNIS/SVM/SVS guideline on the management of patients with extracranial carotid and vertebral artery disease. *J Am Coll Cardiol.* 2011;57:16-94.

and its physiology of the ICA must be interrogated along its full extracranial course. More than 50% stenosis of the proximal ICA renders the flow turbulent in the middle and often in the distal ICA as well. Severe stenosis of the proximal ICA renders the distal ICA flow profile "parvus et tardus." High-grade obstruction or occlusion in the distal ICA or intracranial ICA makes the flow pattern of the proximal/middle ICA high resistance. Proximal ICA stenosis severity is established on the basis of grayscale appearance, the PSV of the ICA, the end-diastolic velocity of the ICA, and the PSA of the CCA.

Grayscale imaging in long axis view is performed to localize and characterize plaque severity as less than 50%, greater than or equal to 50%, or occlusion. Optimized color Doppler flow mapping is useful to define the lumen, because hypoechoic plaque and restenosis material may by inapparent by regular grayscale imaging (Fig. 2-11).

Scanning of the External Carotid Artery

The ECA is scanned with grayscale, color Doppler, and pulsed-wave Doppler recording of the proximal, middle, and distal portions. Stenosis, when present, is generally

---

BOX 2-3 Recommendations for Carotid Artery Evaluation and Revascularization Before Cardiac Surgery

Class IIa

1. Carotid duplex ultrasound screening is reasonable before elective CABG surgery in patients older than 65 years of age and in those with left main coronary stenosis, PAD, a history of cigarette smoking, a history of stroke or TIA, or carotid bruit. (*Level of Evidence: C*)
2. Carotid revascularization by CEA or CAS with embolic protection before or concurrent with myocardial revascularization surgery is reasonable in patients with

greater than 80% carotid stenosis who have experienced ipsilateral retinal or hemispheric cerebral ischemic symptoms within 6 months. (*Level of Evidence: C*)

Class IIb

1. In patients with asymptomatic carotid stenosis, even if severe, the safety and efficacy of carotid revascularization before or concurrent with myocardial revascularization are not well established. (*Level of Evidence: C*)

From 2011 ASA/ACCF/AHA/AANN/AANS/ACR/ASNR/CNS/SAIP/SCAI/SIR/SNIS/SVM/SVS guideline on the management of patients with extracranial carotid and vertebral artery disease. *J Am Coll Cardiol.* 2011;57:16-94.

BOX 2-4 Recommendations for Selection of Patients for Carotid Revascularization

Class I

1. Patients at average or low surgical risk who experience nondisabling ischemic stroke or transient cerebral ischemic symptoms, including hemispheric events or amaurosis fugax, within 6 months (symptomatic patients) should undergo CEA if the diameter of the lumen of the ipsilateral internal carotid artery is reduced more than 70% as documented by noninvasive imaging (20,83) (*Level of Evidence: A*) or more than 50% as documented by catheter angiography (*Level of Evidence: B*) and the anticipated rate of perioperative stroke or mortality is less than 6%.
2. CAS is indicated as an alternative to CEA for symptomatic patients at average or low risk of complications associated with endovascular intervention when the diameter of the lumen of the internal carotid artery is reduced by more than 70% as documented by noninvasive imaging or more than 50% as documented by catheter angiography and the anticipated rate of periprocedural stroke or mortality is less than 6%. (*Level of Evidence: B*)
3. Selection of asymptomatic patients for carotid revascularization should be guided by an assessment of comorbid conditions, life expectancy, and other individual factors and should include a thorough discussion of the risks and benefits of the procedure with an understanding of patient preferences. (*Level of Evidence: C*)

Class IIa

1. It is reasonable to perform CEA in asymptomatic patients who have more than 70% stenosis of the internal carotid artery if the risk of perioperative stroke, MI, and death is low. (*Level of Evidence: A*)
   It is reasonable to choose CEA over CAS when revascularization is indicated in older patients,

particularly when arterial pathoanatomy is unfavorable for endovascular intervention. (*Level of Evidence: B*)
3. It is reasonable to choose CAS over CEA when revascularization is indicated in patients with neck anatomy unfavorable for arterial surgery. (*Level of Evidence: B*)
4. When revascularization is indicated for patients with TIA or stroke and there are no contraindications to early revascularization, intervention within 2 weeks of the index event is reasonable rather than delaying surgery. (*Level of Evidence: B*)

Class IIb

1. Prophylactic CAS might be considered in highly selected patients with asymptomatic carotid stenosis (minimum 60% by angiography, 70% by validated Doppler ultrasound), but its effectiveness compared with medical therapy alone in this situation is not well established. (*Level of Evidence: B*)
2. In symptomatic or asymptomatic patients at high risk of complications for carotid revascularization by either CEA or CAS because of comorbidities, the effectiveness of revascularization versus medical therapy alone is not well established. (*Level of Evidence: B*)

Class III: No Benefit

1. Except in extraordinary circumstances, carotid revascularization by either CEA or CAS is not recommended when atherosclerosis narrows the lumen by less than 50%. (*Level of Evidence: A*)
2. Carotid revascularization is not recommended for patients with chronic total occlusion of the targeted carotid artery. (*Level of Evidence: C*)
3. Carotid revascularization is not recommended for patients with severe disability caused by cerebral infarction that precludes preservation of useful function. (*Level of Evidence: C*)

From 2011 ASA/ACCF/AHA/AANN/AANS/ACR/ASNR/CNS/SAIP/SCAI/SIR/SNIS/SVM/SVS guideline on the management of patients with extracranial carotid and vertebral artery disease. *J Am Coll Cardiol.* 2011;57:16-94.

---

located in the proximal portion, often contiguous with plaque of the CCA and ICA. Stenosis is not established by category as it is with ICA stenosis. A PSV of the ECA two times greater than the PSA of the CCA constitutes a hemodynamically significant stenosis. A PSV of the

ECA that is less than two times greater than the PSA of the CCA constitutes a nonhemodynamically significant stenosis. An absence of flow constitutes occlusion. The temporal tap maneuver is modestly successful in distinguishing the ECA from the ICA (Fig. 2-12).

TABLE 2-2 Scanning Protocol		
ANATOMIC SEGMENT	**TECHNIQUE**	**DUPLEX MODALITY**
Common carotid	SAX sweep	Grayscale
		Color Doppler
	LAX sweep	Grayscale
		Color Doppler
	LAX	
	Proximal	Grayscale
		Color Doppler
		Pulsed-wave spectral
	Mid	Grayscale
		Color Doppler
		Pulsed-wave spectral
	Distal	Grayscale
		Color Doppler
		Pulsed-wave spectral
Internal carotid	LAX	
	Proximal	Grayscale
		Color Doppler
		Pulsed-wave spectral
	Mid	Grayscale
		Color Doppler
		Pulsed-wave spectral
	Distal	Grayscale
		Color Doppler
		Pulsed-wave spectral
External carotid	LAX	Grayscale
		Color Doppler
		Pulsed-wave spectral
Brachiocephalic	LAX	Grayscale
		Color Doppler
		Pulsed-wave spectral
Subclavian	LAX	Grayscale
		Color Doppler
		Pulsed-wave spectral
Vertebral	LAX	
	Ostial	Color Doppler
		Pulsed-wave spectral
	Mid	Color Doppler
		Pulsed-wave spectral
Brachial blood pressure recording		

LAX, long-axis imaging; SAX, short-axis imaging.

Scanning of the Vertebral Artery

The vertebral artery is scanned with grayscale, color Doppler, and pulsed-wave Doppler at its ostium—a common site of stenosis—and in its mid-portion. Hemodynamically significant stenosis is present when there is a focal 100% increase in PSV (Fig. 2-13). Flow in the mid-portion is recorded with respect to its pattern and directionality; anterograde is normal, retrograde establishes subclavian steal syndrome, and a high-resistance pattern might indicate a distal high-grade stenosis or occlusion or hypoplastic/atretic vessel. There is often a disparity in size identified on grayscale (Figs. 2-14 to 2-16).

Recommendations for vascular imaging in patients with vertebral artery disease are given in Box 2-6.

Scanning of the Subclavian Artery

The subclavian arteries, the normal inflow to the vertebral arteries, are scanned with grayscale, color Doppler, and pulsed-wave Doppler. Hemodynamically significant subclavian artery stenosis, the substrate of subclavian steal (from the vertebral circulation), is evident as a focal 100% increase in PSV.

Recording of the Brachial Blood Pressure

The brachial blood pressure is recorded bilaterally to identify cases of unilateral subclavian artery stenosis.

Assessment of Stenosis

Distinguishing mild from severe stenoses is not that difficult by duplex or other imaging modality and has low intraobserver and interobserver variability. Correct "categorization" of moderately severe lesions to within 10% severity (50% to 60%, 60% to 70%) is feasible but requires careful attention to technique and is associated with a higher intraobserver and interobserver variability.

The ability to detect and accurately record low volume of flow through near-total occlusions has historically been a technical challenge and often a significant clinical failure of duplex imaging. An inadequate flow signal may be mistaken for no flow. Current imaging equipment and persistence of effort are able to distinguish most total from subtotal carotid lesions. CEA is not indicated for complete occlusion of a carotid artery and is generally unsuited to it, and carotid stenting, whose role is evolving, is also unsuitable for the complete occlusion lesion, because passage of a wire across a complete stenosis is difficult and entails risk. Conversely, CEA is indicated for a symptomatic (non-disabling stroke, transient ischemic attack, or amaurosis fugax) ipsilateral high-grade carotid lesion in a patient with acceptable operative risk.

Plaque Characterization

The ultrasonographic appearance of plaque also predicts clinical events. In asymptomatic patients, echolucent plaques are associated with two to four times the risk of stroke than is associated with echogenic plaques.[19,32,33]

Criteria for Categorizing Plaque Severity

Initially, conventional angiography was clearly the established and standard test by which carotid stenosis severity was detailed and from which endarterectomy

BOX 2-5 Recommendations for Duplex Ultrasonography to Evaluate Asymptomatic Patients with Known or Suspected Carotid Stenosis

Class I

1. In asymptomatic patients with known or suspected carotid stenosis, duplex ultrasonography, performed by a qualified technologist in a certified laboratory, is recommended as the initial diagnostic test to detect hemodynamically significant carotid stenosis. (*Level of Evidence: C*)

Class IIa

1. It is reasonable to perform duplex ultrasonography to detect hemodynamically significant carotid stenosis in asymptomatic patients with carotid bruit. (*Level of Evidence: C*)

2. It is reasonable to repeat duplex ultrasonography annually by a qualified technologist in a certified laboratory to assess the progression or regression of disease and response to therapeutic interventions in patients with atherosclerosis who have had stenosis greater than 50% detected previously. Once stability has been established over an extended period or the patient's candidacy for further intervention has changed, longer intervals or termination of surveillance may be appropriate. (*Level of Evidence: C*)

Class IIb

1. Duplex ultrasonography to detect hemodynamically significant carotid stenosis may be considered in asymptomatic patients with symptomatic PAD, coronary artery disease (CAD), or atherosclerotic aortic aneurysm, but because such patients already have an indication for medical therapy to prevent ischemic symptoms, it is unclear whether establishing the additional diagnosis of ECVD in those without carotid bruit would justify actions that affect clinical outcomes. (*Level of Evidence: C*)

2. Duplex ultrasonography might be considered to detect carotid stenosis in asymptomatic patients without clinical evidence of atherosclerosis who have two or more of the following risk factors: hypertension, hyperlipidemia, tobacco smoking, a family history in a first-degree relative of atherosclerosis manifested before age 60 years, or a family history of ischemic stroke. However, it is unclear whether establishing a diagnosis of ECVD would justify actions that affect clinical outcomes. (*Level of Evidence: C*)

Class III: No Benefit

1. Carotid duplex ultrasonography is not recommended for routine screening of asymptomatic patients who have no clinical manifestations of or risk factors for atherosclerosis. (*Level of Evidence: C*)

2. Carotid duplex ultrasonography is not recommended for routine evaluation of patients with neurological or psychiatric disorders unrelated to focal cerebral ischemia, such as brain tumors, familial or degenerative cerebral or motor neuron disorders, infectious and inflammatory conditions affecting the brain, psychiatric disorders, or epilepsy. (*Level of Evidence: C*)

3. Routine serial imaging of the extracranial carotid arteries is not recommended for patients who have no risk factors for development of atherosclerotic carotid disease and no disease evident on initial vascular testing. (*Level of Evidence: C*)

From 2011 ASA/ACCF/AHA/AANN/AANS/ACR/ASNR/CNS/SAIP/SCAI/SIR/SNIS/SVM/SVS guideline on the management of patients with extracranial carotid and vertebral artery disease. *J Am Coll Cardiol.* 2011;57:16-94.

BOX 2-6 Recommendations for Vascular Imaging in Patients with Vertebral Artery Disease

Class I

1. Noninvasive imaging by CTA or MRA for detection of vertebral artery disease should be part of the initial evaluation of patients with neurological symptoms referable to the posterior circulation and those with subclavian steal syndrome. (*Level of Evidence: C*)

2. Patients with asymptomatic bilateral carotid occlusions or unilateral carotid artery occlusion and incomplete circle of Willis should undergo noninvasive imaging for detection of vertebral artery obstructive disease. (*Level of Evidence: C*)

3. In patients whose symptoms suggest posterior cerebral or cerebellar ischemia, MRA or CTA is recommended rather than ultrasound imaging for evaluation of the vertebral arteries. (*Level of Evidence: C*)

Class IIa

1. In patients with symptoms of posterior cerebral or cerebellar ischemia, serial noninvasive imaging of the extracranial vertebral arteries is reasonable to assess the progression of atherosclerotic disease and exclude the development of new lesions. (*Level of Evidence: C*)

2. In patients with posterior cerebral or cerebellar ischemic symptoms who may be candidates for revascularization, catheter-based contrast angiography can be useful to define vertebral artery pathoanatomy when noninvasive imaging fails to define the location or severity of stenosis. (*Level of Evidence: C*)

3. In patients who have undergone vertebral artery revascularization, serial noninvasive imaging of the extracranial vertebral arteries is reasonable at intervals similar to those for carotid revascularization. (*Level of Evidence: C*)

From 2011 ASA/ACCF/AHA/AANN/AANS/ACR/ASNR/CNS/SAIP/SCAI/SIR/SNIS/SVM/SVS guideline on the management of patients with extracranial carotid and vertebral artery disease. *J Am Coll Cardiol.* 2011;57:16-94.

was planned. The techniques and technology of duplex ultrasound developed steadily, and at some centers, especially those with the ability to achieve imaging or surgical correlation, duplex succeeded conventional angiography, because it was without the 1% stroke/death risk associated with conventional angiography, and it generated sufficiently reliable preoperative results. At other centers, duplex never developed into a stand-alone test. Other forms of angiography—magnetic resonance angiography (MRA) and computed tomography angiography (CTA)—have become widely available and are also utilized in the evaluation of carotid disease. The practice of carotid disease evaluation is variable, depending on a center's interests, expertise, and access. There is an increasing trend to perform duplex and either MRA or CTA as a paired initial evaluation. Unless both generate a consistent determination of the presence/severity of disease, conventional angiography is performed to optimally evaluate potentially surgical lesions.

Achieving ready equivalence of stenosis determination between duplex and conventional angiography is challenged by the historical differences in the vessel's reference standard used to establish percent stenosis and the uncommon situation that ICA stenoses generally develop in the bulb segment of the vessel, which is anatomically larger than the ongoing ICA. The North American Symptomatic Carotid Endarterectomy Trial (NASCET) standard is the first nondiseased portion of the ongoing ICA. The European Carotid Surgery Trial (ECST) standard is different from the NASCET standard and uses the visually estimated dimension of the bulb. Duplex criteria were initially developed on basis of velocity correlations with bulb standard (measured by high-resolution radiograph), but later, to achieve more ready correlation with angiography, developed on basis of velocity correlations with ongoing ICA standards.

Adding to the confusion, the initial (Washington) duplex categories expressed by bulb standard differed from angiographic categories expressed by ongoing ICA standard that were adopted from endarterectomy trials. Washington categories were as follows: no disease, less than 50%, 51% to 79%, 80% to 99% and 100%. Surgical categories were 70% to 99% (NASCET), 60% to 99% (Asymptomatic Carotid Atherosclerosis Study [ACAS]), and greater than 50%

(Figs. 2-17 to 2-20). Angiography entails technical challenges (Figs. 2-21 and 2-22).

Current duplex criteria represent an amalgam of different criteria, and they vary between laboratories and often within laboratories. To attempt to standardize duplex categories and criteria, a Consensus Conference document was published in 2003, which is increasingly adopted (Tables 2-3 to 2-5).[34] The basis for these categories is to respect the standard surgical thresholds and the following validation studies (Tables 2-6 and 2-7). The current Doppler criteria for carotid stenting to detect a residual stenosis greater than 20% are PSV greater than or equal to 150 cm/sec and ICA:CCA greater than or equal to 2.16 (sensitivity 100%, specificity 98%, positive predictive value 75%, negative predictive value 100%).[35] These criteria and clinical examples are illustrated in Figures 2-23 to 2-31.

The sensitivity and specificity of duplex ultrasound as a function of degree of stenosis are presented in Table A-8, and the sensitivity and specificity of computed tomographic angiography as a function of degree of carotid stenosis are presented in Table A-9.

COMMON TECHNICAL PROBLEMS

Disease states affecting areas remote from the extracranial carotid and peripheral vessels can nevertheless cause atypical flow patterns to exist, conferring a challenge for the sonographer. Knowledge and understanding of disease entities that alter flow patterns leads to more accurate interpretation. Some cases remain equivocal, and complementary noninvasive imaging or conventional catheter angiography are needed.

Aortic Insufficiency

In the presence of aortic insufficiency or regurgitation, there is regurgitant flow into the left ventricle from the aorta during diastole. Mild aortic insufficiency and even moderate aortic insufficiency are unlikely to considerably change carotid artery waveforms. However, moderate to severe and severe aortic insufficiency may result in two possible changes in the normal carotid velocity contour.
1. A bisferiens ("twice-beating") peak, two prominent systolic peaks, separated by brief midsystolic velocity decay, is seen in approximately 50% of cases.

TABLE 2-3 Carotid Duplex Consensus Criteria Accuracy					
STENOSIS SEVERITY	PSV (cm/sec)	SENSITIVITY	SPECIFICITY	OVERALL ACCURACY
50–69%	125–230	93%	68%	85%
	140–230	94%	92%	92%
>70%	>230	99%	86%	95%

From AbuRahma AF, Srivastava M, Stone PA, Mousa AY, Jain A, Dean LS, Keiffer T, Emmett M. Critical appraisal of the Carotid Duplex Consensus criteria in the diagnosis of carotid artery stenosis. *J Vasc Surg.* 2011; 53(1):53-59; discussion 59-60.

TABLE 2-4   Receiver Operating Characteristic-Area Under the Curve

	PSV	EDV	ICA/CCA RATIO
ROC AUC (Area Under the Curve)	0.97	0.94	0.84

From AbuRahma AF, Srivastava M, Stone PA, Mousa AY, Jain A, Dean LS, Keiffer T, Emmett M. Critical appraisal of the Carotid Duplex Consensus criteria in the diagnosis of carotid artery stenosis. *J Vasc Surg.* 2011;53(1):53-59; discussion 59-60.

This should be present for multiple beats of the cardiac cycle.[36] It is seen in the CCA, ECA, and ICA.

2. Pandiastolic reversal is a reversal of flow through more than 50% of diastole (Fig. 2-32). Lesser duration of reversal is seen even in mild cases of regurgitation. Pandiastolic flow[37] reversal is most often seen in the CCA and ECA only, presumably because they supply vascular beds of high resistance, whereas the ICA flow pattern is dominated by the low resistance of arteriolar vessels.

Flow reversal due to aortic insufficiency is seldom seen in the ICA; such reversal is unlikely to be a problem for disease assessment of the ICA.

Mixed Aortic Stenosis and Insufficiency

Carotid artery flow patterns may be complex in the presence of mixed aortic stenosis and insufficiency, representing a combination of abnormal waveform changes (Fig. 2-33).

Aortic Stenosis

Mild and moderate aortic stenoses are unlikely to affect carotid artery velocity profiles. Severe aortic stenosis is likely to affect the velocity profile of the common and eternal carotid arteries, but not of the ICA.[38] Concomitant aortic insufficiency further alters the spectral pattern.

The most definitive carotid waveform patterns associated with aortic stenosis are: (1) increased acceleration time (i.e., angle of upstroke), or the so-called "parvus tardus" spectral profile (a borrowed observation from the pressure waveform being diminished and delayed—"parvus et tardus"); and (2) a rounded systolic peak. Severe and critical aortic stenosis may reduce the PSV recorded in the CCA and ECA.

Distal Lesions of the Internal Carotid Artery

Until recently, it was seldom possible to differentiate subtotal stenosis and total occlusion reliably by duplex imaging. With current high-resolution digital scanners and beam-forming technology, there is improved sensitivity and greater ability to scan into the distal segment of the extracranial ICA. Doppler findings in the extracranial/cervical ICA in the presence of an occlusion distal to the ophthalmic artery, the first major ICA branch, or in the case of dissection, show a high-resistance/low-velocity flow pattern. In the case of occlusion of the ICA, it may remain open by virtue of inflow through patent branch vessels (see Fig. 2-26).[39]

In dissection, the false lumen is often not visualized if the false lumen is thrombosed or if the lesion is in fact an intramural hematoma. Dissection and intramural hematoma may result in a sudden and dramatic tapering of the lumen beyond the origin of the ICA (Fig. 2-34).[40] Power imaging may be useful if flow rate is reduced (see Fig. 2-28).

Intra-Aortic Balloon Counterpulsation

Doppler waveforms generated during intra-aortic balloon counterpulsation (IABP) include two peaks; one is systolic and the other, typically the higher one, is

TABLE 2-5   Consensus Panel Grayscale and Doppler Ultrasound Criteria for Diagnosis of Internal Carotid Artery Stenosis

DEGREE OF STENOSIS	PRIMARY PARAMETERS		ADDITIONAL PARAMETERS	
	ICA PSV (cm/sec)	Plaque Estimate (%)*	ICA/CCA PSV Ratio	ICA EDV (cm/sec)
Normal	<125	None	<2.0	<40
<50%	<125	<50	<2.0	<40
50%–69%	125–230	≥50	>4.0	40–100
≥70% but less than near occlusion	>230	≥50	>4.0	>100
Near occlusion	High, low, or undetectable	Visible	Variable	Variable
Total occlusion	Undetectable	Visible, no detectable lumen	Not applicable	Not applicable

*Plaque estimate (diameter reduction) with grayscale and color Doppler ultrasound.
CCA, common carotid artery; EDV, end-diastolic velocity; ICA, internal carotid artery; PSV, peak systolic velocity.
From Grant EG, Benson CB, Moneta GL, et al. Carotid artery stenosis: gray-scale and Doppler US diagnosis—Society of Radiologists in Ultrasound Consensus Conference. *Radiology.* 2003;229(2):340-346; used with permission.

TABLE 2-6   Literature Review of Doppler Ultrasound Thresholds and Performance in Diagnosis of Internal Carotid Artery Stenosis

STUDY AND YEAR	Stenosis (%)	THRESHOLD PSV (cm/sec)	EDV (cm/sec)	Ratio	PERFORMANCE Sensitivity (%)	Specificity (%)	PPV (%)	NPV (%)	Accuracy (%)
Huston et al. (2000)	50	130	—	1.6	92	90	90	91	91
	70	230	70	3.2	86	90	83	92	89
Grant et al. (1999)	60	200	—	3	AP	AP	AP	AP	AP
	70	175	—	2.5	SP	SP	SP	SP	SP
AbuRahma et al. (1998)	50	140	—	—	92	95	97	89	93
	60	150	65	—	82	97	96	86	90
	70	150	90	—	85	95	91	92	92
Carpenter et al. (1995)	70	210	—	—	94	77	68	96	83
	70	—	70	—	92	60	73	86	77
	70	—	—	3.3	100	65	65	100	79
Hood et al. (1996)	70	130	100	—	78	97	88	94	93
Carpenter et al. (1995)	60	170	—	—	98	87	88	98	92
	60	—	40	—	97	52	86	86	86
	60	—	—	2.0	97	73	78	96	76
	60	230	40	2.0	100	100	100	100	100
Browerman et al. (1995)	70	175	—	—	91	60	—	—	—
Moneta et al. (1995)	60	260	70	3.2-3.5	84	94	92	88	90
Neale et al. (1994)	70	270	110	—	96	91	—	—	93
Moneta et al. (1993)	70	325	130	—	83	90	80	92	88

Ratio is internal carotid artery PSV to distal common carotid artery PSV. Thresholds are based on outcome > sensitivity/specificity > sensitivity/specificity > accuracy.
AP, asymptomatic patients; EDV, end-diastolic velocity; NPV, negative predictive value; PPV, positive predictive value; PSV, peak systolic velocity; SP, symptomatic patients.
From Grant EG, Benson CB, Moneta GL, et al. Carotid artery stenosis: gray-scale and Doppler US diagnosis—Society of Radiologists in Ultrasound Consensus Conference. *Radiology.* 2003;229(2):340-346.
Studies cited in this table:

Huston J 3rd, James EM, Brown RD Jr, et al. Redefined duplex ultrasonographic criteria for diagnosis of carotid artery stenosis. *Mayo Clin Proc.* 2000;75(11):1133-1140.
Grant EG, Duerinckx AJ, El Saden S, et al. Doppler sonographic parameters for detection of carotid stenosis: is there an optimum method for their selection? *AJR Am J Roentgenol.* 1999;172:1123-1129.
AbuRahma AF, Robinson PA, Strickler DL, et al. Proposed new duplex classification for threshold stenoses used in various symptomatic and asymptomatic carotid endarterectomy trials. *Ann Vasc Surg.* 1998;12(4):349-358.
Carpenter JP, Lexa FJ, Davis JT. Determination of sixty percent or greater carotid artery stenosis by duplex Doppler ultrasonography. *J Vasc Surg.* 1995;22(6):697-703; discussion 703-705.
Hood DB, Mattos MA, Mansour A, et al. Prospective evaluation of new duplex criteria to identify 70% internal carotid artery stenosis. *J Vasc Surg.* 1996;23(2):254-261; discussion 261-262.
Browerman MW, Cooperberg PL, Harrison PB, et al. Duplex ultrasonography criteria for internal carotid stenosis of more than 70% diameter: angiographic correlation and receiver operating characteristic curve analysis. *Can Assoc Radiol J.* 1995;46:291-295.
Moneta GL, Edwards JM, Papanicolaou G, et al. Screening for asymptomatic internal carotid artery stenosis: duplex criteria for discriminating 60% to 99% stenosis. *J Vasc Surg.* 1995;21(6):989-994.
Neale ML, Chambers JL, Kelly AT, et al. Reappraisal of duplex criteria to assess significant carotid stenosis with special reference to reports from the North American Symptomatic Carotid Endarterectomy Trial and the European Carotid Surgery Trial. *J Vasc Surg.* 1994;20:642-649.
Moneta GL, Edwards JM, Chitwood RW, et al. Correlation of North American Symptomatic Carotid Endarterectomy Trial (NASCET) angiographic definition of 70% to 99% internal carotid artery stenosis with duplex scanning. *J Vasc Surg.* 1993;17:152-159.

TABLE 2-7   Other Pertinent Literature on Internal Carotid Artery Stenosis

STUDY AND YEAR	THRESHOLD CHOSEN			ASSESSMENT AND RESULTS
	Stenosis (%)	PSV (cm/sec)	Ratio*	
Umemura and Yamada (2001)	NA	NA	NA	Evaluated results of B-flow imaging without Doppler
Perkins et al. (2000)	NA	NA	NA	Survey results show that laboratories use inconsistent thresholds
Grant et al. (2000)	NA	NA	NA	Doppler ultrasound cannot be used to estimate a single degree of stenosis but is better for differentiating less than or more than a single degree of stenosis
Beebe et al. (1999)	NA	NA	NA	Color and gray scale perform well alone: Doppler helps for midrange lesions
Soulez et al. (1999)	70, 60	NA	3.4, 2.9	Ratio of ICA PSV at and distal to stenosis performs better than ICA:CCA ratio
Ranke et al. (1999)	70	NA	NA	Ratio of ICA PSV at and distal to stenosis: sensitivity, 97%, specificity, 98%
Derdeyn and Powers (1996)	60	230	NA	Evaluation of cost-effectiveness of asymptomatic screening
Griewing et al. (1996)	NA	NA	NA	Power Doppler better than color Doppler (not quantified)
Srinivasan et al. (1995)	NA	NA	NA	Doppler poor for differentiating degree of <50% stenosis
Hunink et al. (1993)	70	230	NA	PSV best parameter for predicting >70% stenosis
Bluth et al. (1988)	NA	NA	NA	End-diastolic volume best Doppler parameter; did not use NASCET angiography criteria

*Ratio is ICA PSV to distal CCA PSV.

NA, not applicable; ICA, internal carotid artery; NASCET, North American Symptomatic Carotid Endarterectomy Trial; PSV, peak systolic velocity.
From Grant EG, Benson CB, Moneta GL, et al. Carotid artery stenosis: gray-scale and Doppler US diagnosis—Society of Radiologists in Ultrasound Consensus Conference. *Radiology.* 2003;229(2):340-346.

Studies cited in this table:

Umemura A, Yamada K. B-mode flow imaging of the carotid artery. *Stroke.* 2001;32(9):2055-2057.

Perkins JM, Galland RB, Simmons MJ, Magee TR. Carotid duplex imaging: variation and validation. *Br J Surg.* 2000;87(3):320-322.

Grant EG, Duerinckx AJ, El Saden SM, et al. Ability to use duplex US to quantify internal carotid arterial stenoses: fact or fiction? *Radiology.* 2000;214(1):247-252.

Beebe HG, Salles-Cunha SX, Scissons RP, et al. Carotid arterial ultrasound scan imaging: a direct approach to stenosis measurement. *J Vasc Surg.* 1999;29(5):838-844.

Soulez G, Therasse E, Robillard P, et al. The value of internal carotid systolic velocity ratio for assessing carotid artery stenosis with Doppler sonography. *AJR Am J Roentgenol.* 1999;172(1):207-212.

Ranke C, Creutzig A, Becker H, Trappe HJ. Standardization of carotid ultrasound: a hemodynamic method to normalize for interindividual and interequipment variability. *Stroke.* 1999;30(2):402-406.

Derdeyn CP, Powers WJ. Cost-effectiveness of screening for asymptomatic carotid atherosclerotic disease. *Stroke.* 1996;27(11):1944-1950.

Griewing B, Morgenstern C, Driesner F, et al. Cerebrovascular disease assessed by color-flow and power Doppler ultrasonography. Comparison with digital subtraction angiography in internal carotid artery stenosis. *Stroke.* 1996;27(1):95-100.

Srinivasan J, Mayberg MR, Weiss DG, Eskridge J. Duplex accuracy compared with angiography in the Veterans Affairs Cooperative Studies Trial for Symptomatic Carotid Stenosis. *Neurosurgery.* 1995;36(4):648-653; discussion 653-655.

Hunink MG, Polak JF, Barlan MM, O'Leary DH. Detection and quantification of carotid artery stenosis: efficacy of various Doppler velocity parameters. *AJR Am J Roentgenol.* 1993;160(3):619-625.

Bluth EI, Stavros AT, Marich KW, et al. Carotid duplex sonography: a multicenter recommendation for standardized imaging and Doppler criteria. *Radiographics.* 1988;8(3):487-506.

diastolic and due to the inflation of the intra-aortic balloon in diastole and the aortic pressure rise ("augmentation"). IABP typically reduces the systolic pressure and the waveform. IABP may be set with fixed but different relation to the cardiac cycles: 1:1, 1:2, or 1:3, influencing the cycle pattern of diastolic augmentation (Fig. 2-35). IABP influences the common carotid flow patterns, and may confuse the internal carotid flow patterns.[41] The systolic velocity ratio can be used, or more simply, putting the pump to standby, if safe, during sampling, simplifies waveforms and their interpretation.

Bilateral Significant Stenosis of the Internal Carotid Artery

It has been established that in the presence of bilateral severe stenosis/occlusion of the ICA, there can be a compensatory flow increase in the contralateral (asymptomatic) ICA that is variable and entirely dependent on the particular collateralization pathways. In the context of significant bilateral disease, the systolic velocity ratio diagnostic criteria should be emphasized.

Tandem Lesions

Although rare, tandem lesions involving both distal CCA and proximal ICA do occur. The poststenotic flow disturbance from the more proximal lesion may extend into the flow pattern of the distal lesion, confounding its assessment using PSV alone and making it unreliable. In this situation the ICA:CCA systolic velocity ratio[42] may be more useful in determining if the stenosis is less than or greater than 70%. Use of complementary imaging is advisable in the context of tandem lesions.

Cardiac Arrhythmia

Arrhythmias, such as atrial fibrillation, that result in widely varying cardiac cycle lengths can result in systolic peaks of varying heights. This renders accurate measurement of the true PSV difficult and necessitates the averaging of a minimum of four or five successive spectral profiles to determine the local velocity measurement (Fig. 2-36).

Paragangliomas

Originally referred to as chemodectomas, paragangliomas are rare (<1% of neck tumors),[43] slow-growing tumors, that are unilateral in 95% of cases.[40,44] They most commonly occur in the carotid body (Fig. 2-37).[43] Approximately 6% to 12.5% of cases are malignant.[41,45] They are often first noticed as a palpable, painless neck mass. On ultrasound, their appearance is that of a well-defined, heterogeneous, and hypervascularized mass resulting in splaying of the ECA:ICA bifurcation and displacement of the ICA and ECA.[46] Parangliomas can be distinguished from other neck masses by their position in the carotid bifurcation together with their solitary nature. In most cases, the ascending pharyngeal artery[44] feeds the tumor, but increased ECA end-diastolic flow has been identified by duplex.[45]

OTHER LESIONS AND DISEASES OF THE CAROTID AND VERTEBRAL ARTERIES

Fibromuscular Dysplasia

Fibromuscular dysplasia is a nonatherosclerotic disease of unknown cause that most often affects young women with early onset of hypertension and involves most commonly the renal and distal ICAs (25% to 30%).[47] From 7% to 51% of the carotid cases are associated with intracranial aneurysm. They may be asymptomatic and detected only by their generation of a carotid bruit or may result in transient ischemic attack or cerebrovascular accident.

The distal extracranial/cervical ICA is usually accessible by duplex, and grayscale resolution can be limited, especially if it is necessary to use a nonlinear transducer. However, the typical appearance of distal color and Doppler flow velocity elevation can be readily seen and easily distinguished from the more typical proximal atherosclerotic disease (Fig. 2-38).

Tortuosity

Tortuosity of the middle and distal ICA is commonplace and causes disturbed flow generally along the inner wall distal to the curve, with subsequent normalization of flow shortly downstream. In nondiseased but tortuous carotid arteries, the streaming and eddies are complex as is readily noted by color Doppler flow mapping, and true velocity measurements can be a technical challenge to record with spectral Doppler, because optimal angle of insonation (≤60 degrees) may be difficult or ambiguous to obtain.

It has been suggested[48] that the most reliable velocity recording be gathered from the inner wall distal to the curve and that the angle of insonation be recorded, to be adopted in any subsequent studies.

Hoskins and colleagues[49] demonstrated in a study involving 220 consecutive patients (440 vessels) that although occlusive disease in the ICA occurs most frequently in the first 3 cm of the cervical ICA, tortuosity occurs most commonly distal to this, suggesting that the presence of significant atherosclerosis in the tortuous segment is uncommon. Furthermore, it has long been established and should be emphasized that current diagnostic criteria are reliable only for the proximal first 2 to 3 cm of the ICA.

Postcarotid Endarterectomy

Duplex scanning is best performed several weeks after surgery when edema and incisional tenderness have resolved and the endothelium has undergone repair. CEA involves the excision of plaque by arteriotomy, beginning just proximal to the plaque and ending immediately distal to it. Intimal irregularities are apparent by ultrasound following CEA (Fig. 2-39). Recurrent stenosis is caused by myointimal hyperplasia rather than atherosclerosis and usually occurs at either the proximal or distal arteriotomy site.[48] The incidence of recurrent stenosis is 10% to 20%, and it generally occurs within 2 years of surgery. The lesion is typically fibrous, smooth, and stable; rarely with stenosis exceeding 80%; and is often asymptomatic (Fig. 2-40). On duplex imaging, the lesion appears noncalcified and smooth-surfaced. Increased flow velocity may occur depending on the severity but usually without the typical poststenotic turbulence associated with more irregular-surfaced and generally shorter atherosclerotic plaques (Figs. 2-41 and 2-42). Total occlusion due to restenosis is rare. A double wall can be seen at the arteriotomy site as remodeling progresses, and this should not be interpreted as recurrent disease.

Postcarotid Stenting

As with the endarterectomized vessel, if restenosis occurs, it will be because of myointimal hyperplasia ingrowth through the stent struts. Although the stent strut material is highly reflective, the sections between the wires enable some visualization beyond the stent, unless multiple stents are overlapping and provide an effective barrier to visualization. Most carotid artery restenosis tissue is uncalcified and seldom appears obvious within the stent and beyond the near stent wall. Unlike post-CEA where the plaque is removed, poststenting where the plaque still remains, calcified plaque may impair visualization by conferring acoustical shadowing postsurgery (Fig. 2-43). Several investigators have identified an increase in PSV in some stents in the absence of any other sign of disease (Fig. 2-44).[50] It has been suggested that the traditional criteria used for native vessels not be used for stents, where there might be reduced compliance because the plaque still remains adjacent to the vessel wall, and that greater emphasis should be placed on such findings as focal flow velocity elevation and poststenotic turbulence, rather than solely on the PSV.

Carotid Artery Fistula

Most carotid artery fistulas are the result of penetrating trauma, especially central line insertion. Most carotid artery fistulas occur between the CCA and the internal jugular vein. The fistula imparts a low-resistance outflow from the carotid artery. Color flow mapping generally readily depicts the fistulous flow, and pulsed-wave sampling confirms the continuous pattern of the flow. If the volume of fistulous flow is large, it imparts a low-resistance pattern to the CCA proximal to it and reduced velocity distal to it (Fig. 2-45).

Carotid Intima-Medial Thickness

Measurement of the carotid artery intimal plus medial thickness has been shown to stratify cardiovascular (usually myocardial infarction) risk.[51] The threshold of greater than 1 mm or less than 1 mm of IMT has variable prediction of risk. The nature of the thickening—atherosclerotic or smooth muscle—has not been established. The IMT of the CCA is most commonly used rather than the ICA or bulb IMT, because imaging of the CCA is almost always feasible. Measurement of the far wall is preferred over use of the near wall. Grayscale imaging and M-mode may both be used. For serial studies (intervention investigation), measurement off the same part of the cardiac cycle is necessary.

In general, the presence of actual plaques is far more predictive of atherosclerotic risk (e.g., myocardial infarction) than is IMT.[52]

The presence of carotid plaques, stenosis, or IMT affords some predictiveness (96% sensitivity, 89% specificity) of the distinction of ischemic versus nonischemic cardiomyopathy.[53] Similarly, absence of carotid IMT (>0.55 mm) is predictive of the absence of coronary artery disease in patients undergoing heart valve surgery.[54]

Spontaneous Carotid or Vertebral Artery Dissection

The incidence of spontaneous carotid artery dissection is 1 to 3 per 100,000 per year. Spontaneous carotid and vertebral artery dissection together account for only approximately 2% of cases of stroke overall but 10% to 25% of stroke cases in younger and middle-aged patients. There is no gender predilection, but women present an average of 5 years earlier than men.

By either imaging or microscopy, an intimal tear is far more difficult to identify in the case of carotid artery dissection than in aortic dissection. A significant proportion of cases may be frank intramural hematomas. Flow within the false lumen is notoriously difficult to demonstrate.

As with aortic dissection, particularly when looking at younger patients, spontaneous carotid dissection is common as a manifestation of an underlying disorder of medial degeneration or defective synthesis. Ehlers-Danlos syndrome type IV, Marfan syndrome, and other hereditary syndromes are examples. Five percent of cases have a family history of carotid dissection.

Presentations vary. Minor preceding trauma occurs in many cases. It is estimated that one in 20,000 cervical chiropractic manipulations causes a stroke. Pain involving the face, neck, or head is common in carotid artery dissection. Oculosympathetic palsy/partial Horner syndrome (miosis, ptosis) occurs in 50% of cases. Cerebral or retinal ischemic symptoms also occur in 50% of cases. Vertebral artery dissection is associated with pain in the posterior neck or head and posterior circulation problems.

Forms of angiography (conventional, MRA, and CTA) have been the standard diagnostic tests. An intimal flap is seldom demonstrated. Carotid artery dissection usually begins 2 to 3 cm distal to the bulb and extends no further than the base of the skull. Tapered beginning and endings are characteristic. Angiographic findings of vertebral artery dissection are less specific than for carotid artery dissection. Multiple dissections may occur simultaneously.

Ultrasound is useful in establishing abnormality of the carotid artery morphology and flow in the case of carotid artery dissection, but frank and specific demonstration of dissection (intimal flap/true dissection and false lumens/intramural hematoma) is far more difficult than for aortic dissection. In more than 90% of cases, flow is abnormal, typically high resistance, with a low amplitude triphasic pattern. Confirmatory

TABLE 2-8   2007 ICAVL* Standards for Accreditation: Extracranial Carotid Testing

- Cerebrovascular testing is performed for appropriate clinical indications.
- The indication for testing must be documented.
- A complete extracranial study is bilateral and evaluates the entire course of the accessible portions of the common carotid arteries (CCAs) and internal carotid arteries (ICAs). The external carotid arteries (ECAs) and vertebral arteries are identified, and Doppler spectral analysis is performed.
- The laboratory must have a written protocol to determine the anatomic extent of the study.
- Measurement of bilateral arm systolic blood pressures and/or recording of subclavian artery velocity waveforms are recommended as a part of the complete examination.
- A written protocol must be in place that defines the components and documentation of the extracranial cerebrovascular examination. The entire course of the accessible portions of the CCA and ICA must be evaluated.
- The protocol must also describe how color-coded Doppler is utilized to supplement grayscale imaging and spectral Doppler. If other flow imaging modes (e.g., power Doppler) are used, the protocol must describe how they are utilized.
- Representative long-axis grayscale images must be documented as required by the protocol and must include at a minimum images of the:
  - CCA
  - ICA
  - Carotid bifurcation
- Representative spectral Doppler waveforms must be documented as required by the protocol and must include at a minimum waveforms taken from:
  - Proximal CCA
  - Mid/distal CCA
  - Proximal ICA
  - Distal ICA, sampling as distally as possible
  - One site in the ECA
  - One site in the vertebral
  - Documentation of areas of suspected stenosis must include representative waveforms recorded at and distal to the stenosis.
- Representative color-coded Doppler images must be documented as required by the protocol.
- Diagnostic criteria for interpretation of grayscale images, spectral Doppler, and when reported, plaque description and color-coded Doppler images must be laboratory specific and documented. These criteria can be based on published reports or internally generated and internally validated.
- The interpretation and report that is generated from the examination findings and diagnostic criteria must state the absence or presence of abnormalities in the vessels that were investigated. Disease, if present, must be characterized according to its location, etiology, extent, and severity.
- In general, a laboratory should perform a minimum of 100 complete examinations annually.
- The laboratory must have a written procedure for regular correlation of carotid duplex examinations with angiographic findings produced by digital subtraction arteriography, contrast-enhanced computed tomography, or magnetic resonance angiography. The correlation must be reported using the categories of stenosis defined by the diagnostic criteria utilized by the laboratory. Surgical correlations may be used when angiographic correlation is not available.
- A minimum of 30 internal carotid arteries must be correlated every 3 years.
- The correlation matrix should demonstrate greater than 70% agreement.

*Intersocietal Commission for the Accreditation of Vascular Laboratories.
From the Intersocietal Commission for the Accreditation of Vascular Laboratories (ICAVL). ICAVL standards. <http://www.icavl.org/icavl/main/standards.htm>

testing with angiography is standard (Figs. 2-46 and 2-47).[55] The 2007 Intersocietal Commission for the Accreditation of Vascular Laboratories (ICAVL) accreditation standards for extracranial carotid testing are summarized in Table 2-8.[56]

Carotid and Vertebral Artery Dissection from Aortic Dissection

The intimal flap and false lumen of aortic dissection involving the aortic arch may extend into the branches of the carotid or vertebral arteries. In some cases, this condition may be responsible for cerebral ischemia. Syncope, coma, and "painless" aortic dissection are more common with carotid/vertebral extension; delayed diagnosis, confusion with other more common forms of

ischemic stroke, and worse outcomes occur with acute aortic dissection that present with cerebrovascular branch vessel compromise. Dissection extension into the common carotid artery is more common than into the ICA. The right carotid artery may be involved via brachiocephalic dissection and the left carotid artery by direct extension of aortic dissection. Vertebral artery dissection may also result from aortic dissection.

Temporal Artery Disease (Temporal Arteritis)

Temporal arteritis (giant cell arteritis) in the active phase can be imaged by vascular ultrasound. Diffuse and regular hypoechoic wall thickening is usual. Focal increase of velocity may be seen, but more usually the velocities are increased throughout the segments affected by disease within narrowed sections (Fig. 2-48).

Incidental Lesions

Carotid ultrasound may hazard across many relevant incidental lesions within the neck, including thyroid cysts, thyroid nodules and tumors, jugular venous disease, and lymph nodes (Fig. 2-49).

REFERENCES

1. Strandness Jr DE. *Collateral Circulation in Clinical Surgery.* Philadelphia: WB Saunders; 1969.
2. Layton KF, Kallmes DF, Cloft HJ, Lindell EP, Cox VS. Bovine aortic arch variant in humans: clarification of a common misnomer. *AJNR Am J Neuroradiol.* 2006;27(7): 1541-1542.
3. Maybody M, Uszynski M, Morton E, Vitek JJ. Absence of the common carotid artery: a rare vascular anomaly. *AJNR Am J Neuroradiol.* 2003;24(4):711-713.
4. Given CA, Baker MD, Chepuri NB, Morris PP. Congenital absence of the internal carotid artery: case reports and review of the collateral circulation. *AJNR Am J Neuroradiol.* 2001;22(10):1953-1959.
5. Ghilardi G. The priliminary experience of the OPI program. The Obiettivo prevenzione ictus (stroke prevention objective). *Minerva Cardioangiol.* 1994;42(6): 269-273.
6. Keagy BA, Battaglini JW, Lucas CL, Thomas DD, Wilcox BR. Identification of internal carotid artery stenosis in coronary artery bypass candidates. *South Med J.* 1983;76(8):996-999.
7. Sauve JS, Thorpe KE, Sackett DL, et al. Can bruits distinguish high-grade from moderate symptomatic carotid stenosis? The North American Symptomatic Carotid Endarterectomy Trial. *Ann Intern Med.* 1994;120(8):633-637.
8. de Virgilio C, Arnell T, Lewis RJ, et al. Asymptomatic carotid artery stenosis screening in patients with lower extremity atherosclerosis: a prospective study. *Ann Vasc Surg.* 1997;11(4):374-377.
9. Qureshi AI, Alexandrov AV, Tegeler CH, Hobson RW, Dennis BJ, Hopkins LN. Guidelines for screening of extracranial carotid artery disease: a statement for healthcare professionals for the multidisciplinary practice guidelines committee of the American Society of Neuroimaging: cosponsored by the Society of Vascular and Interventional Neurology. *J Neuroimaging.* 2007; 17(1):19-47.
10. Collaborative overview of randomized trials of antiplatelet therapy—I: Prevention of death, myocardial infarction, and stroke by prolonged antiplatet therapy in various categories of patients. Antiplatelet Trialists' Collaboration. *BMJ.* 1994;308(6921):81-106.
11. Algra A, van Gign J. Aspirin at any dose above 30 mg offers only modest protection after cerebral ischaemia. *J Neurol Neurosurg Psychiatry.* 1996;60(2):197-199.
12. Gent M, Blakely JA, Easton JD, et al. The Canadian American Ticlopidine Study (CATS) in thromboembolic stroke. *Lancet.* 1989;1(8649):1215-1220.
13. Hass WK, Easton JD, Adams HPJ, et al. A randomized trial comparing ticlopidine hydrochloride with aspirin for the prevention of stroke in high-risk patients. Ticlopidine Aspirin Stroke Study Group. *N Engl J Med.* 1989;321(8):501-507.
14. A randomized, blinded trial of clopidogrel versus aspirin in patients at risk of ischaemic events (CAPRIE). CAPRIE Steering Committee. *Lancet.* 1996;348(9038): 1329-1339.
15. The European Stroke Prevention Study (ESPS). Principal end-points. The ESPE Group. *Lancet.* 1987;2(8572): 1351-1354.
16. Diener HC, Cunha L, Forbes C, Sivenius J, Smets P, Lowenthal A. European Stroke Prevention Study 2. Dipyridamole and acetylsalicyclic acid in the secondary prevention of stroke. *J Neurol Sci.* 1996;143(1-2): 1-13.
17. Sacco RL, Diener HC, Yusef S, et al. Aspirin and extended-release dipyridamole versus clopidogrel for recurrent stroke. For the PRoFESS study group. *N Engl J Med.* 2008;359:1238-1251.
18. Cote R, Battista R, Abrahamowicz M, Langlois Y, Bourque F, Mackey A. Lack of effect of aspirin in asymptomatic patients with carotid bruits and substantial carotid narrowing. *Ann Intern Med.* 1995;123(9):649-655.
19. Bock RW, Gray-Waele AC, Mock PA, et al. The natural history of asymptomatic carotid artery disease. *J Vasc Surg.* 1993;17(1):160-169.
20. Beneficial effect of carotid endarterectomy in symptomatic patients with high-grade carotid stenosis. North American Symptomatic Carotid Endarterectomy Trial Collaborators. *N Engl J Med.* 1991;325(7):445-453.
21. MRC European Carotid Surgery Trial: interim results for symptomatic patients with severe (70-99%) or with mild (0-29%) carotid stenosis. European Carotid Surgery Trialists' Collaborative Group. *Lancet.* 1991; 337(8752):1235-1243.
22. Mayberg MR, Wilson SE, Yatsu F, et al. Carotid endarterectomy and prevention of cerebral ischemia in symptomatic carotid stenosis. Veterans Affairs Cooperative Studies Program 309 Trialist Group. *JAMA.* 1991; 266(23):3289-3294.
23. Carotid surgery versus medical therapy in asymptomatic carotid stenosis. The CASANOVA study group. *Stroke.* 1991;10:1229-1235.
24. Hobson RW, Weiss DG, Fields WS, et al. Efficacy of carotid endarterectomy for asymptomatic carotid stenosis. The Veterans Affairs Cooperative Study Group. *N Engl J Med.* 1993;328(4):221-227.
25. Endarterectomy for asymptomatic carotid artery stenosis. Executive Committee for the Asymptomatic Carotid Atherosclerosis Study. *JAMA.* 1995;273(18):1421-1428.
26. Yadev JS, Wholey MH, Kuntz RE, et al. Protected carotid-artery stenting versus endarterectomy in high-risk patients. *N Engl J Med.* 2004;351(15):1493-1501.

27. McPhee JT, Schanzer A, Messina L, Eslami M. Carotid artery stenting has increased rates of postprocedure stroke, death and resource utilization than does carotid endarterectomy in the United States, 2005. *J Vasc Surg.* 2008;48(6):1442-1450.

28. Hallett Jr JW, Pietropaoli Jr JA, Ilstrup DM, Gayari MM, Williams JA, Meyer FB. Comparison of North American Symptomatic Carotid Endarterectomy Trial and population-based outcomes for carotid endarterectomy. *J Vasc Surg.* 1998;27(5):845-850:discussion 851.

29. Gorelick PB. Carotid endarterectomy: where do we draw the line? *Stroke.* 1999;30(9):1745-1750.

30. Chassin MR. Appropriate use of carotid endarterectomy. *N Engl J Med.* 1998;339(20):1468-1471.

31. Morey SS. AHA updates guidelines for carotid endarterectomy. *Am Fam Physician.* 1998;58(8):1898:1903–1894.

32. Mathiesen EB, Bonaa KH, Joakimsen O. Echolucent plaques are associated with high risk of ischemic cerebrovascular events in carotid stenosis: the Tromso study. *Circulation.* 2001;103(17):2171-2175.

33. Gronholdt ML, Nordestgaard BG, Schroeder TV, Vorstrup S, Sillesen H. Ultrasonic echolucent carotid plaques predict future strokes. *Circulation.* 2001;104(1):68-73.

34. Grant EG, Benson CB, Moneta GL, et al. Carotid artery stenosis: gray-scale and Doppler US diagnosis—Society of Radiologists in Ultrasound Consensus Conference. *Radiology.* 2003;229(2):340-346.

35. Lal BK, Hobson RW, Goldstein J, Chakhtoura EY, Duran WN. Carotid artery stenting: is there a need to revise ultrasound velocity criteria? *J Vasc Surg.* 2004;39(1):58-66.

36. Kallman CE, Gosink BB, Gardner DJ. Carotid duplex sonography: bisferious pulse contour in patients with aortic valvular disease. *AJR Am J Roentgenol.* 1991;157(2):403-407.

37. Kervancioglu S, Davutoglu V, Ozkur A, et al. Duplex sonography of the carotid arteries in patients with pure aortic regurgitation: pulse waveform and hemodynamic changes and a new indicator of the severity of aortic regurgitation. *Acta Radiol.* 2004;45(4):411-416.

38. O'Boyle MK, Vibhakar NI, Chung J, Keen WD, Gosink BB. Duplex sonography of the carotid arteries in patients with isolated aortic stenosis: imaging findings and relation to severity of stenosis. *AJR Am J Roentgenol.* 1996;166(1):197-202.

39. Lee TH, Ryu SJ, Chen ST, Chan JL. Carotid ultrasonographic findings in intracranial internal carotid artery occlusion. *Angiology.* 1993;44(8):607-613.

40. Sidhu PS, Jonker ND, Khaw KT, et al. Spontaneous dissections of the internal carotid artery: appearances on color Doppler ultrasound. *Br J Radiol.* 1997;70:50-57.

41. Horrow MM, Stassi J, Shurman A, Brody JD, Kirby CL, Rosenberg HK. The limitations of carotid sonography: interpretive and technology-related errors. *AJR Am J Roentgenol.* 2000;174(1):189-194.

42. Moneta GL, Edwards JM, Chitwood RW, et al. Correlation of North American Symptomatic Carotid Endarterectomy Trial (NASCET) angiographic definition of 70% to 99% internal carotid artery stenosis with duplex scanning. *J Vasc Surg.* 1993;17(1):152-157:[discussion 157-159].

43. Rao AB, Koeller KK, Adair CF. From the archives of the AFIP. Paragangliomas of the head and neck: radiologic-pathologic correlation. Armed Forces Institute of Pathology. *Radiographics.* 1999;19(6):1605-1632.

44. Mansour MA, Labropolous N. *Vascular Diagnosis.* Philadelphia: Elsevier-Saunders; 2005.

45. Singh D, Pinjala RK, Reddy RC, Satya Vani PV. Management for carotid body paragangliomas. *Interact Cardiovasc Thorac Surg.* 2006;5(6):692-695.

46. Stoeckli SJ, Schuknecht B, Alkadhi H, Fisch U. Evaluation of paragangliomas presenting as a cervical mass on color-coded Doppler sonography. *Laryngoscope.* 2002;112(1):143-146.

47. Olin JW. Recognizing and managing fibromuscular dysplasia. *Cleve Clin J Med.* 2007;74(4):273-274:277-282.

48. Strandness Jr DE. *Duplex Scanning in Vascular Disorders.* 3rd ed. Philadelphia: Lippincott Williams & Wilkins; 2002.

49. Hoskins MS, Scissons RP. Hemodynamically significant carotid disease in duplex ultrasound patients with carotid artery tortuosity. *J Vasc Ultrasound.* 2007;31(1):11-15.

50. Kupinski MA, Khan AM, Stanton JE, et al. Duplex ultrasound follow-up of carotid stents. *J Vasc Ultrasound.* 2004;28(2):71-75.

51. O'Leary DH, Polak JF, Kronmal RA, Manolio TA, Burke GL, Wolfson Jr SK. Carotid-artery intima and media thickness as a risk factor for myocardial infarction and stroke in older adults. Cardiovascular Health Study Collaborative Research Group. *N Engl J Med.* 1999;340(1):14-22.

52. Roman MJ, Naqvi TZ, Gardin JM, Gerhard-Herman M, Jaff M, Mohler E. Clinical application of noninvasive vascular ultrasound in cardiovascular risk stratification: a report from the American Society of Echocardiography and the Society of Vascular Medicine and Biology. *J Am Soc Echocardiogr.* 2006;19(8):943-954.

53. Androulakis AE, Andrikopoulos GK, Richter DJ, et al. The role of carotid atherosclerosis in the distinction between ischaemic and non-ischaemic cardiomyopathy. *Eur Heart J.* 2000;21(11):919-926.

54. Belhassen L, Carville C, Pelle G, et al. Evaluation of carotid artery and aortic intima-media thickness measurements for exclusion of significant coronary atherosclerosis in patients scheduled for heart valve surgery. *J Am Coll Cardiol.* 2002;39(7):1139-1144.

55. Schievink WI. Spontaneous dissection of the carotid and vertebral arteries. *N Engl J Med.* 2001;344(12):898-906.

56. Intersocietal Commission for the Accreditation of Vascular Laboratories (ICAVL). ICAVL standards. <http://www.icavl.org/icavl/main/standards.htm>; Accessed March 26, 2009.

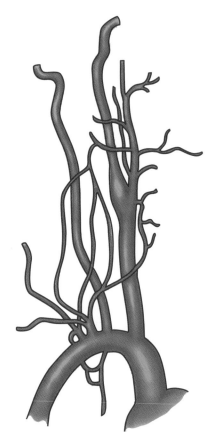

Figure 2-1. The vertebral and carotid arteries and their branches are only some of the arteries within the neck. Note the appearance of the normal proximal internal carotid artery, which is bulb-shaped. The external carotid artery branch to subclavian branch collaterals are normal.

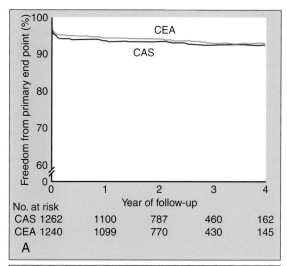

A

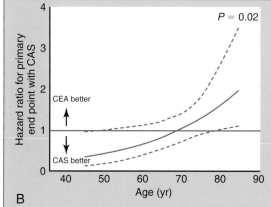

B

Figure 2-3. Primary end point, according to treatment group. The primary end point was a composite of stroke, myocardial infarction, or death from any cause during the periprocedural period or ipsilateral stroke within 4 years after randomization. Panel A shows the Kaplan-Meier curves for patients undergoing carotid artery stenting (CAS) and those undergoing carotid endarterectomy (CEA) in whom the primary end point did not occur, according to year of follow up, Panel B shows the hazard ratios for the primary end points, as calculated for the CAS group versus the CEA group, according to age at the time of the procedure. The hazard ratios were estimated from the proportional-hazards model with adjustment for sex and symptomatic status. Dashed lines indicate the 95% confidence intervals. (From Brott et al. Stenting versus endarterectomy for treatment of carotid-artery stenosis. *N Engl J Med.* 2010;363:11-23; used with permission.)

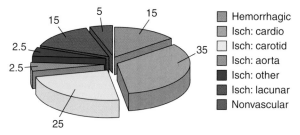

Hemorrhagic
Isch: cardio
Isch: carotid
Isch: aorta
Isch: other
Isch: lacunar
Nonvascular

Figure 2-2. Carotid artery disease accounts for approximately 25% of all stroke cases and is the second largest cause of ischemic stroke. Cardio, cardio-embolic; Isch, ischemic.

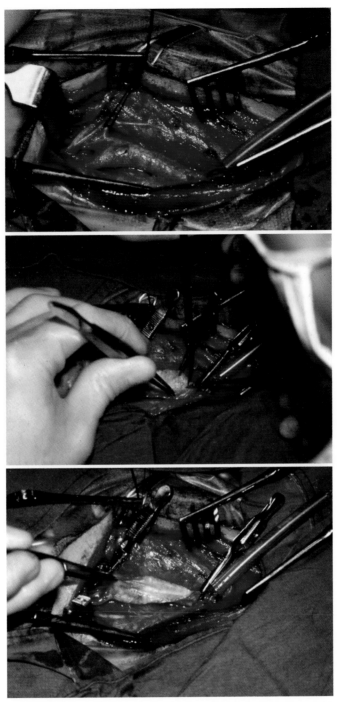

Figure 2-4. Carotid endarterectomy. *Top,* The internal carotid artery (ICA) is exposed either by an incision that is longitudinal to the body of the sternocleido-mastoid muscle or by an incision that is oblique and within an available skin crease. The incision is followed by dissection through the platysma muscle and beneath it to the vessels. The longitudinal relation of the common carotid artery (CCA) to the internal jugular vein is established. The common facial vein, a major branch of the internal jugular artery that fairly consistently overlies the internal carotid artery bulb, is ligated, and then the internal jugular vein mobilized laterally to expose the common carotid artery. The CCA is mobilized with tape and extended toward the internal and external carotid arteries. The ICA must be mobilized well above the extent of intimal plaque (so that all of it is cleanly removed). The level at which the resuming ICA is normal is established by palpation of the artery, often against a clamp on the posterior aspect of the vessel. The twelfth cranial (hypogloassal) nerve is identified, usually superior to the bulb. Inadvertant damage to it results in sensory and motor dysfunction of the ipsilateral tongue. Hemostatic control is achieved at the lingual artery of the nearby external carotid artery (ECA). *Middle,* The ICA is dissected open after proximal and distal clamps have been put on to it. The atherosclerotic plaque is yellow and firm. *Bottom,* The atherosclerotic plaque has been removed from the ICA, which has now collapsed onto itself due to the lack of inflow of blood from either the proximal or distal ends because of the surgical clamps.

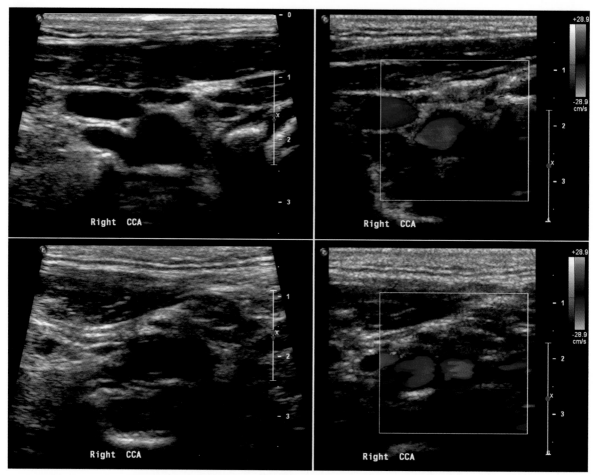

Figure 2-5. Grayscale images (*left*) and color Doppler flow mappings (*right*) of a short-axis sweep of the common carotid artery in cross-section from its origin to its bifurcation.

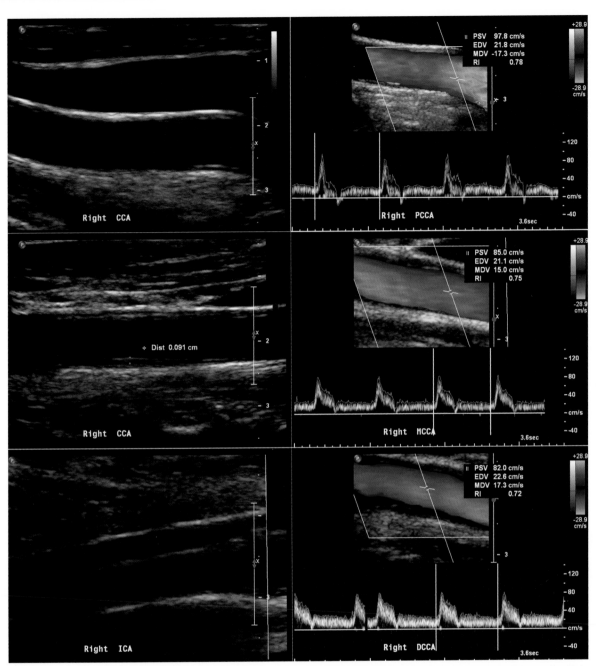

Figure 2-6. *Left*, Grayscale images of the proximal, mid-, and distal common carotid artery (CCA) with ongoing internal carotid artery (ICA) extension. *Right*, Corresponding spectral recordings guided by color flow mapping of these three different segments of the CCA.

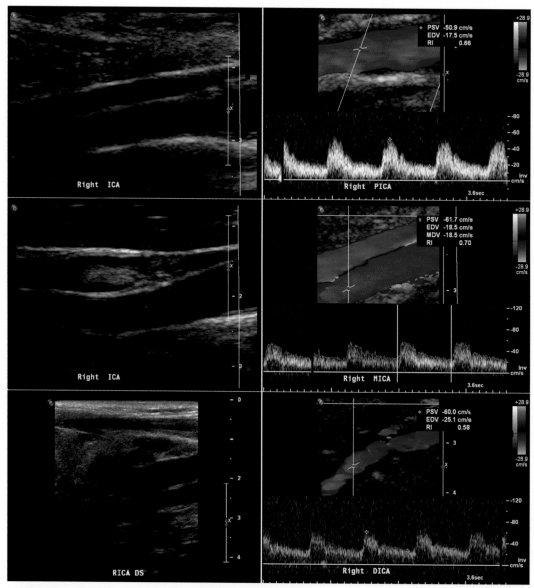

Figure 2-7. Normal exam. Grayscale images (*left*) and corresponding color Doppler flow mapping–guided spectral profiles (*right*) characterizing the anatomy and the flow physiology in the proximal, mid-, and distal extracranial internal carotid artery.

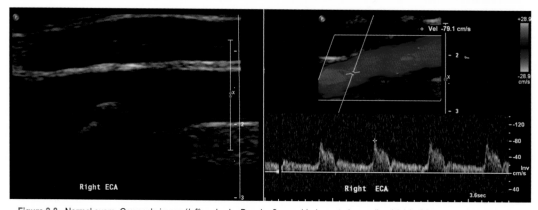

Figure 2-8. Normal exam. Grayscale image (*left*) and color Doppler flow–guided spectral recording (*right*) of the external carotid artery.

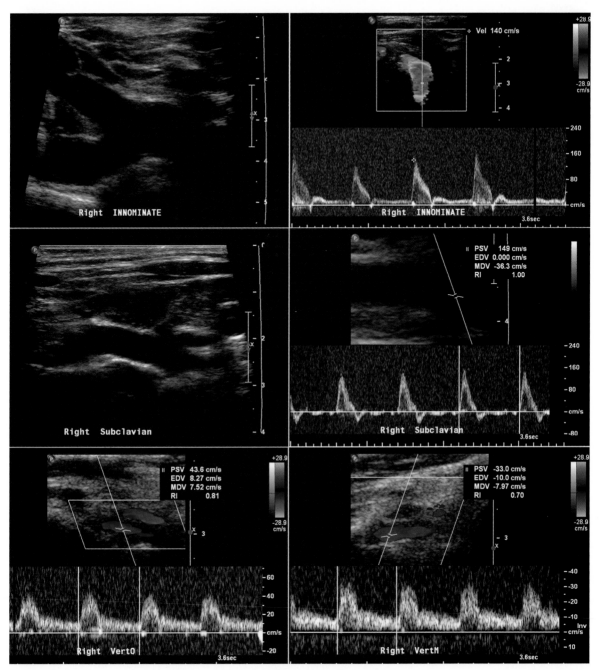

Figure 2-9. Normal exam. Innominate artery grayscale imaging and spectral flow recording (*top*), subclavian artery grayscale and spectral flow recordings (*middle*), and vertebral origin and mid-vertebral color Doppler flow mapping guided spectral flow recordings (*bottom*).

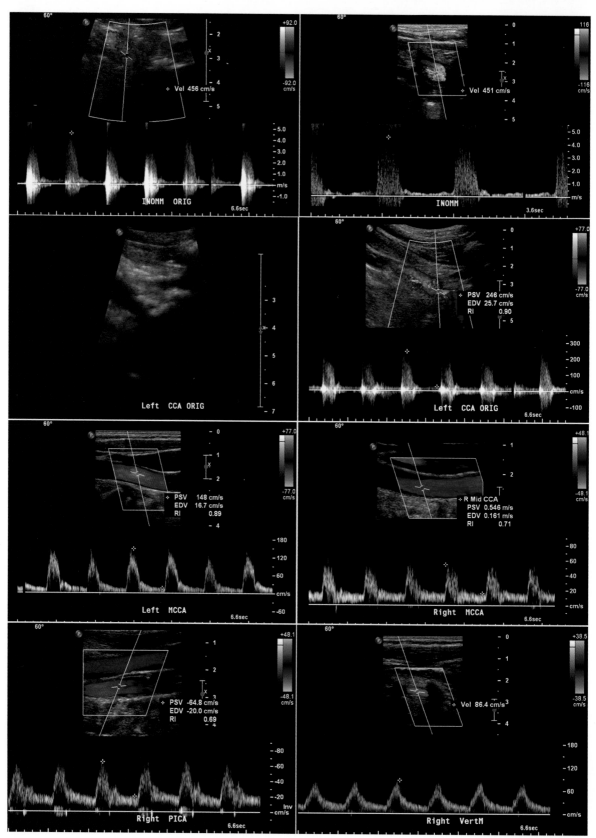

Figure 2-10. *First (top) row,* At the site of flow acceleration and turbulence denoted by color Doppler, spectral recording demonstrates severely elevated velocities with the monophasic pattern and turbulence consistent with innominate artery stenosis. *Second row,* Vaguely revealed plaque at the origin of the left common carotid artery (CCA). There is flow acceleration at the left CCA origin, and turbulence of flow consistent with stenosis. *Third row,* Wave forms of CCA flow velocities, normal bilaterally. The flow pattern had recovered from the effect of the innominate artery stenosis and left common carotid origin stenoses by within the mid-CCA. *Fourth (bottom) row, left,* Normal flow pattern within the proximal right internal carotid artery (ICA). *Fourth (bottom) row, right,* Delayed upstroke (tardus) pattern consistent with the presence of the severe upstream stenosis. In this patient, the flow patterns within the CCAs in the mid- and distal portions and within the ICAs were entirely normal. Significant stenoses were present within the innominate artery and the origin left CCA and as well the origin at the right vertebral artery, underscoring the need for complete assessment of the carotid arteries and the vertebral arteries through their entire length.

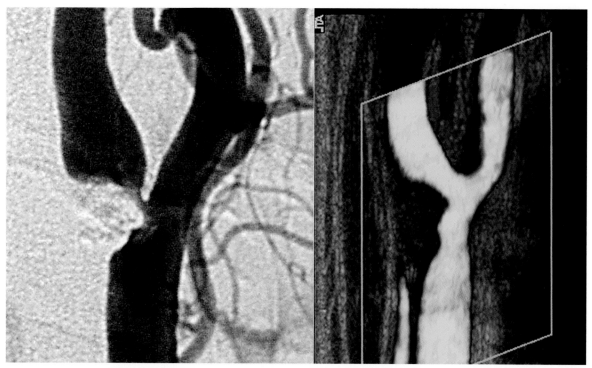

Figure 2-11. Conventional catheter angiography and power angiography Doppler imaging of distal common carotid artery and proximal internal carotid artery stenosis. The projections are approximately the same.

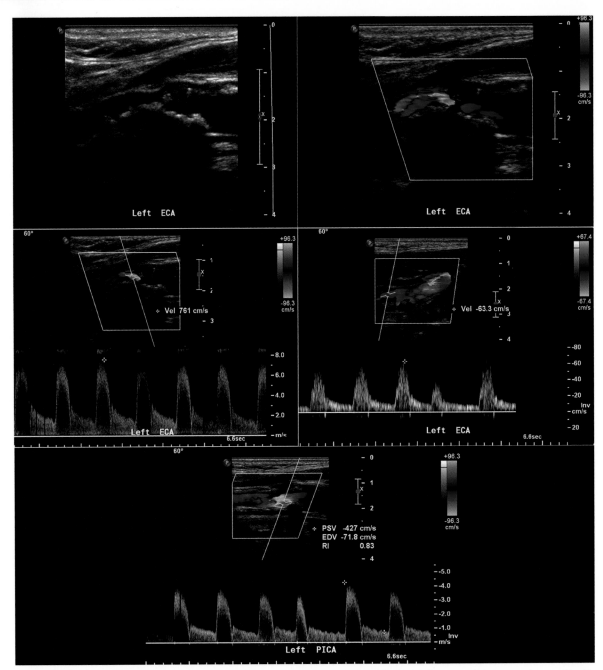

Figure 2-12. Hemodynamically significant stenosis at the origin of the external carotid artery (ECA). *Top left,* The grayscale image reveals a considerable volume of calcified atherosclerotic plaque. *Top right,* Color Doppler flow mapping demonstrates reduction of the lumen as well, in addition to turbulence. *Middle left,* Spectral flow recording at the site of turbulence and narrowing establishes severely elevated velocities at the site of narrowing at the origin of the ECA. *Middle right,* Flow velocities more distally in the ECA have normalized. *Bottom,* There is one spectral profile with lower systolic peak velocity due to the shorter cardiac cycle preceding it. Conversely, the spectral profile following it is higher due to the longer cardiac cycle preceding it.

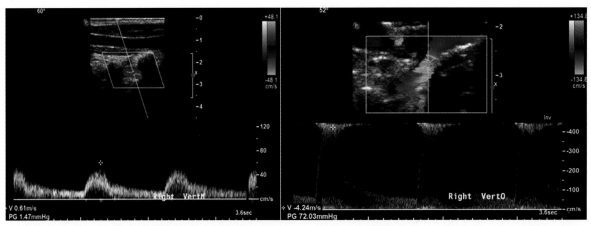

Figure 2-13. Ostial vertebral artery stenosis. *Left,* Spectral recording from the mid-right vertebral artery with normal velocities and no turbulence. *Right,* Spectral flow recording at the ostial level of the same artery. The upper box reveals the site of flow acceleration and turbulence. The spectral display demonstrates severely increased velocities and turbulence. The jet of accelerated flow from the stenosis had recovered by the site of sampling in the mid-right vertebral artery.

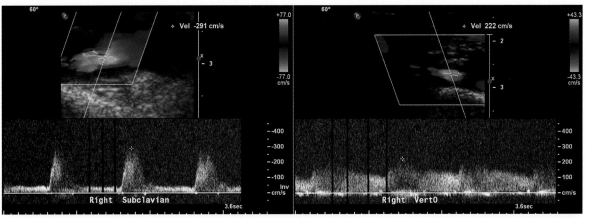

Figure 2-14. *Left,* At the site of flow turbulence seen by color Doppler within the right subclavian artery, spectral display reveals high velocity as well as turbulence. The flow pattern is biphasic. This is consistent with borderline subclavian artery stenosis. In fact, the sampling here was too distal from what was severe subclavian stenosis more proximally in the artery. *Right,* Spectral flow pattern of the origin of the right vertebral artery. The upstroke of the wave form is tardus, consistent with and due to severe stenosis at the origin of the vertebral artery.

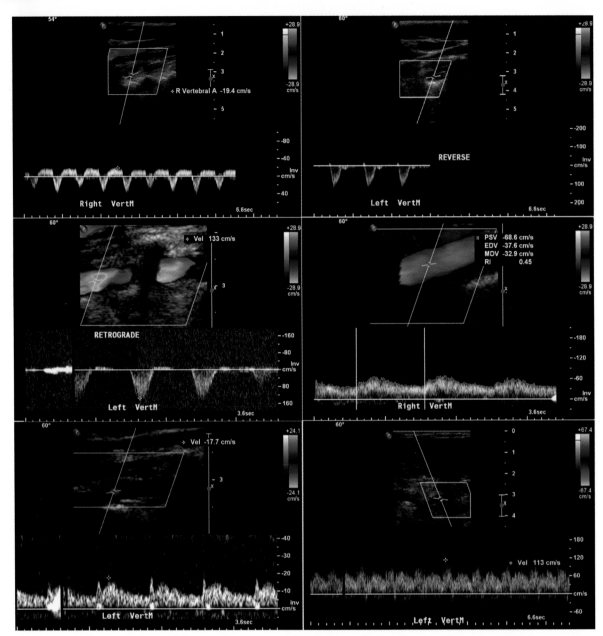

Figure 2-15. Abnormal wave forms within the vertebral arteries due to disease. The flow patterns are recorded in different patients. *Top left and right, middle left,* Flow reversal of varying degrees and patterns in the mid-portion of vertebral arteries consistent in three cases of subclavian steal physiology. *Middle right,* A flow pattern is tardus and there is turbulence, consistent with upstream severe stenosis. *Bottom left and right,* "Spike and dome" or "bunny rabbit" patterns of flow recorded in the mid-vertebral arteries consistent with borderline subclavian steal physiology.

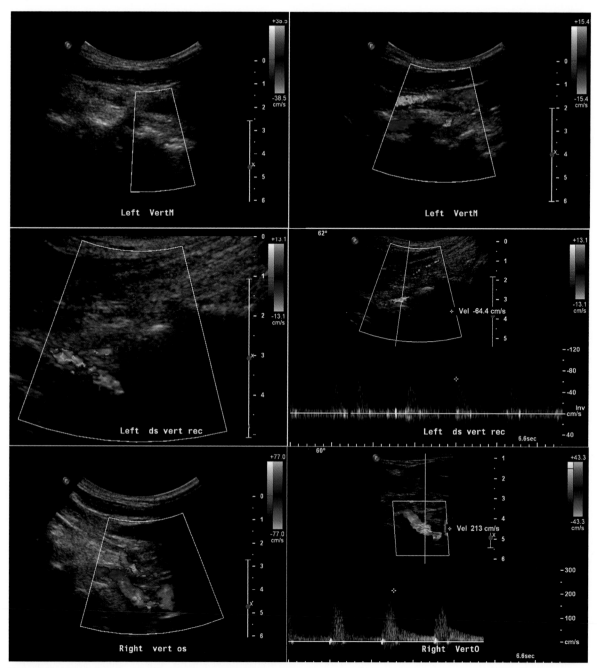

Figure 2-16. *Top left,* Color flow mapping does not depict any flow within the mid-portion of the left vertebral artery. *Top right,* Flow mapping of the more distal mid-portion of the mid left vertebral artery. In the more nearfield part of the carotid artery, flow is revealed. A collateral vessel in the mid-field appears to be returning to the vertebral artery. *Middle left,* A collateral vessel is in fact seen returning to reconstitute the distal left vertebral artery. *Middle right,* Spectral flow recording of pulsatile flow in the reconstituted distal vertebral artery, distal to the total occlusion in the mid-portion. *Bottom left and right,* Turbulence and mildly elevated but biphasic flow patterns, nonetheless, within the origin at the right vertebral artery, consistent with nonsevere stenosis. This patient, like many, had bilateral vertebral disease.

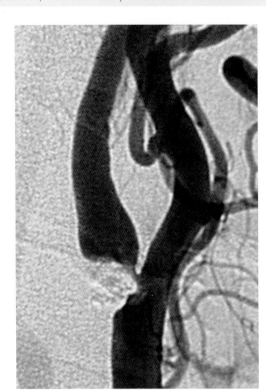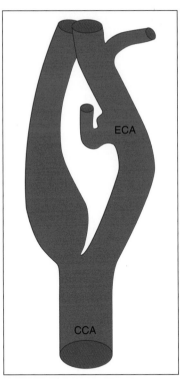

Figure 2-17. The proximal internal carotid artery (ICA) is larger in diameter than the ongoing portion. The proximal portion of the ICA, usually the posterior wall, is the usual site of plaque accumulation. Therefore, the stenosis is tending to occur in what would normally be a wider diameter segment of the vessel.

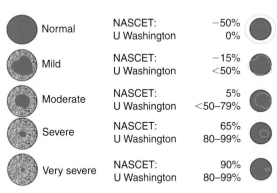

	NASCET:	
Normal	NASCET:	−50%
	U Washington	0%
Mild	NASCET:	−15%
	U Washington	<50%
Moderate	NASCET:	5%
	U Washington	<50–79%
Severe	NASCET:	65%
	U Washington	80–99%
Very severe	NASCET:	90%
	U Washington	80–99%

Figure 2-18. The NASCET (North American Symptomatic Carotid Endarterectomy Trial) and Washington reference standards to describe the luminal dimension ("diameter") differ significantly. The NASCET standard is the ongoing internal carotid artery of lesser size than the true bulb dimension. *Top left,* Cross-sectional schematics through internal carotid vessels (normal on top and worsening severity of stenosis below), with lumen depicted in gray and plaque depicted in marbled gray. The remaining lumen is demarcated by a yellow line. *Top right,* The luminal diameters are drawn on the NASCET standards (gray circles). In the absence of stenosis, the bulb diameter is greater than that of the ongoing ICA. Therefore, normal and mild stenosis within the bulb would actually yield a negative stenosis calculation when the ongoing ICA is used as the standard. Thus NASCET and Washington determinations of stenosis are inherently dissimilar. They differ most in the absence of stenosis or in the presence of very mild stenosis and agree increasingly as the severity of the stenosis increases. The graph below the illustration shows how the relation of the bulb standard and distal ICA standard are nonlinear and away from a line of identity.

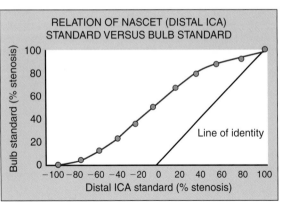

RELATION OF NASCET (DISTAL ICA)
STANDARD VERSUS BULB STANDARD

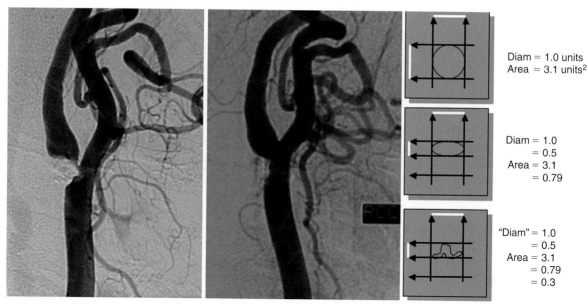

Diam = 1.0 units
Area = 3.1 units^2

Diam = 1.0
= 0.5
Area = 3.1
= 0.79

"Diam" = 1.0
= 0.5
Area = 3.1
= 0.79
= 0.3

Figure 2-19. Projection/eccentricity issues. Varying rotation and projections of plaque and lumen give a variable depiction of the stenosis severity. The convention is to take the most severe projection. Eccentricity of the lumen is responsible for the variable depiction according to projection. In the case of a very irregular and eccentric lumen, almost no angiographic technique is optimal to express what would be the hemodynamic consequence of the stenosis using linear measurement to describe the nonlinear orifice. The schematics on the right depict how a 90 degree difference in the incident x-ray beam does not vary the impression of the cross-sectional area of a round lumen (upper schematic), but does for the eccentric lesions. Symmetric (middle schematic) and asymmetric (bottom schematic) lumens may have the same dimensions as depicted by projection but different areas.

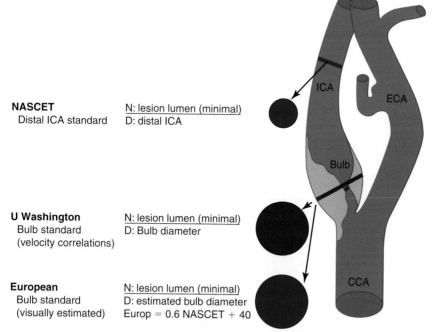

NASCET
Distal ICA standard

N: lesion lumen (minimal)
D: distal ICA

U Washington
Bulb standard
(velocity correlations)

N: lesion lumen (minimal)
D: Bulb diameter

European
Bulb standard
(visually estimated)

N: lesion lumen (minimal)
D: estimated bulb diameter
Europ = 0.6 NASCET + 40

Figure 2-20. The expression of carotid artery stenosis is performed according to distal internal carotid artery (ICA) standards and to bulb standard. The Washington/Strandness ultrasound technique correlated different velocities with different stenosis severity according to bulb standard. The European angiographic standard uses best attempt to measure bulb standard as seen on angiography. The North American Symptomatic Carotid Endarterectomy Trial (NASCET) angiographic standard uses the ongoing ICA as a reference standard. ECA, external carotid artery.

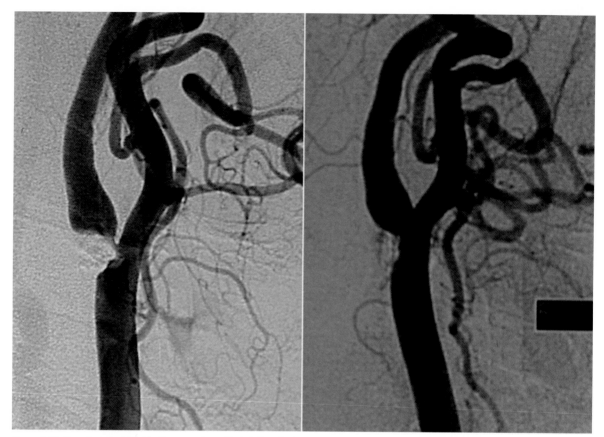

Figure 2-21. The effect of rotation/ejection on angiographic depiction of an internal carotid artery stenosis. *Left,* Optimally projected, the full severity of the stenosis can be seen. *Right,* Suboptimally projected, the severity of the stenosis is underrepresented. There is also a calcification within the atherosclerotic blockage.

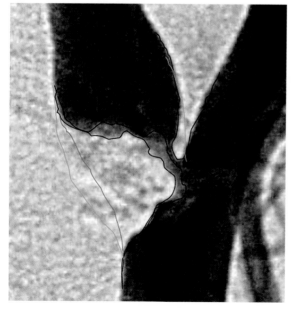

Figure 2-22. Edge delineation challenges an angiography. Both the delineation of the luminal margin to determine by North American Symptomatic Carotid Endarterectomy Trial (NASCET) or European criteria and delineation of the outside vessel margin for the European criteria are subject to some uncertainty and thereby variability. The luminal boundary may be abrupt and definitive or graduated through shades of gray (*black lines*). The outside of the way of the vessel is even more subjectively determined somewhat on the basis of where calcium is visualized but also on the basis of the presumed projection of the curvature of the visualized parts of the artery (*colored lines*).

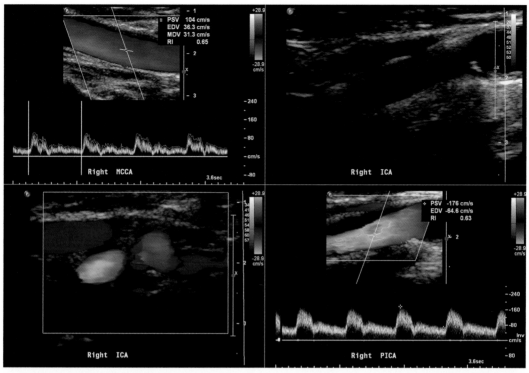

Figure 2-23. Ambiguity in categorization of internal carotid artery (ICA) stenosis using consensus criteria. The ICA peak systolic velocity (PSV) is elevated and consistent with 50% to 69% stenosis. The primary parameters yield discordant categorization by PSVs. The stenosis is 50% to 69%, but the plaque estimate appears to be less than 50%. Additional parameters are also discordant with an ICA-to-common carotid artery (CCA) PSV ratio of less than 2 but an ICA and diastolic velocity between 40 and 100 cm/sec.

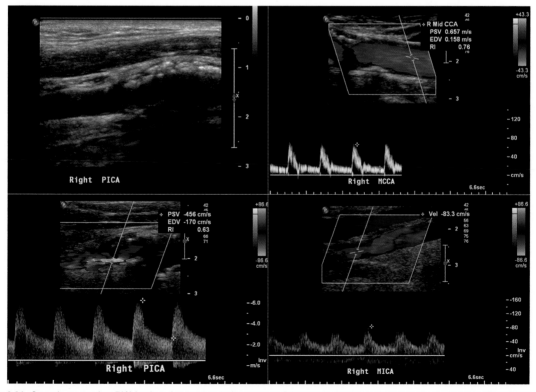

Figure 2-24. Stenosis greater than 70% but less than near-occlusion category. Primary and additional parameters are all consistent. The internal carotid artery (ICA) peak systolic velocity (PSV) is greater than 230 cm/sec, the plaque estimate in the most severe portion is greater than 50%, the ICA-to-common carotid artery (CCA) PSV ratio is greater than 4, and the end-diastolic velocity is greater than 100 cm/sec.

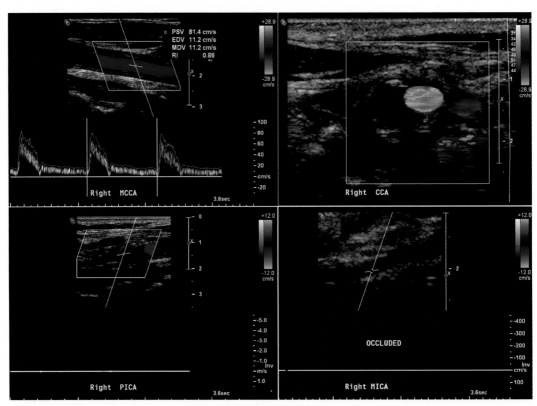

Figure 2-25. A total occlusion of the internal carotid artery (ICA). *Top left,* Normal flow in the middle portion of the common carotid artery (CCA). *Top right,* Above the level of the carotid artery bifurcation, there is flow seen in the external carotid artery (ECA) but not in the ICA. *Bottom left and right,* Images demonstrating an absence of flow in the proximal and mid-ICA, without flow depiction by color flow mapping or by spectral display of pulsed-wave Doppler sampling.

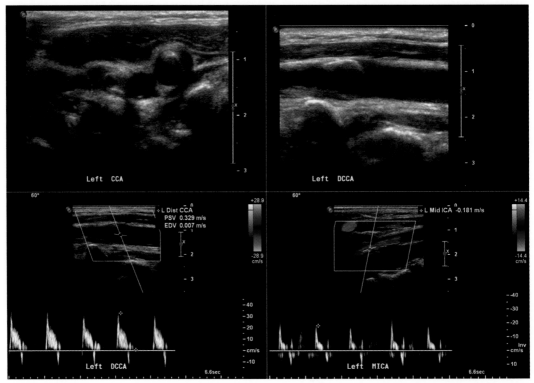

Figure 2-26. *Top left and right,* Grayscale imaging demonstrates that approximately 50% plaque is occupying the distal common carotid artery (CCA) and proximal internal carotid artery (ICA). *Bottom left,* The flow pattern within the CCA was high resistance, with brief reversal. *Bottom right,* The same pattern is seen within the ICA, sampled in the mid-portion. This was due to the complete occlusion of the distal ICA, resulting in high resistance.

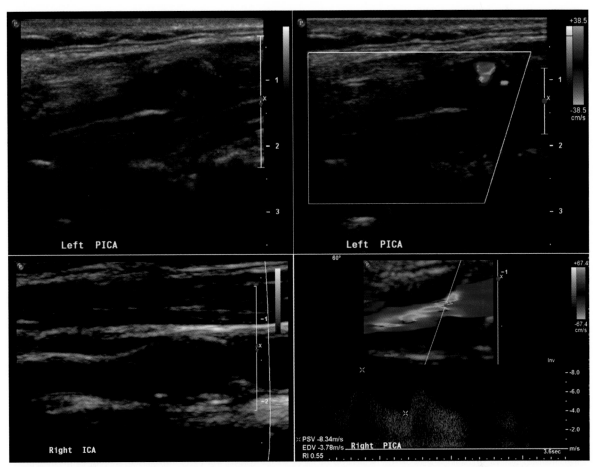

Figure 2-27. Upper images depict occlusion of the proximal left internal carotidartery (ICA), with complete absence of flow seen within it. Bottom images depict a greater than 70% but less than near-occlusion severity stenosis of the contralateral right ICA with a peak systolic velocity greater than 200 cm/sec. There is a plaque estimate greater than 50%, an ICA-to-common carotid artery (CCA) peak systolic velocity ratio of 7:1, and end-diastolic velocity greater than 100 cm/sec.

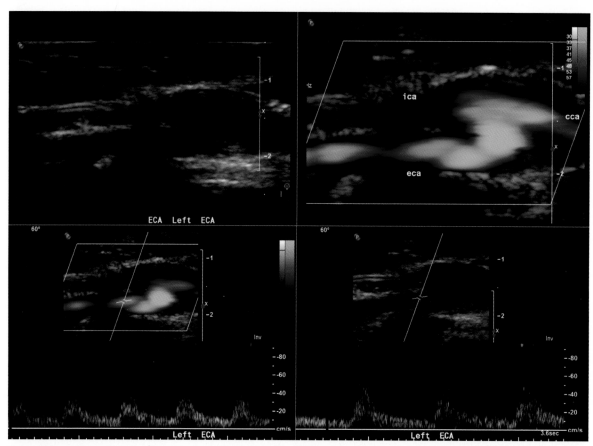

Figure 2-28. Occlusion of the internal carotid artery (ICA). Grayscale (*top left*) and power angiography Doppler imaging (*top right*), revealing occlusion of the proximal carotid artery. Lower images show flow recording within the patent but diseased external carotid artery (ECA). Spectral recording of flow within the ECA; the pattern is "internalized" as collaterals from the ECA have conferred a low-resistance pattern (*bottom left*). Temporal tap effect confirming that the vessel is the ECA (*bottom right*).

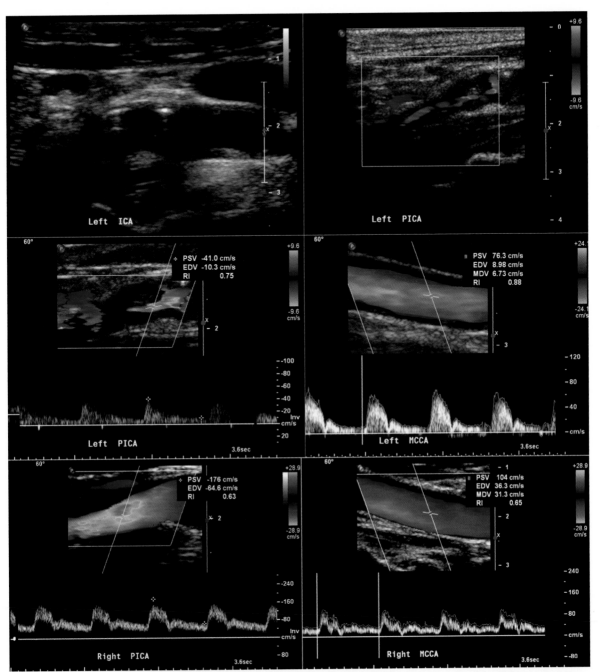

Figure 2-29. *Top left,* By grayscale imaging plaque is apparent within the left internal carotid artery (ICA). The severity is ambiguous, but it does appear to be significant. *Top right,* Color flow mapping of the same segment depicts a significantly reduced lumen. *Middle left,* Spectral flow recording from the proximal ICA, yielding reduced velocities. *Middle right,* The left common carotid artery (CCA) flow velocities are normal or slightly reduced. There was occlusion of the distal left ICA. *Bottom left and right,* The images describe the probable 50% to 69% stenosis of the contralateral right proximal ICA. The peak systolic velocity is between 125 and 230 cm/sec. The plaque estimate is about 50%. The ICA:CCA peak systolic velocity ratio is less than 2, more consistent with a less than 50% stenosis, which is in keeping with the plaque estimate as well. The ICA end-diastolic velocity is 65 cm/sec, more consistent with 50% to 69% stenosis than less than 50% stenosis. Internally inconsistent estimation of the grade of severity is regularly encountered.

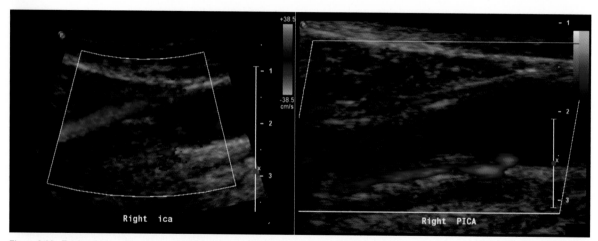

Figure 2-30. Total occlusion of the right proximal internal carotid artery (ICA). *Left,* Color Doppler flow mapping does not demonstrate any continuity of flow through the ICA. A large volume of plaque is present, seemingly filling the vessel and leaving it without a lumen. *Right,* Power angiography Doppler flow mapping cannot detect any flow within the ICA, only in the adjacent external carotid artery (ECA).

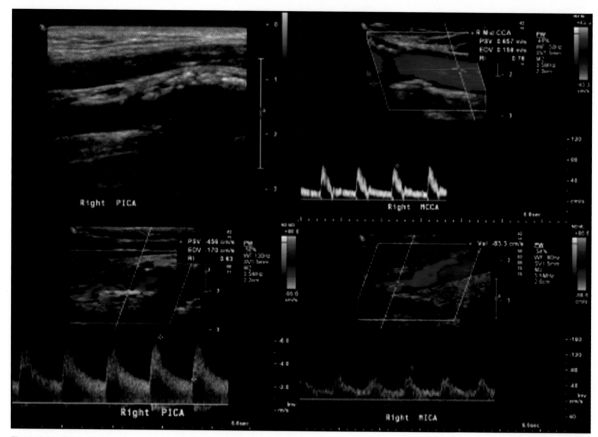

Figure 2-31. Bilaterally there is greater than 70% but less than near-occlusion of the internal carotid arteries (ICAs). Peak systolic velocities in the ICA vary 230 cm/sec, and plaque estimates are greater than 50%. ICA-to-common carotid artery (CCA) peak systolic velocity ratios are greater than 4, and diastolic velocities are greater than 100 cm/sec.

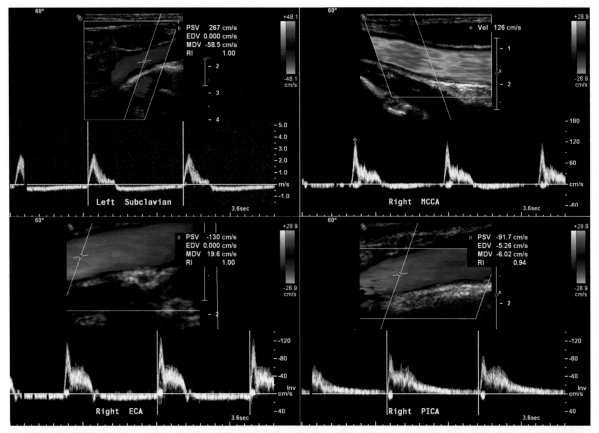

Figure 2-32. The effect of severe aortic insufficiency on subclavian and carotid flow patterns. Spectral flow recording from within the left subclavian artery. There is abnormal diastolic flow reversal due to diastolic regurgitation of aortic blood volume into the left ventricle (*top left*). The same abnormal pattern of diastolic flow reversal is seen within the common carotid arteries (*top right*) and also within (*bottom left*) the external carotid arteries. The spectral flow pattern within the internal carotid artery (*bottom right*) remains biphasic with anterograde diastolic flow.

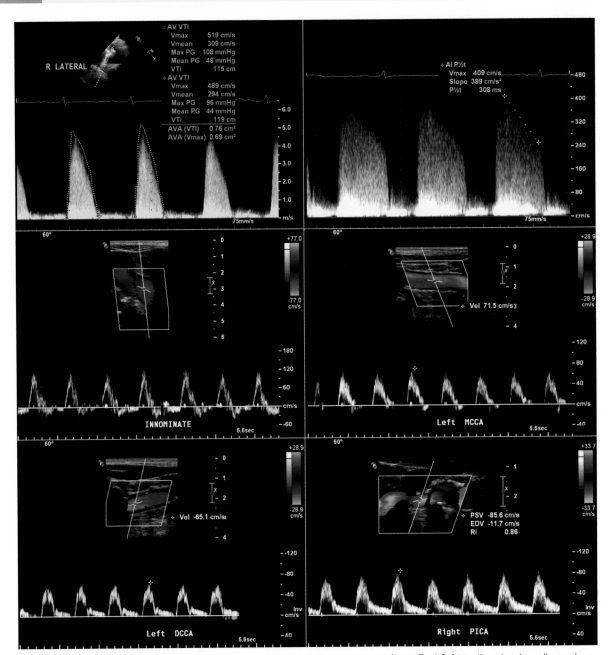

Figure 2-33. The effect of mixed severe aortic stenosis and insufficiency on carotid artery wave forms. *Top left,* A transthoracic echocardiogram image demonstrates the presence of severe aortic stenosis, with a peak gradient across the aortic valve of nearly 100 mm Hg and a mean gradient of 48 mm Hg. *Top right,* The spectral display of the associated 3+ aortic insufficiency. *Middle left,* The innominate spectral flow pattern is notable for vibratory artifact of the systolic waveform due to transmission of the thrill from the aortic stenosis. As well, the innominate spectral flow pattern is abnormal with pandiastolic flow reversal due to the aortic insufficiency. *Middle right,* The left mid-common carotid artery (CCA) spectral flow pattern is abnormal with a brief diastolic reversal and no appreciable anterograde diastolic flow. *Bottom left,* The left distal CCA spectral flow pattern is largely normalized with anterograde diastolic flow. *Bottom right,* There is preservation of the normal biphasic spectral flow pattern in the internal carotid arteries (ICAs), despite the presence of 3+ aortic insufficiency. The systolic spectral patterns in the innominate CCAs and ICAs are all unusually coarse due to the transmission of the thrill of the aortic stenosis jet.

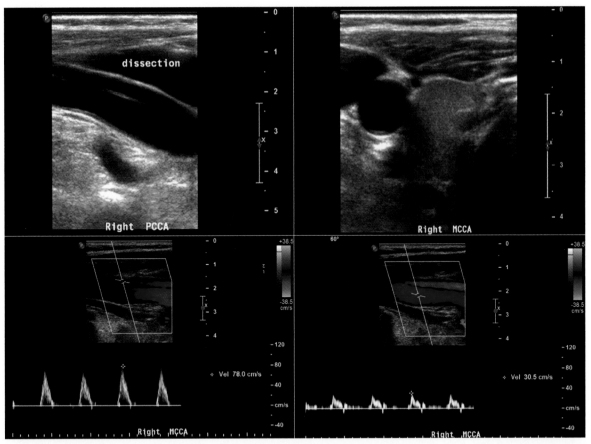

Figure 2-34. Common carotid artery (CCA) dissection due to branch vessel involvement by acute aortic dissection. *Top left,* The common carotid artery is depicted in long axis. There is an obvious intimal flap along the full length of the common carotid artery partitioning true and false lumens. *Top right,* The common carotid artery is seen cross-section and again the intimal flap is revealed. *Bottom left and right,* The spectral display depicts the difference in the flow profile in the true and false lumens.

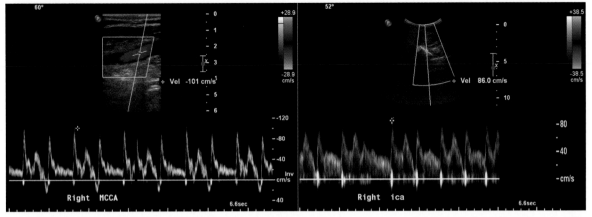

Figure 2-35. The effect of intra-aortic balloon counterpulsation on carotid artery waveforms. The intra-aortic balloon is set on a 1:2 mode of alternating cardiac cycles. *Left,* Common carotid artery spectral recording, the intra-aortic balloon is inflating in diastole, resulting in an anterograde flow profile and also in brief diastolic late flow reversal due to late diastolic deflation of the balloon. In alternating cardiac cycles, the flow pattern is normal with a biphasic pattern. Of note, the peak systolic velocity alternates between cardiac cycles with counterpulsation and cardiac cycles without counterpulsation. The cardiac cycles that are preceded by intra-aortic balloon deflation are of lower peak systolic velocity than the cardiac cycles that are "native." *Right,* The internal carotid artery (ICA) waveforms are different from the common carotid artery (CCA) waveforms during intra-aortic balloon counterpulsation. The anterograde diastolic flow pattern is still present; however, there is no late diastolic flow reversal with balloon deflation. Anterograde diastolic flow is preserved in all cardiac cycles. With balloon pump–augmented cardiac cycles, the diastolic flow becomes abnormally reduced but is not reversed, as it was in the CCA.

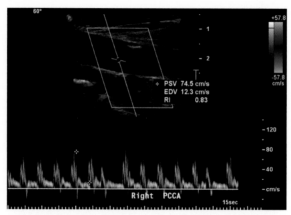

Figure 2-36. The effect of irregular cardiac intervals on carotid artery flow patterns. This patient was in atrial fibrillation. In addition to resulting in varying the intervals between successive spectral profiles, the amplitude of the profiles varies. When the cardiac cycle is shorter, the peak systolic velocity is less, and when the cardiac cycle length is longer, the peak systolic velocity is higher.

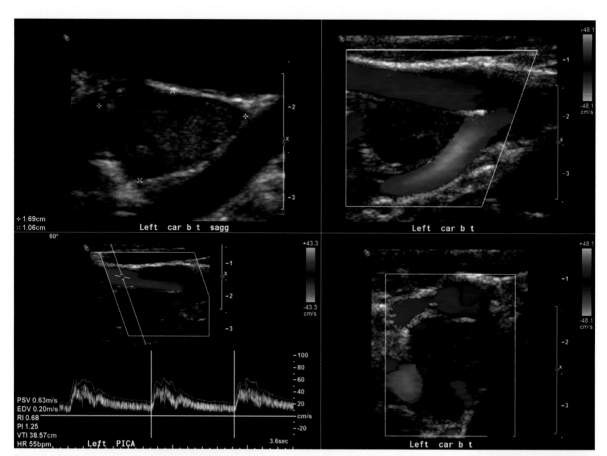

Figure 2-37. Paraganglioma. *Top left,* Soft tissue mass measuring 1.7 × 1.1 cm presents within the carotid bifurcation, slightly splaying the proximal internal carotid artery (ICA) and external carotid artery (ECA). *Top right,* The flow within the ICA and ECA remains laminar in spite of the interposed soft tissue mass. *Bottom left,* Left proximal ICA flow is again seen to be undisturbed with normal velocities and no turbulence. *Bottom right,* The paraganglioma seen in cross-section with the ECA anterior to it and the ICA right lateral to it.

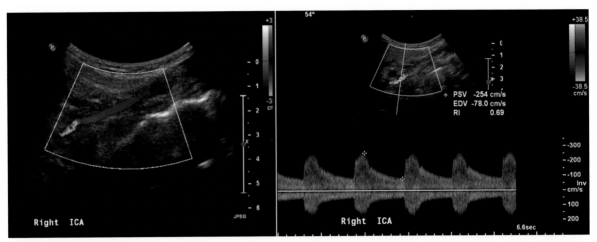

Figure 2-38. Fibromuscular dysplasia of the internal carotid artery (ICA). *Left,* There is slight tapering of the ICA without any intimal surface irregularities. Color flow mapping denotes the beginning of turbulent flow within the ICA. *Right,* Spectral display at the site of flow turbulence, revealing elevation of the peak systolic velocity and turbulence caused by stenosis.

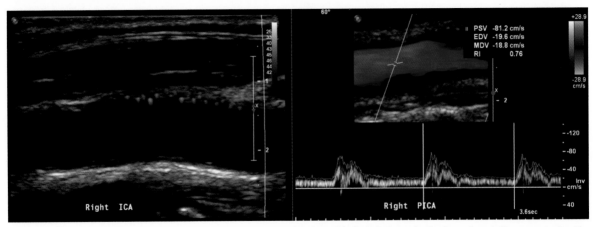

Figure 2-39. Post–carotid endarterectomy. *Left,* The internal carotid artery has been debulked of atherosclerotic plaque. Irregularities are present on the near-field wall and are exaggerated by discrete reverberation artifacts. *Right,* Color Doppler and spectral Doppler representation of normal systolic and diastolic velocities.

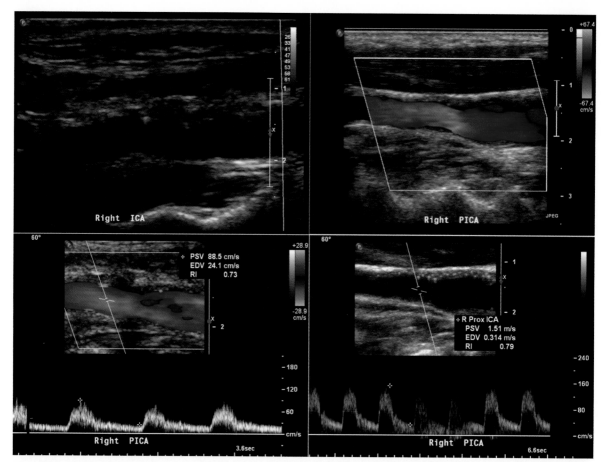

Figure 2-40. Mild restenosis post–carotid endarterectomy. *Top left,* There are irregularities of the near-field wall with some localized reverberation artifacts. *Top right,* Color Doppler flow mapping demonstrates laminar flow within the central lumen of the internal carotid artery (ICA) at the site of endarterectomy. *Bottom left,* Flow in the distal proximal ICA has a normal pattern and normal velocity. *Bottom right,* At the site of the intimal irregularities and slight luminal waist, the flow velocity is increased but not quite double increased. Spectral flow analysis, which suggests less than 50% residual stenosis, corroborates the conclusion that the endarterectomy, which appears incomplete in the top left image, is actually incomplete.

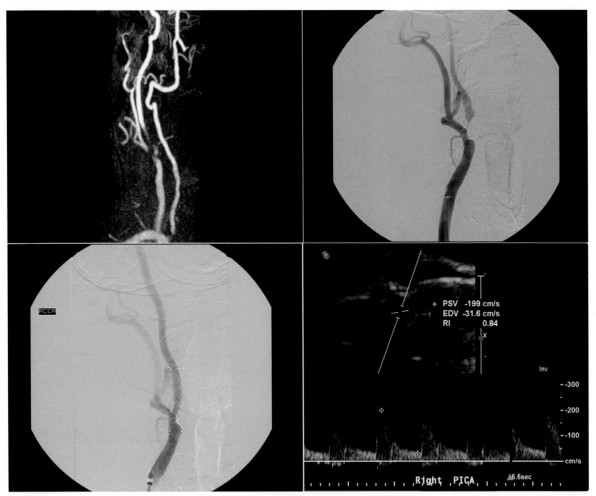

Figure 2-41. Restenosis. *Top left,* Magnetic resonance imaging reveals tight narrowing of the internal carotid artery (ICA) and suggests a narrowing of the external carotid artery (ECA) as well. *Top right,* Conventional catheter angiography delineates a tight stenosis of the proximal ICA and no stenosis of the ECA. *Bottom left,* Following stenting of the ICA lesion, a significant increase in the ICA diameter is present, although the residual bulk of the atherosclerotic lesion still intrudes into the lumen. *Bottom right,* Spectral recordings within the recently stented ICA demonstrates normal ICA velocities and flow pattern following steuting.

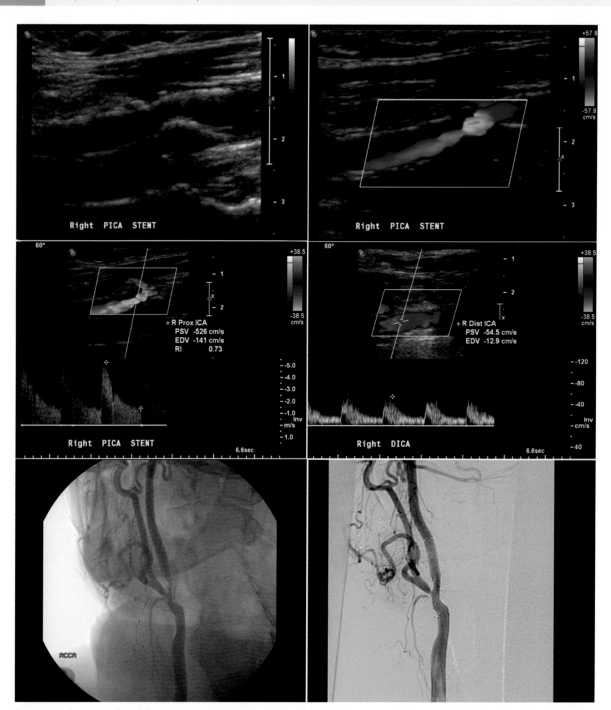

Figure 2-42. Restenosis. *Top left,* One year post–carotid stenting. This two-dimensional image reveals the stent within the internal carotid artery (ICA) but does not well detail the lumen. *Top right,* Color flow mapping within the stented segment. The color Doppler depiction of flow suggests that there is significant narrowing of the lumen due to hypoechoic material within the stent. *Middle left,* Spectral Doppler recording within the stent. There is a prominent elevation of the systolic and also the diastolic flow velocities. This is consistent with significant restenosis. *Middle right,* The distal portion of the ICA has normal flow velocities and pattern. *Bottom left,* Conventional catheter angiography for presumed restenosis. There is significant narrowing of the ICA at the previously stented site. *Bottom right,* Following restenting of the site, the lumen of the ICA is nearly normalized, although there is slight pinching of the external carotid artery (ECA) origin.

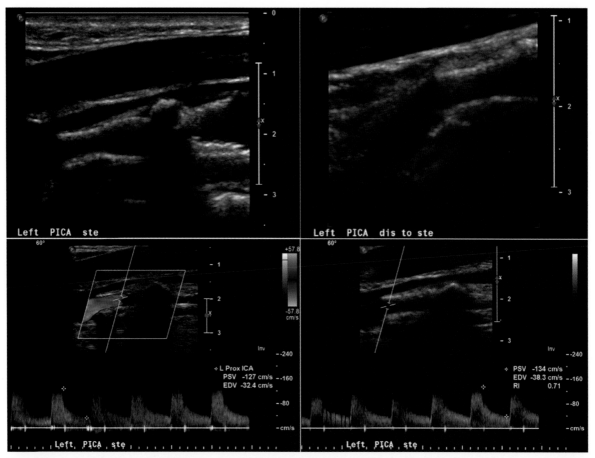

Figure 2-43. Post–carotid artery stenting without restenosis. *Top left,* The stent is apparent in the internal carotid artery (ICA) by its mesh appearance. Also apparent is its variably complete deployment. The proximal and distal margins are well apposed to the arterial vessel wall. In the mid-portion at the site of the prior severe carotid artery stenosis, where there was a large bulk of calcium, the stent is less convincingly maximally deployed. Also, the calcification within the preexisting atherosclerotic plaque (which unlike following carotid endarterectomy has not been removed), now confers an extensive area of shadowing. Whether restenosis has occurred within the zone of shadowing cannot be determined in this case by two-dimensional imaging because of the severity of shadowing. *Top right,* The distal marginal stent and its relation to the ongoing ICA is readily apparent. *Bottom left,* Flow velocities within the stent are slightly increased, and turbulence is present within the stent. *Bottom right,* Turbulence is present both within the stent and at the distal extent of the stent.

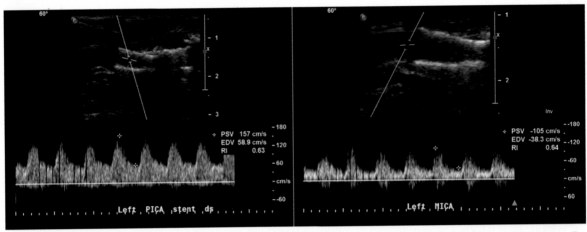

Figure 2-44. Spectral flow pattern within and distal to an internal carotid artery (ICA) stent. *Left,* Spectral flow pattern at the distal end of the ICA stent. The peak systolic velocity is mildly increased, and there is turbulence. The associated two-dimensional image depicts complete deployment of the stent and displacement of the large bulk of atheroma. *Right,* Spectral flow pattern immediately distal to the stent. There remains turbulence of flow, but the peak systolic velocity within the ongoing ICA has recovered to normal.

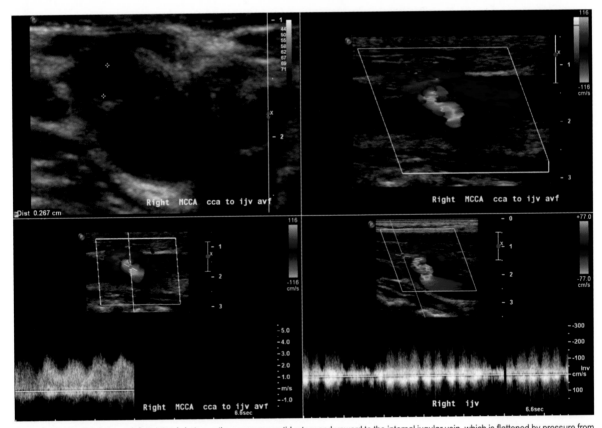

Figure 2-45. *Top left,* A tissue defect extends between the common carotid artery and upward to the internal jugular vein, which is flattened by pressure from the transducer. *Top right,* Color Doppler flow mapping. *Bottom left,* Spectral flow recording through the fistula showing continuous flow, typical of an arteriovenous fistula. *Bottom right,* The flow within the receiving internal jugular vein exhibits respiratory phase variation consistent with central venous flow patterns.

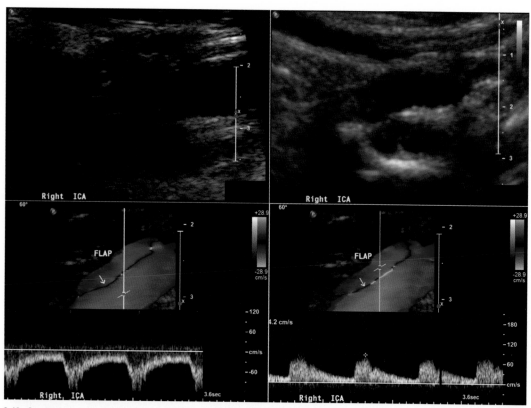

Figure 2-46. Spontaneous internal carotid artery (ICA) dissection. *Top left,* The intimal flap of the dissection of the ICA is only barely visible and only for part of its length. *Top right,* The intimal flap is more readily seen on this cross-sectional image of the ICA and the resulting true and false lumens. *Bottom left and right,* Color flow mapping of the ICA in long axis and spectral recording of the false and true lumens. In this case, the spectral recordings corroborate the color flow mapping depiction of oppositely directed flow in the true and false lumens.

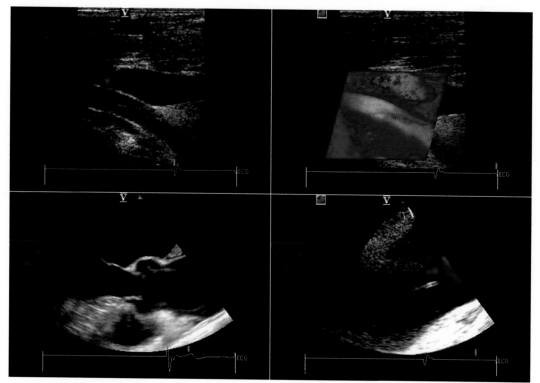

Figure 2-47. Acute aortic dissection with extension into the right common carotid artery (CCA). The patient had a malperfusion syndrome due to the involvement of the CCA and was having cerebral ischemia. *Top left,* An intimal flap is faintly visible within the CCA. *Top right,* Power angiography imaging reveals the true and false lumens and somewhat better depicts the intimal flap in this case. *Bottom left,* Transesophageal view of the intimal flap of the aortic dissection in the aortic root level. *Bottom right,* Transesophageal view of the intimal flap at aortic arch level.

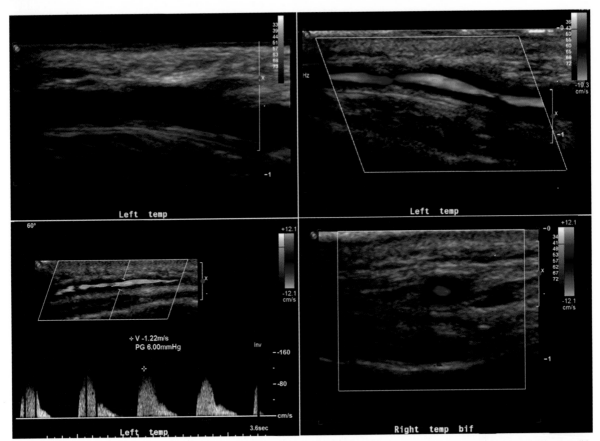

Figure 2-48. *Top left,* Grayscale imaging of a section of the temporal artery in long axis. All in all, the vessel does not look remarkable, other than possible wall thickening on the deep side. *Top right,* However, color Doppler flow mapping does delineate a narrower lumen than anticipated by the grayscale imaging due to the presence of hypoechoic thickening uniformly along the walls. *Bottom left,* Spectral display of flow within the temporal artery, revealing elevation of the systolic velocity and the nearly monophasic pattern consistent with stenosis. *Bottom right,* The halo sign of wall thickening in temporal arteritis nicely demarcated by luminal depiction by color flow mapping.

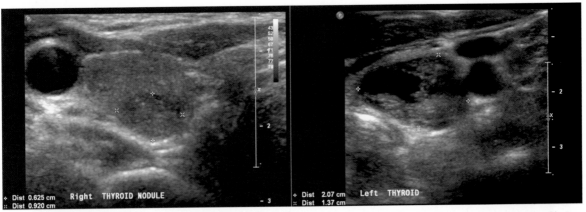

Figure 2-49. Incidental thyroid lesions identified during carotid ultrasound. *Left,* A 6 × 9 mm thyroid nodule is present lateral to the common carotid artery. *Right,* A cystic lesion is present within a left lobe of the thyroid gland.

3

Upper Extremity Arterial Disease

Key Points

■ Knowledge of normal and variant anatomy of the upper extremity arterial vasculature is critical.
■ A standardized and comprehensive duplex examination protocol is critical.
■ Knowledge of possible diseases/lesions potentially within the upper extremity arterial vasculature, and how to maximize their recognition, is critical.

ARTERIAL ANATOMY OF THE UPPER EXTREMITY

The arterial anatomy of the arm and the hand is depicted schematically in Figures 3-1 and 3-2. The subclavian artery on the right side usually arises along with the common carotid artery from the innominate artery at the level of the sternoclavicular joint and in its distal extent rises slightly above the clavicle. However, variation may occur, such as the anomalous origin of the right subclavian artery directly from the descending aorta distal to the left subclavian artery and independently of the right common carotid artery.

On the left side, the subclavian artery arises from the distal arch of the aorta at the level of the fourth thoracic vertebra, and then arches laterally.

The main trunk of the subclavian artery is considered to be divided into three parts. The first part extends from the origin to the medial border of the scalene muscle. The second part lies behind the muscle. The third part extends from the lateral border of the scalene muscle and then over the first rib.

From the first segment and posterosuperior aspect of the subclavian artery arises the vertebral artery, the most constant of all its branches. The internal mammary artery arises from its inferior aspect, courses downward parasternally in a pedicle alongside its accompanying nerve and vein, and can become a useful collateral pathway along with its many vascular connections.

The thyrocervical trunk and its three branches, the inferior thyroid, transverse scapular, and superficial cervical arteries, the most important and variable of collateral pathways, supply flow around subclavian and innominate artery occlusive disease. These structures display the textbook configuration of a main

trunk and three branches in only 46% of cases. The trunk is absent in 17% of cases.[1]

Arising from the posterior aspect of the second part of the subclavian artery is the costocervical trunk, which passes above the pleura to the first rib, dividing into the deep cervical and superior intercostal to supply the first and second intercostal spaces. These vessels are small and are not considered to be significant collateral pathways. The third segment of the subclavian artery usually has no branches.

On each side of the body, the subclavian artery becomes the axillary artery at the level of the outer border of the first rib and the inferior border of the teres major muscle and then descends into the axilla. As with the subclavian artery, the axillary is divided into three parts: the first part lies medial to the pectoralis minor muscle, the second part behind it, and the third part on the lateral side of the muscle.

From 6 to 11 arteries may arise from the axillary artery and anastomose with each other to form a meshlike network that is effective as a collateral pathway in the presence of thoracic-scapular-humoral trauma. Although the configuration is fairly consistent, there is some variation related to the origin of these arteries. These arteries are the superior thoracic, thoracoacromial, lateral thoracic, subscapular, upper subscapular, and anterior and posterior circumflex humeral arteries.

At the level of the lower border of the teres major muscle, the brachial artery begins, leaving the axilla and running downward and medially to the humerus. Where this artery reaches the elbow joint, where it is positioned midway between the epicondyles, it comes in front of the humerus.

The brachial artery has several branches along its course, forming important potential pathways around the elbow and, occasionally, a superficial brachial artery[2] (9% incidence). When present, the superficial brachial artery may either replace the brachial artery or parallel it down the arm and continue as the radial or rarely, the ulna artery. Smaller branch vessels supply the muscles of the arm, and the majority of them are nameless.

The brachial artery bifurcates into the ulnar artery and the radial artery at approximately 1.5 cm distal to the radiohumeral line, with the ulnar artery most often being the deeper and more dominant vessel.

In 13% to 25% of cases, the radial artery has a variable origin arising from the axillary artery or from the proximal, mid-, or distal brachial artery. It is most often unilateral and is then called the brachioradial artery.[2] In this same sample of patients, a brachioulnar artery was present in 5% with the same pattern of origin as the brachioradial artery.

Other anomalous vessel origins of lesser significance have been identified in both the upper arm and forearm, and absent or rudimentary ulnar and radial arteries have been reported but is considered rare. When either the radial or ulnar arteries are absent, there function is replaced by anterior interosseous artery.[3]

The ulnar artery is the more dominant of the two forearm arteries. Although the radial artery gives off only small branches that supply the musculature of the forearm, the ulna artery has a large branch, the common interosseous artery, which divides and delivers branches to both sides of the interosseous membrane.

The more superficial radial artery runs downward beneath the brachioradialis muscle and extends into the hand, where the deep palmar arch is formed by the anastomosis of a deep palmar branch of the ulna artery with the radial artery. This arch is complete in 97% of cases, and this results in an excellent collateral network for the hand.[4]

The ulnar artery lies between the deep and superficial flexor muscles and continues down the arm to the hand, where it joins the superficial palmar branch of the radial artery to form the superficial palmar arch. The arch is incomplete in 20% of cases.[5] The perforating branches of the deep palmar arch are thought to be responsible for blood supply to the dorsum of the hand, and the recurrent branches from the deep arch are thought to be the collateral supply when the radial and ulnar arteries are ligated.

The digital arteries are formed by the volar metacarpal arteries from the deep arch, the dorsal metacarpals from the perforating arteries, the common volar digitals from the superficial arch, and the dorsal branch of the radial artery.

Recommendations for the management of patients with occlusive disease of the subclavian and brachiocephalic arteries are given in Box 3-1.

DUPLEX EVALUATION OF THE UPPER EXTREMITY ARTERIES

The purpose of duplex evaluation is to identify the presence or absence of occlusive or aneurysmal disease and, subsequently, to determine extent and degree. Common indications include:

- ❐ Upper extremity ischemia
- ❐ Asymmetrical brachial systolic blood pressure readings
- ❐ Suspected upper extremity arterial embolism
- ❐ Reduced pulses
- ❐ Bruit
- ❐ Suspected subclavian "steal"
- ❐ Evaluation of arterial trauma
- ❐ Thoracic outlet syndrome (evaluation is under a separate protocol)

The most common contraindication to duplex examination is the presence of wound dressings.

Several examples of normal and abnormal scans are shown in Figures 3-3 to 3-12.

BOX 3-1 Recommendations for the Management of Patients with Occlusive Disease of the Subclavian and Brachiocephalic Arteries

Class IIa

1. Extra-anatomic carotid-subclavian bypass is reasonable for patients with symptomatic posterior cerebral or cerebellar ischemia caused by subclavian artery stenosis or occlusion (subclavian steal syndrome) in the absence of clinical factors predisposing to surgical morbidity or mortality (690–692). (*Level of Evidence: B*)

2. Percutaneous endovascular angioplasty and stenting is reasonable for patients with symptomatic posterior cerebral or cerebellar ischemia caused by subclavian artery stenosis (subclavian steal syndrome) who are at high risk of surgical complications. (*Level of Evidence: C*)

3. Revascularization by percutaneous angioplasty and stenting, direct arterial reconstruction, or extra-anatomic bypass surgery is reasonable for patients with symptomatic ischemia involving the anterior cerebral circulation caused by common carotid or brachiocephalic artery occlusive disease. (*Level of Evidence: C*)

4. Revascularization by percutaneous angioplasty and stenting, direct arterial reconstruction, or extra-anatomic bypass surgery is reasonable for patients with symptomatic ischemia involving upper-extremity claudication caused by subclavian or brachiocephalic artery occlusive disease. (*Level of Evidence: C*)

5. Revascularization by either extra-anatomic bypass surgery or subclavian angioplasty and stenting is reasonable for asymptomatic patients with subclavian artery stenosis when the ipsilateral internal mammary artery is required as a conduit for myocardial revascularization. (*Level of Evidence: C*)

Class III: No Benefit

1. Asymptomatic patients with asymmetrical upper-limb blood pressure, periclavicular bruit, or flow reversal in a vertebral artery caused by subclavian artery stenosis should not undergo revascularization unless the internal mammary artery is required for myocardial revascularization. (*Level of Evidence: C*)

From 2011 ASA/ACCF/AHA/AANN/AANS/ACR/ASNR/CNS/SAIP/SCAI/SIR/SNIS/SVM/SVS guideline on the management of patients with extracranial carotid and vertebral artery disease. *J Am Coll Cardiol.* 2011;57:16-94.

Equipment
- ❏ Color duplex imaging system
- ❏ 5- to 15-MHz linear transducers
- ❏ 2- to 6-MHz sector/curved array transducers
- ❏ Selection of blood pressure cuffs (one suitable for the size of the patient's arms)
- ❏ Sphygmomanometer (manual/automatic)
- ❏ Continuous-wave probe, 8 MHz/5 MHz
- ❏ Digit cuffs, 1.6 × 8 cm
- ❏ Photoplethysmographic sensors
- ❏ Chart recorder
- ❏ Stethoscope
- ❏ Coupling gel
- ❏ Digital reporting

Procedure
- ❏ Explain the procedure to the patient and answer any questions.
- ❏ Obtain and document applicable patient history.
- ❏ Verify that the procedure requested correlates with the patient's symptoms.
- ❏ Ascertain whether the patient is taking medications.
- ❏ Perform a limited physical examination of the limbs in question.
- ❏ Review any previous duplex studies available.
- ❏ Select appropriate test preset values.
- ❏ Select appropriate annotation throughout the test.
- ❏ Record images digitally on video and print film.
- ❏ Complete the technologist's preliminary report when necessary.

Technique
- ❏ The patient lies supine for at least 10 minutes before testing.
- ❏ The technologist stands or sits beside the patient.
- ❏ Gloves should be worn by the technologist when there is a threat of contamination by infected body fluids.

Physiologic Testing
- ❏ Blood pressure readings: taken at the level upper arms bilaterally
- ❏ Interpretation: normal range is 2 to 20 mm Hg difference between cuffs; abnormal entails greater than a 20–mm Hg difference
- ❏ Note: stenosis distal to the lower cuff is not discernible.

Duplex Scan
The symptomatic arm is supinated and abducted slightly. The subclavian artery in its distal and mid-segment can be scanned subclavicularly through the anterior chest wall. The most proximal segment and the innominate artery can be imaged by angling caudad into the sternal notch. To scan the axillary artery, the patient's arm is bent at a 90-degree angle and raised toward the head. The vessel can easily be followed from mid-clavicle into the axilla. The arm is then lowered to its original position to scan the remainder of the vessels. From the axilla, the brachial artery can be followed along the medial aspect of the upper arm. Approximately 1 to 2 cm distal to the antecubital fossa, the brachial bifurcation is seen, and from there the radial artery is scanned along the anterolateral part of the forearm and the ulnar artery along the anteromedial aspect.

Views
Identify all the vessels listed below in the transverse plane, and where applicable (if aneurysm is suspected) take representative diameter measurements.
- ❏ Subclavian artery
- ❏ Axillary artery
- ❏ Brachial artery
- ❏ Radial artery
- ❏ Ulnar artery

Next, in the sagittal plane, use grayscale, color, and pulsed-wave Doppler, and perform spectral Doppler measurements using an angle of 60 degrees to the vessel wall where possible and a sample volume of 1.5 mm. Attempt to classify pathology (e.g., wall thickening, calcification (medial calcinosis) and plaque appearance, length, location, and extent).

If aneurysmal dilatation was apparent in the transverse plane, now measure its depth, length, and, the diameter of the aneurysmal neck.

Obtain representative peak systolic velocity (PSV) measurements along the vessels every 2 to 3 cm.

When a lesion is detected, take PSV measurements immediately proximal to the site of stenosis, within the stenosis and immediately distal to it. Note any obvious collateral vessel formation associated with a significant lesion. Document any retrograde flow identified.

Interpretation and Reporting
Plaque Characteristics
- ❏ Calcified: hyperechoic lesion causing acoustical shadowing
- ❏ Heterogeneous or complex: lesion of mixed echogenicity causing no acoustical shadowing
- ❏ Anechoic: hypoechoic, poorly delineated lesion but possibly with flow disturbance
- ❏ Smooth: surface contour of lesion is smoothly defined
- ❏ Irregular: surface contour lesion is rough and irregular—thought to be related to ulceration
- ❏ Aneurysm: focal dilation of arterial wall

Normal Study
- ❏ Typical triphasic/biphasic Doppler waveform
- ❏ No evidence of plaque, calcification, or aneurysmal dilatation on grayscale
- ❏ Normal flow velocities

Abnormal Study
- ❏ Intraluminal echoes identified
- ❏ Abnormal waveforms
- ❏ Flow velocity changes

Classification of Stenosis

❏ Less than 50%
  • Plaque visualized on grayscale
  • Triphasic/biphasic waveforms
  • From a 30% to 100% increase in PSV compared with that immediately proximal
❏ Between 50% and 99%
  • Plaque visualized
  • Loss of reverse flow component (variable)
  • Greater than 100% increase in PSV velocity compared with that immediately proximal
  • Evidence of true poststenotic turbulence
  • Color flow representation of narrowed flow channel
❏ Complete occlusion
  • Intraluminal echoes observed throughout vessel
  • Absence of Doppler and color Doppler signals
  • Reconstitution postocclusion
  • Resumption of flow visualized by color Doppler
  • Spectral Doppler flow pattern usually containing both forward and reverse flow
  • Elements (influenced by collateral branch flow)

True Aneurysm

❏ Pulsating mass seen on grayscale
❏ Possible visualization of an intimal flap if dissection is present
❏ Turbulent flow in the aneurysmal sac
❏ Possible intraluminal heterogeneous echoes suggestive of thrombus

Pseudoaneurysm

❏ Pulsating mass identified on grayscale and color and connected to the artery via a "tract"
❏ High-velocity antegrade and retrograde ("to and fro") flow within the "tract"
❏ Turbulent flow in the mass

Arteriovenous Fistula

❏ Connection between artery and vein identified with color Doppler
❏ Pulsatile flow identified in the vein distal to the fistula
❏ Monophasic flow patterns may be present proximal to fistula
❏ High-velocity turbulent flow seen in arteriovenous connection

DIGITAL STUDY

A digital study of the fingers is added to the arterial duplex scan if specifically requested (Fig. 3-13).

Physiologic Testing

❏ Perform an Allen test.
  • Have the patient sit with the arm to be examined resting in the lap, palm up, comfortably. Obtain a Doppler signal from the radial artery while manually compressing the ulnar artery at the wrist level and then vice versa (to assess patency of the palmar arch prior to harvesting of the radial artery for coronary artery bypass grafting)
  • Interpretation: diminution or obliteration of the Doppler pulse suggests a complete palmar arch.
❏ Digits
  • If the hands are cold they should be warmed to room temperature.
  • Finger pneumatic cuffs are wrapped around the proximal phalanx of each second digit.
  • If requested or indicated by symptoms, other digits should be examined.
  • Photoplethysmographic sensors are attached to the pad of each finger with double-sided adhesive tape/straps.
  • A pulsatile plethysmographic waveform is displayed on a chart recorder and amplitude adjusted where necessary (calibration is not required).
  • The cuffs are inflated above arterial pressure until the waveform disappears.
  • The chart paper is marked at 10–mm Hg increments while the cuffs are slowly deflated—until the waveform reappears.
  • Both waveform and pressure are documented.
  • A digit-to-brachial pressure ratio is obtained (finger pressure divided by the ipsilateral brachial pressure).
  • Interpretation: normal digit pressure is greater than 80 mm Hg and the normal digit-to-brachial ratio is greater than or equal to 0.65.

THORACIC OUTLET SYNDROME TESTING

Signs and symptoms caused by extrinsic compression of the neurovasculature of the thoracic outlet region (Fig. 3-14) include paresthesias, coldness, pain, swelling, tingling, and numbness of the upper limb while in motion and are indications for duplex ultrasound study.

Technique

❏ A full upper extremity arterial scan is performed first.
❏ Both upper limbs are scanned.
❏ The scan is performed with the patient in the sitting or standing position.
❏ The arm is placed in the symptomatic position while both the subclavian and axillary arteries are scanned in the sagittal plane.
❏ In addition, the patient is asked to move his or her arm through abduction into hyperabduction while the scan continues.
❏ The subclavian and axillary veins are also scanned (as described in the upper extremity venous protocol) while the patient performs these same maneuvers.
❏ Any change in flow identified during the process is documented.

Interpretation
Normal Study
❏ PSV: 50 to 120 cm/sec
❏ No change with maneuvers

Abnormal Study
❏ Focal area of doubling of PSV in subclavian artery with abduction
❏ Decrease of PSV in axillary artery with hyper-abduction
❏ Rebound increase of PSV on release of abduction
❏ Dramatic decrease in PSV with maneuvers
❏ Obliteration of flow (venous or arterial) with maneuvers

ACCREDITATION

The Intersocietal Commission for Accreditation of Vascular Laboratories (ICAVL) maintains the standards for testing and accreditation of vascular laboratories. The standards for peripheral arterial testing are summarized in Table 3-1.[6]

TABLE 3-1 ICAVL* Standards for Accreditation: Peripheral Arterial Testing Summary Points

- Peripheral arterial testing is performed for appropriate clinical indications.
- The indication for testing must be documented.
- The laboratory must have a written protocol to determine the anatomic extent of the study. Bilateral testing is considered an integral part of a complete examination.
- Limited examinations may be performed for an appropriate or recurring indication. The reasons for a limited examination must be documented.
- A written protocol must be in place that defines the components and documentation of the peripheral arterial examination, which must include measurement of systolic blood pressure at one or more levels in combination with either Doppler or plethysmographic waveform analysis.
- Grayscale. Representative grayscale images, including spectral and color Doppler images, must be documented as required by the protocol with additional documentation of any abnormalities and must include at a minimum:
  - Subclavian artery
  - Axillary artery
  - Brachial artery
  - Innominate and forearm arteries when appropriate
  - Bypass graft(s) when present, including anastomoses
- Documentation of areas of suspected stenosis must include representative waveforms recorded at and distal to the stenosis.
- Interpretation of the peripheral arterial examination must use validated diagnostic criteria to assess the presence of disease, and to document its location, etiology, extent, and severity.
- There must be criteria for interpretation of continuous-wave Doppler waveform changes related to the anatomic site and hemodynamic severity of disease.
- There must be criteria for interpretation of grayscale images; spectral Doppler; and when reported, plaque morphology, and color-coded Doppler images related to the anatomic site and hemodynamic severity of disease.
- The interpretation and report that is generated from the examination findings and diagnostic criteria must state the absence or presence of abnormalities in the vessels that were investigated. Disease, if present, must be characterized according to its location, extent, and severity.
- In general, a laboratory should perform a minimum of 100 complete (peripheral arterial) primary examinations annually.
- The laboratory must have a written procedure for regular correlation of peripheral arterial examination results with angiographic findings produced by digital subtraction arteriography, contrast-enhanced computed tomography, magnetic resonance angiography, or surgery. The correlation must be reported using the comparison of the results of the arterial examination and the results of the validating study with regard to the location and severity of disease as defined by the diagnostic criteria utilized by the laboratory.
- A minimum of 30 extremities must be correlated every 3 years. These studies must have been done within the 3 years preceding submission of the application.
- The correlation matrix should demonstrate greater than 70% agreement.

*ICAVL, Intersocietal Commission for Accreditation of Vascular Laboratories.
Adapted from Intersocietal Commission for Accreditation of Vascular Laboratories (ICAVL): The Complete ICAVL Standards for Accreditation in Noninvasive Vascular Testing. < http://www.icavl.org/icavl/Standards/2010_ICAVL_Standards.pdf>.

REFERENCES

1. Radke HM. Arterial circulation of the upper extremity. In: Strandness Jr DE, ed. *Collateral Circulation in Clinical Surgery*. Philadelphia: WB Saunders; 1969:294-307.
2. Rodriguez-Niedenfuhr M, Vazquez T, Nearn L, et al. Variations of the arterial pattern in the upper limb revisited: a morphological and statistical study, with a review of the literature. *J Anat*. 2001;199:547-566.
3. Chhatrapati DN. Absence of radial artery. *Ind J Med Sci*. 1964;18:462-465.
4. Strandness Jr DE, ed. *Collateral Circulation in Clinical Surgery*. Philadelphia: WB Saunders; 1969.
5. Coleman SS, Anson BJ. Arterial patterns in the hand based upon a study of 650 specimens. *Surg Gyn Obst*. 1961;4:409-422.
6. Intersocietal Commission for Accreditation of Vascular Laboratories (ICAVL): The Complete ICAVL Standards for Accreditation in Noninvasive Vascular Testing. <http://www.icavl.org/icavl/Standards/2010_ICAVL_Standards.pdf >; Accessed April 20, 2010.

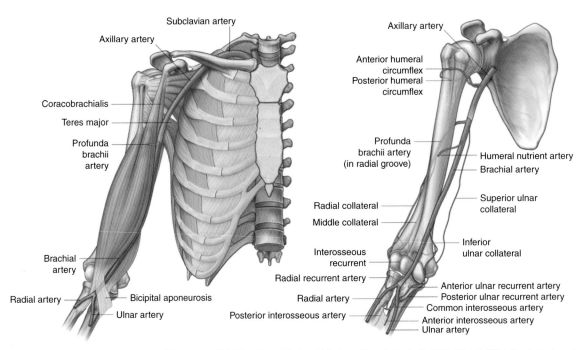

Figure 3-1. Arterial anatomy of the arm. *Left,* In context. *Right,* Branches of the brachial artery. (From Drake R, Vogl AW, Mitchell AWM. *Gray's Anatomy for Students.* 2nd ed. Philadelphia: Elsevier; 2010; Fig. 7-76; used with permission.)

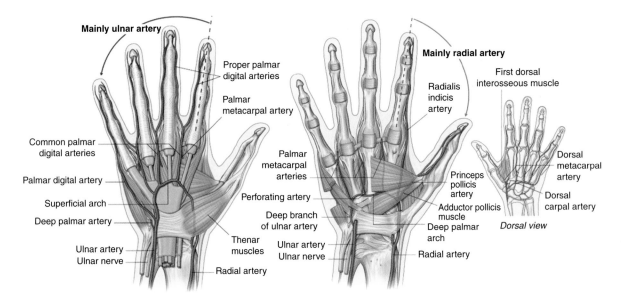

Figure 3-2. Arterial anatomy of the hand. *Left,* Ulnar artery and the superficial palmar arch. *Middle and right,* Radial artery and the deep palmar arch. (From Drake R, Vogl AW, Mitchell AWM. *Gray's Anatomy for Students.* 2nd ed. Philadelphia: Elsevier; 2010; Figs. 7-106 and 7-107; used with permission.)

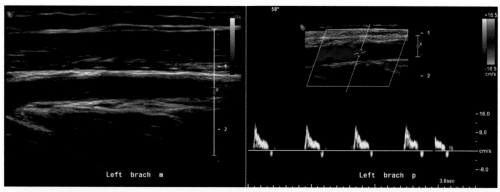

Figure 3-3. Brachial artery embolization and occlusion. *Left,* Grayscale imaging depicts homogenous echogenic material with the typical appearance of thrombus, completely filling the brachial artery. *Right,* The spectral display sampled immediately proximal to the flush occlusion of the brachial artery shows dampened flow at high resistance and faintly triphasic pattern with low amplitude due to the occlusion.

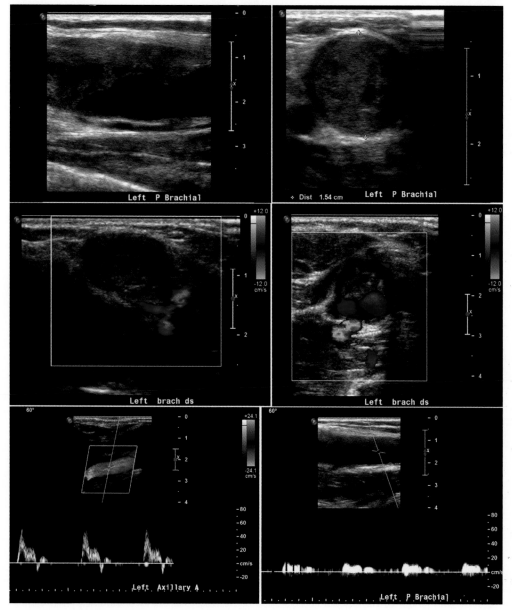

Figure 3-4. Thrombosed brachial artery aneurysm. *Top left and right,* Grayscale images show complex thrombosis within a fusiform aneurysm that is occlusive and non-occlusive at different levels. *Middle left and right,* Occlusion and partial occlusion by color Doppler low mapping. *Bottom left,* Spectral display of flow at the axillary artery level proximal to the aneurysm reveals a high resistance pattern (normal) of abnormally low amplitude. *Bottom right,* Severely dampened flow at the distal end of the thrombus within the ongoing brachial artery.

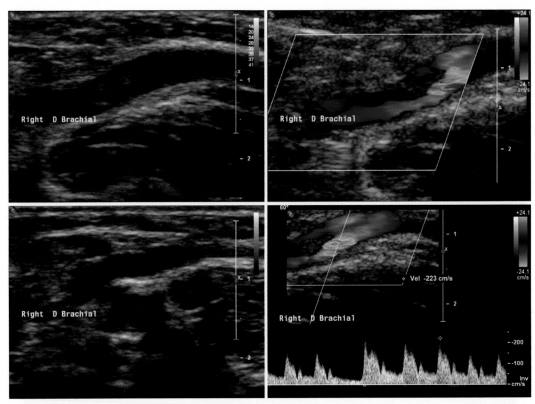

Figure 3-5. The left images demonstrate embolism to the brachial artery and the right views reveal the thrombus to be nearly occlusive and causing significant narrowing of the artery. The irregular cycle length of the Doppler waveform suggests atrial fibrillation, not previously suspected in this patient, and believed to be involved in the etiology of the arterial embolism.

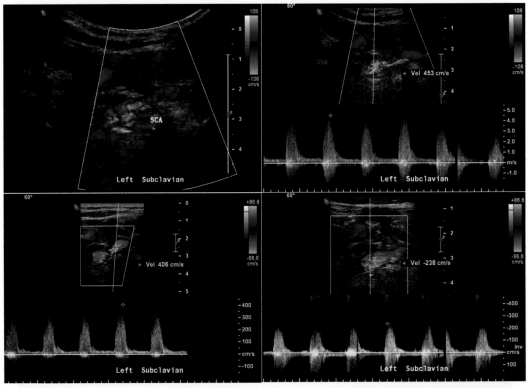

Figure 3-6. Subclavian artery stenosis. Both the grayscale imaging and color Doppler imaging delineate the subclavian artery and the flow within it in this case, but color Doppler flow mapping identifies the artery and depicts turbulence in one segment (*top left*). Spectral displays (*top right and bottom left*) obtained at the site of turbulence reveal high velocity and turbulent flow consistent with stenosis. The image (*bottom right*) shows near recovery of the flow velocities few centimeters distally. The flow pattern though remains turbulent, the only sign at this more distal level of an upstream stenosis.

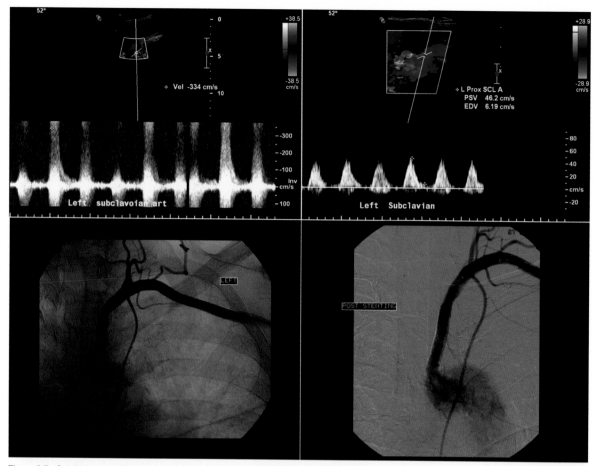

Figure 3-7. Subclavian artery stenosis and stenting. *Top left,* Spectral flow characteristics at the site of turbulence. *Top right,* Spectral flow characteristics further downstream. This patient was scheduled for aortic coronary bypass grafting with the intention of using the left internal mammary artery. Before proceeding to bypass surgery, the patient underwent angiography and stenting of the left subclavian stenosis to preserve benefit from the mammary artery bypass graft. *Bottom left,* The image reveals a short and tight stenosis in a proximal left subclavian artery. *Bottom right,* Following stenting, the vessel lumen is widely patent. On both of the angiographic images, the internal mammary artery can be seen distal to the stenosis site and descending inferiorly.

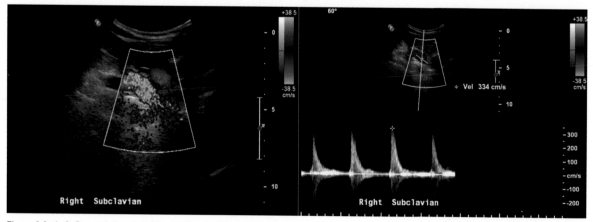

Figure 3-8. *Left,* Grayscale imaging with color Doppler flow mapping that identifies turbulence within the right subclavian artery. *Right,* Spectral display of the flow reveals moderate elevation of the flow velocities consistent with stenosis.

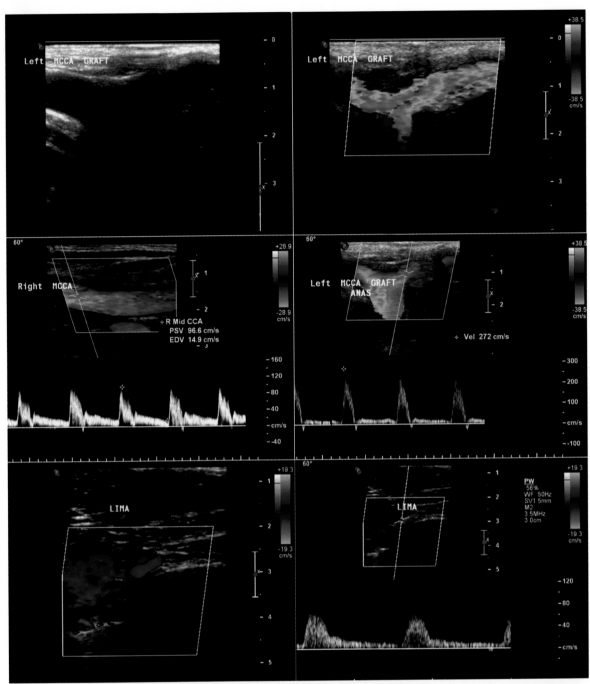

Figure 3-9. Left common carotid artery to left subclavian artery bypass in a patient post–coronary artery bypass grafting in whom occlusion of the left subclavian artery was belatedly recognized (due to ongoing angina post-bypass). *Top left,* A grayscale image demonstrates the anastomosis of the graft to the mid–common carotid artery and its approximately 90-degree takeoff. *Top right,* Color Doppler flow mapping also demonstrates this anastomosis. The flow in the graft is initially laminar and becomes turbulent. Note the crenellated appearance of the walls of the graft. *Middle left,* Color Doppler flow mapping and spectral display of flow within the common carotid artery (normal pattern). *Middle right,* Flow within the proximal graft, which is approximately normal, but with more ongoing diastolic flow than normal. *Bottom left,* Color Doppler flow mapping of the proximal internal mammary/thoracic artery. *Bottom right,* Spectral display of the flow in the internal mammary/thoracic artery (note the higher phasic flow, which is diastolic, and possibly the cause of the higher than normal diastolic flow seen in the proximal graft).

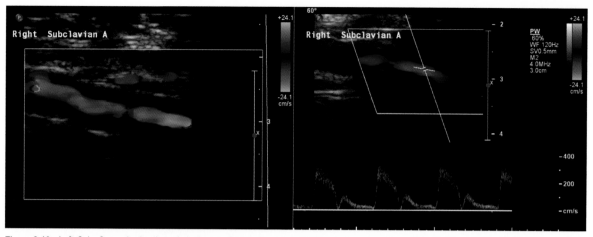

Figure 3-10. *Left,* Color flow reduction through the lumen of a subclavian artery. *Right,* The image corroborates the narrowing by documenting high-velocity flow values.

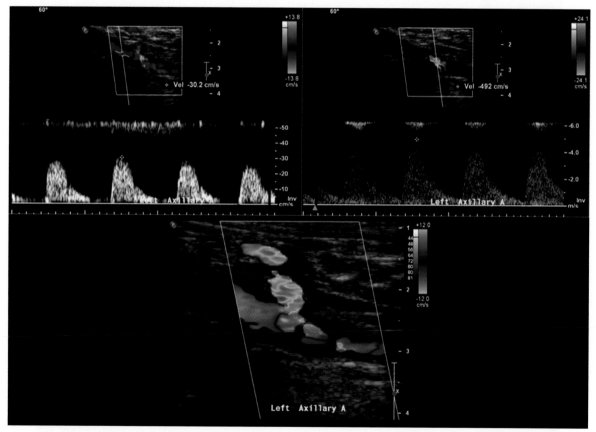

Figure 3-11. Axillary artery stenosis. *Top left and right,* The images demonstrate the spectral waveform proximal to an area of turbulence (the right spectral display confirms high-velocity flow consistent with a stenosis). *Bottom,* The image shows a prominent tributary.

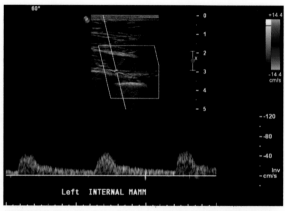

Figure 3-12. Interrogation of the internal thoracic (mammary) artery by pulsed-wave Doppler.

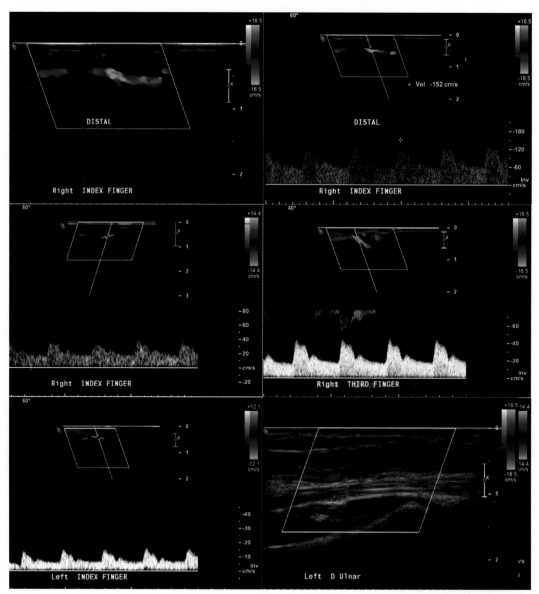

Figure 3-13. Buerger thromboangiitis obliterans. *Top left,* Grayscale imaging of the digital arteries is challenged by their curving/nonplanar course. *Top right,* Color Doppler flow mapping reveals sites of turbulence that can be interrogated by pulsed-wave Doppler, and elevation of flow velocity due to stenosis can be identified. *Middle left,* Flow proximal to the turbulence is of normal velocity. *Middle right and bottom left,* Flow in other digits is normal. *Bottom right,* Occlusion of an ulnar artery.

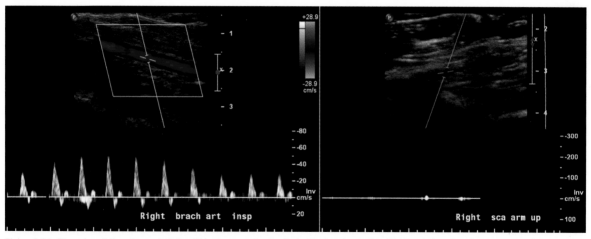

Figure 3-14. Thoracic outlet syndrome. *Left,* Brachial artery sampling is affected by deep inspiration. With inspiration, there is a progressive fall in the peak velocity. *Right,* Cessation of flow in the subclavian artery is achieved by elevation of the right arm.

4 Arteriovenous Fistulas

Key Points

■ An arteriovenous fistula typically lies closer to the skin surface than the native vessel and is therefore more likely to be easily compressed by the probe during scanning, falsely suggesting narrowing. Hence, when scanning, use very light pressure and lots of gel.
■ The flow velocity within a arteriovenous fistula is slower in a mature and well-dilated arteriovenous fistula than in a recently created, smaller diameter vein. Volumetric flow is a more reliable measurement.

Hemodialysis first became available, albeit in a limited fashion, in 1962 in Seattle. The first hemodialysis fistula was created in 1966. Until the 1980s, relatively low median dialysis flow rates were used, and thus even patients with small-veined fistulas could achieve adequate hemodialysis. By the mid-1980s, it was established that urea clearance time could be improved with higher blood flows during dialysis, with very little increase in dialysis time. This, in turn, led to a preference for grafts over fistulas that could more easily handle the increase in flow required and could be used sooner after surgery than fistulas.

In 1997, the National Kidney Foundation Kidney Disease Outcomes Quality Initiative (KDOQI) published a set of evidence-based practice guidelines for vascular access.[1] These guidelines recommended that the primary placement for hemodialysis be autogenous arteriovenous fistula in preference to synthetic grafts. Although arteriovenous fistulas have a higher primary failure rate than arteriovenous grafts, the fistulas are less prone to infection and thrombosis and require less corrective intervention.

There are many different configurations of arteriovenous fistulas. The preferred and most commonly used are created in the upper extremity: radiocephalic, brachiocephalic, and brachiobasilic transposition (Fig. 4-1). Brachiobasilic transposition has been increasingly used in patients possessing veins of insufficient caliber to support the preferred radiocephalic or brachiocephalic fistulas. This involved the transposition of the basilic vein, a vein not used for venipuncture, and therefore much less likely to be diseased than the cephalic vein, to a more superficial level, by dissecting and tunneling the vein to a position that can be more easily reached by the dialysis needle (1 to 1.5 inches in length). The normal volumetric flow through an arteriovenous fistula is held to be >600 mL/min.

Between 20% and 50% of fistulas fail to mature, due principally to the development of stenosis at the venous anastomosis, but also to a lesser extent, due to the presence of large branch veins.[2]

DUPLEX SCANNING

Duplex scanning is used to provide accurate preoperative diameter measurements of the cephalic and basilic veins of the forearm and upper arm (vein diameter > 3 mm is preferred), and also, to determine whether there is stenosis or chronic recanalized thrombosis caused by damage from previous indwelling catheters or venipuncture.

To assess for patency, the veins at the axilla and below are scanned in their entirety and compressed, in short axis, by the transducer at 1- to 2-cm intervals. The subclavian and proximal axillary veins usually collapse briefly if the patient takes in a long "sniff" breath. If the cephalic vein appears to be deeper than usual, the vein is measured with respect to the skin level. Most surgeons also want to know if any significant accessory branch vessels are present (e.g., accessory cephalic vein), which might divert flow away from the main outflow channel.

The scan may be unilateral or bilateral, but the nondominant arm is preferred for access creation. Previously unsuccessful access attempts influence which vessels are most likely to be used for fistula creation.

A full upper extremity arterial scan is also performed to include diameter measurement of the radial artery to uncover any evidence of wall calcification or stenosis that would interfere with the ability of the artery to dilate after surgery. There is a significant prevalence of a high brachial artery bifurcation, and this should be documented when present. Duplex protocol for vein mapping is given in Table 4-1.

TABLE 4-1 Duplex Protocol for Upper Extremity Venous Mapping

VENOUS ANATOMIC SEGMENT	TECHNIQUE	DUPLEX INTERROGATION
Cephalic vein Forearm/upper arm	SAX sweep with or without compression	Grayscale
	Diameter: Distal Mid Proximal	Grayscale
Basilic vein Forearm/upper arm	SAX sweep with or without compression	Grayscale
	Diameter: Distal Mid Proximal	Grayscale
Brachial veins	SAX sweep with or without compression	Grayscale
Axillary vein	SAX sweep with or without compression	Grayscale
	LAX Distal Mid Proximal	Grayscale/color Doppler/pulsed-wave spectral
Subclavian vein	LAX Distal Mid Proximal	Grayscale/color Doppler/pulsed-wave Doppler
Internal jugular vein	SAX sweep	Grayscale
	LAX sweep	Grayscale/color Doppler/pulsed-wave Doppler
Brachiocephalic vein	LAX	Grayscale/color Doppler/pulsed-wave Doppler
Radial artery	SAX sweep	
	Diameter: distal	Grayscale
	LAX sweep	Grayscale/color Doppler/pulsed-wave Doppler
Brachial artery	SAX sweep	Grayscale
	LAX sweep	Grayscale/color Doppler/pulsed-wave Doppler
Axillary artery	LAX sweep	Grayscale/color Doppler/pulsed-wave Doppler
Subclavian artery	LAX sweep	Grayscale/color Doppler/pulsed-wave Doppler
Brachiocephalic artery	LAX sweep	Grayscale/color Doppler/pulsed-wave Doppler

LAX, long-axis; SAX, short-axis.

DUPLEX INTERPRETATION AND REPORTING

Venous Scan: Venous Criteria

Compressibility is the main criterion for the forearm and upper arm veins. Evidence of partial compressibility, accompanied by an intraluminal "cavitational" appearance on grayscale, most likely occurs as a result of thickened walls and recanalized organized residual thrombus. The walls and the thrombus are caused by previous venous cannulation that renders these veins unsuitable for use as a conduit for hemodialysis.

Signs of Deep Vein Thrombosis
Noncompressibility

The venous system is normally distended under low pressure, and as such, veins are compressed easily with very little pressure required from the transducer. With venous thrombosis, the presence of intraluminal thrombus material renders the vein incompletely or noncompressible. Compression maneuvers are best performed in short-axis imaging, because it can be assured that the plane of imaging is not moving off to the side of the vessel, giving a false impression of compressibility as can occur with long-axis imaging. Generally, soft tissue material within the vessel is seen at sites of incompressibility.

TABLE 4-2   Criteria for Arterial Occlusive Disease

DISEASE	PLAQUE	VELOCITY RATIO	WAVEFORM
None	None	60-degree angle of insonation	Triphasic/biphasic
<50%	Yes	<2	Triphasic/biphasic
50–99%	Yes	>2	Biphasic/monophasic with poststenotic turbulence
Occluded	Yes		No flow

Flow Obstruction

Typically, venous flow exhibits spontaneous respiratory variation and in proportion to respiratory effort. In addition, normally, abrupt compression of a muscle bed distally to a site of sampling results in a surge of blood through the vein. With complete obstruction to flow by deep venous thrombosis, the signs of spontaneity, phasicity, and augmentation are lost. With partial obstruction, these signs are attenuated. Therefore, flow signs corroborate some cases of deep venous thrombosis; however, from a diagnostic and therapeutic standpoint, there is no difference between occlusive and nonocclusive thrombosis.

Arterial Scan

Obtain representative peak systolic velocity measurements along the artery every 2 to 3 cm. When a lesion is detected with grayscale scanning and color Doppler flow mapping, record peak systolic velocity measurements immediately proximal to the site of stenosis, within the stenosis, and immediately distal to it. Criteria for arterial occlusive disease are listed in Table 4-2.

POSTOPERATIVE ARTERIOVENOUS FISTULA ASSESSMENT

Duplex scanning is performed postoperatively to identify the presence or absence of occlusive or aneurysmal disease and subsequently to determine its extent and degree of severity, as well as to identify dilated branch vessel formation that could cause a "steal" phenomenon. Common indications include difficulty with cannulation, high venous pressures during hemodialysis, postangioplasty/thrombolytic therapy, pain over access site, extremity swelling, localized redness (possible infection), and palpable mass (hematoma, seroma, lymphocele).

Duplex scanning for an arteriovenous fistula is generally performed 4 to 6 weeks after surgery and then repeated at regular intervals, depending on the preference of the surgeon. If the patient has not been scanned preoperatively, full upper extremity venous and arterial duplex scans are performed.

Spectral Doppler interrogation using an angle of insonation less than or equal to 60 degrees and a sample volume of 1.5 mm is performed where

TABLE 4-3   Duplex Protocol for Scanning for Arteriovenous Fistulas

ANATOMIC SEGMENT	TECHNIQUE	DUPLEX INTERROGATION
Host artery	SAX sweep Distal Mid	Grayscale/color/ pulsed-wave spectral
	LAX Distal Mid	Grayscale/color/ pulsed-wave Doppler
Outflow vein	SAX sweep	Grayscale/color/ pulsed-wave Doppler
	LAX Anastomosis Distal Mid Proximal	Grayscale/color/ pulsed-wave Doppler

LAX, long-axis; SAX, short-axis.

possible. Representative measurements of the peak systolic and end-diastolic velocity are obtained. Volume flow in the distal artery as well as the vein above the anastomosis and distal to any stenosis identified is measured.[3] Duplex protocol for an arteriovenous fistula is presented in Table 4-3.

FISTULA COMPLICATIONS

The most common complications include thrombosis and stenosis. Early thrombosis is often due to an error in surgical technique and can also be due to unknown occlusion of a proximal outflow vein. Stenosis can be caused by inadequate anastomosis, intimal hyperplasia at the anastomosis in the outflow vein, or a protruding valve or fibrosis at the site of previous venipuncture.

True Aneurysm

True aneurysm represents focal dilation of arterial wall. It is a pulsating mass seen on grayscale imaging. If dissection is present, an intimal flap may be visualized. There is turbulent flow in the aneurysmal sac, and intraluminal heterogeneous echoes suggestive of thrombus may be present.

TABLE 4-4   Duplex Criteria of Stenosis Severity for Arteriovenous Fistulas

DISEASE	GRAYSCALE INTRALUMINAL ECHOES	PEAK SYSTOLIC VELOCITY	VELOCITY RATIO	FLOW VOLUME
Anastomosis				
Normal	No	<4 m/sec	<3	
<50% stenosis	Yes	<4 m/sec	<3	
>50% stenosis	Yes	>4 m/sec	>3	
Occluded	Yes throughout	No flow	—	
Outflow Vein and Inflow Artery				
Normal	No	<4 m/sec	<2	>500 mL/min
<50% stenosis	Yes	<4 m/sec	<2	>500 mL/min
>50% stenosis	Yes	>4 m/sec	>2	<500 mL/min
Occluded	Yes throughout	No flow	—	—

False Aneurysm (Pseudoaneurysm)

Pseudoaneurysm is a pulsating mass identified on grayscale and color Doppler imaging that is connected to the artery via a "tract." A pattern of reciprocating high-velocity anterograde and retrograde ("to and fro") flow is present within the tract. Turbulent flow is present within the body of the false aneurysm (apparent on color and spectral Doppler).

Scanning Protocol

The diameter, length, and depth of any aneurysmal lesion identified are measured. Color Doppler is used where appropriate to identify anastomosis and kinked or tortuous sections of vein. Volume flow in the distal artery, in the vein above the anastomosis and distal to any stenosis identified, is measured. It has been found that a blood flow volume greater than 500 mL/min is required for adequate dialysis.[4] Flow volume is followed mostly as a trend. Duplex criteria of stenosis severity for arteriovenous fistulas are listed in Table 4-4.

"Steal" from the palmar arch, by the fistula outflow tract, is thought to occur in 75% to 90% of patients after creation of access, and reverse flow in the radial artery distal to the anastomosis is a common finding on duplex scanning.[5] However, in most cases, the "steal" is asymptomatic, although some patients have a severe enough reduction of flow as to lead to rest pain in the hand, and sometimes, in extreme cases, ischemia. It is thought that these patients most likely have concurrent underlying vascular occlusive disease, and patients with diabetes are at particular risk.

ARTERIOVENOUS GRAFT

The most common site of narrowing is in the host vein proximal to the venous anastomosis. The body of the graft, anastomoses, host artery, and vein are scanned.

TABLE 4-5   Scanning Protocol for Arteriovenous Grafts

GRAFT	SHORT-AXIS SWEEP	DUPLEX INTERROGATION
	LAX: Venous anastomosis Arterial anastomosis Body of graft	Grayscale, color/ spectral Doppler
Host artery	LAX: proximal to graft	Grayscale, color/ spectral Doppler
Host vein	LAX: proximal to graft	Grayscale, color/ spectral Doppler

Scanning protocol for arteriovenous grafts is presented in Table 4-5.

Diameter, depth, and length of any perigraft abscess identified are measured. Percent diameter reduction measurements are performed where appropriate. Length, diameter, and depth of any aneurysm identified are measured.

Failure of graft access is most commonly caused by infection (delays maturity), pseudoaneurysm, distal extremity ischemia (a direct result of chronic "steal"), proximal venous stenosis, steal via large collaterals, or thrombosis. Proximal venous stenosis is predictive of failure and probably to be considered for remedial intervention in both arteriovenous fistulas and prosthetic grafts. Duplex crtieria for arteriovenous grafts are listed in Table 4-6.

Other Diagnostic Criteria

These criteria include:

❏ **Aneurysm** of the outflow vein may occur as a result of the sudden outflow demands placed on the native vein. There is a focal dilation of the vein, and thrombus may be present within the aneurysmal sac.

TABLE 4-6 Duplex Criteria for Arteriovenous Grafts

DISEASE	GRAYSCALE INTRALUMINAL ECHOES	PEAK SYSTOLIC VELOCITY	VELOCITY RATIO	FLOW VOLUME
Anastomotic Stenosis				
Normal	No	<4 m/sec	—	—
>50% stenosis	Yes	>4 m/sec	>3	—
Graft Body				
Normal	No	<4 m/sec	—	>500 mL/min
>50% stenosis	Yes	4 m/sec	>2	

❏ **Pseudoaneurysms** may form at the site of graft puncture.
❏ **Wall irregularities** manifest as a discontinuity of vessel lumen, with possible intimal flap formation (not to be confused with retained venous valves).
❏ **Thrombus** may or may not be occlusive.
❏ **Infection** requires looking for perigraft fluid collections, central venous stenosis, or loss of pulsatility.
❏ **Hematoma** may manifest as a complex or cystic mass lying superficial to vessel.

REFERENCES

1. NKF-DOQ1 clinical practice guidelines for hemodialysis adequacy. National Kidney Foundation. *Am J Kidney Dis.* 1997;30(3 suppl 2):S15-S66.

2. Allon M, Robbin M. Increasing arteriovenous fistulas in hemodialysis patients: problems and solutions. *Kidney Int.* 2002;62:1109-1124.

3. Barbour M, Tinkler K, Boutin A. Duplex ultrasound evaluated against fistulogram findings in patients with renal dialysis arterial-venous fistula: a validation study at the Royal Free Hospital. Presented at the 13th Annual General Meeting of the Society for Vascular Technology of Great Britain. *Harrogate.* 2004.

4. Singh P, Robbin M, Lockhart ME. Clinically immature arteriovenous hemodialysis fistulas: effect of US on salvage. *Radiology.* 2008;246:299-305.

5. Goldfield M, Koifman B, Loberant N, et al. Distal arterial flow in patients undergoing upper extremity dialysis shunting: a prospective study using Doppler sonography. *AJR Am J Roentgen.* 2000;175:513-516.

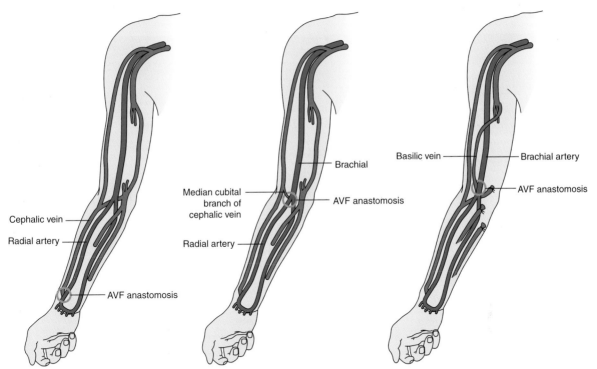

Figure 4-1. Common types of arteriovenous fistulas. *Left,* Radiocephalic fistula. *Middle,* Brachiocephalic fistula. *Right,* Brachiobasilic transposition. (Redrawn from Allon M, Robbin ML. Increasing arteriovenous fistulas in hemodialysis patients: problems and solutions. *Kidney Int.* 2002;62:1109-1124; figures 5 to 7; used with permission.)

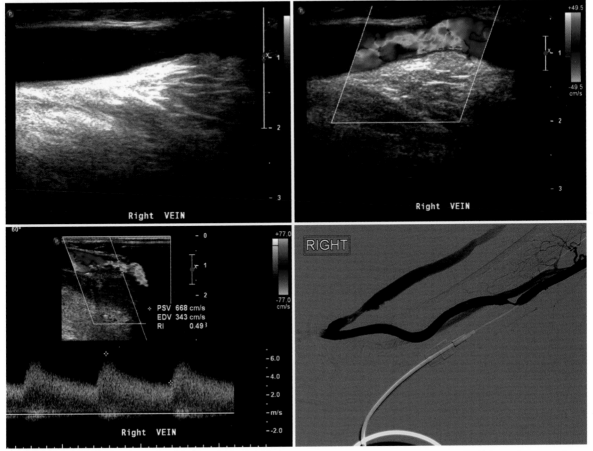

Figure 4-2. *Top left,* Grayscale imaging at site of focal narrowing of what appears to be a protruding valve cusp in the right cephalic outflow vein. *Top right,* Color Doppler flow mapping at same site. *Bottom left,* Severe flow acceleration at the site consistent with stenosis. *Bottom right,* A venogram corroborates the presence of stenosis.

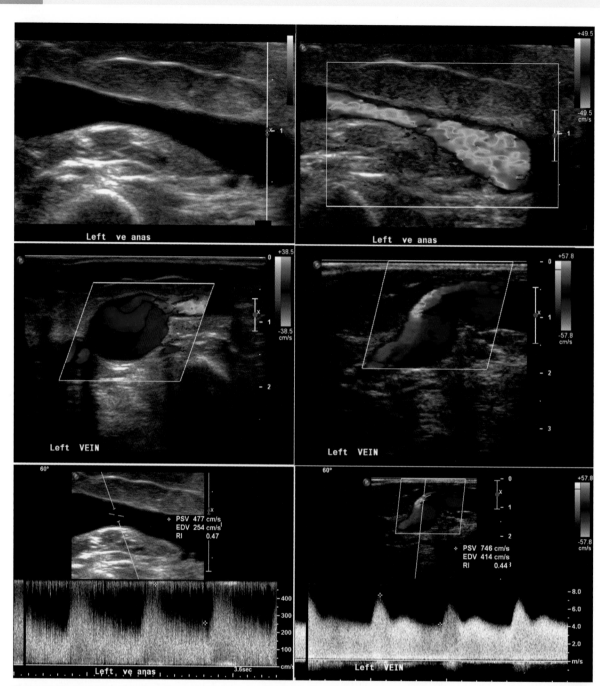

Figure 4-3. Duplex interrogation of arteriovenous dialysis fistula with stenosis. *Top left and right,* Grayscale and color Doppler flow mapping in the longitudinal axis show narrowing near the arteriovenous anastomosis. *Middle left and right,* The vein and turbulent flow near its anastomosis are depicted in the short-axis view. *Bottom left and right,* Spectral display with pulsed-wave Doppler sampling along the longitudinal and transverse plane reveals markedly elevated flow consistent with stenosis.

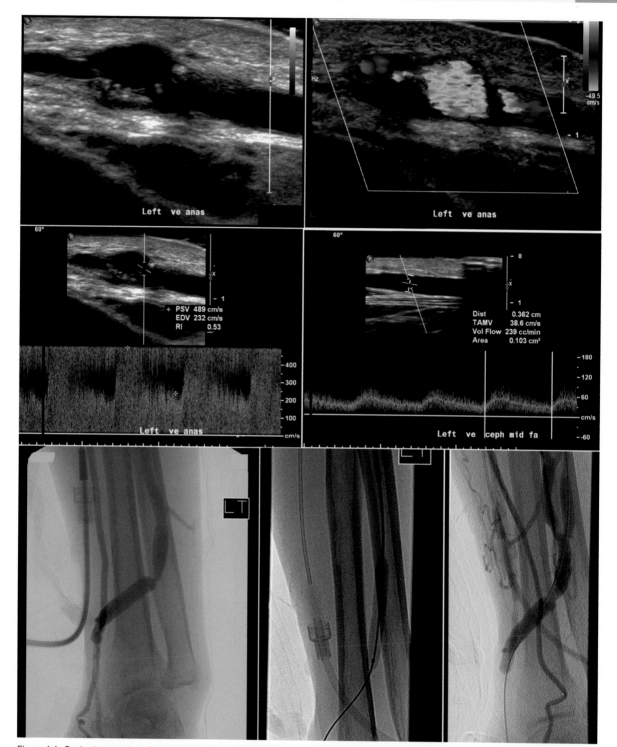

Figure 4-4. Duplex interrogation of arteriovenous dialysis fistula with stenosis. *Top left and right,* Long-axis grayscale and with color Doppler flow mapping show a narrowing along the course of the vein. *Middle left,* Turbulent and accelerated flow within the vein is seen. *Middle right,* Reduced volumetric flow. *Bottom left,* Angiographic image depicts the site of narrowing within the vein. *Bottom middle and right,* Dilation is seen during and following angioplasty of the stenotic site.

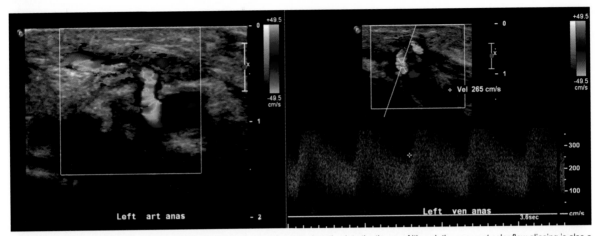

Figure 4-5. *Left,* A narrowed fistula anastomosis is suggested by color flow reverberation into the tissues. Although the apparent color flow aliasing is also a sign of a high-flow velocity state, it is not a definitive finding at an anastomotic site due to pressure from the adjacent attached arterial conduit. *Right,* Severely elevated flow velocity well above the normal range is seen.

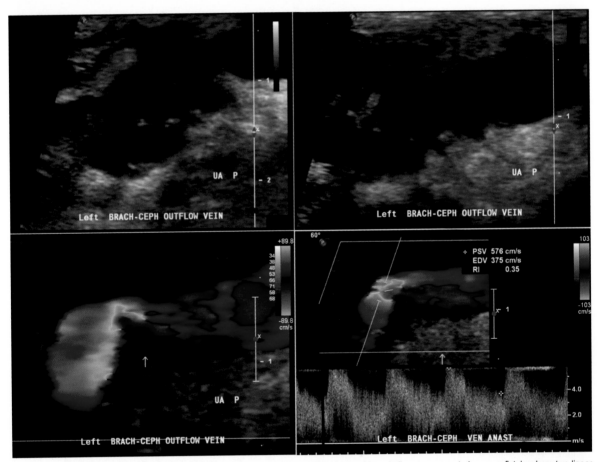

Figure 4-6. *Top left and right,* Short-axis and long-axis views show the outflow vein of a brachiocephalic upper arm arteriovenous fistula where two linear echoes are seen to extend into the lumen of the vessel. This most likely represents valve protrusion. *Bottom left,* Color flow convergence and turbulent flow, corresponding to the site of one of those valves, is seen. *Bottom right,* Spectral Doppler waveform at the site of one of the valves identifies high peak and diastolic flow velocities consistent with significant stenosis.

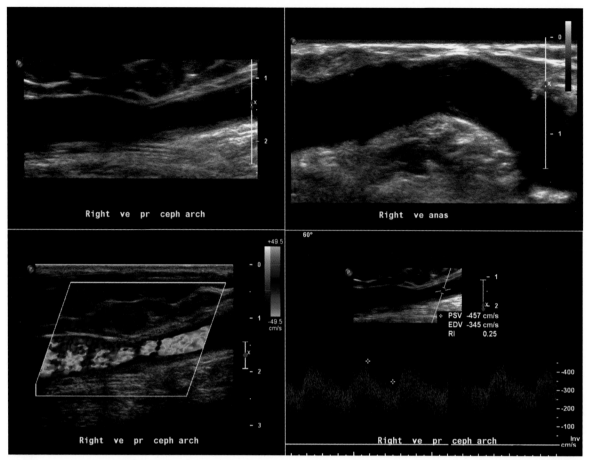

Figure 4-7. *Top left,* Mild wall thickening in the outflow vein at the anastomosis of a brachiocephalic fistula. *Top right,* An image taken in the proximal cephalic vein of the fistula shows wall thickening and narrowing with obvious poststenotic dilation. *Bottom left,* Color Doppler view defines the narrowing further and also depicts reverberation into the tissues, suggesting high velocity flow. *Bottom right,* Flow velocity elevation is consistent with significant stenosis.

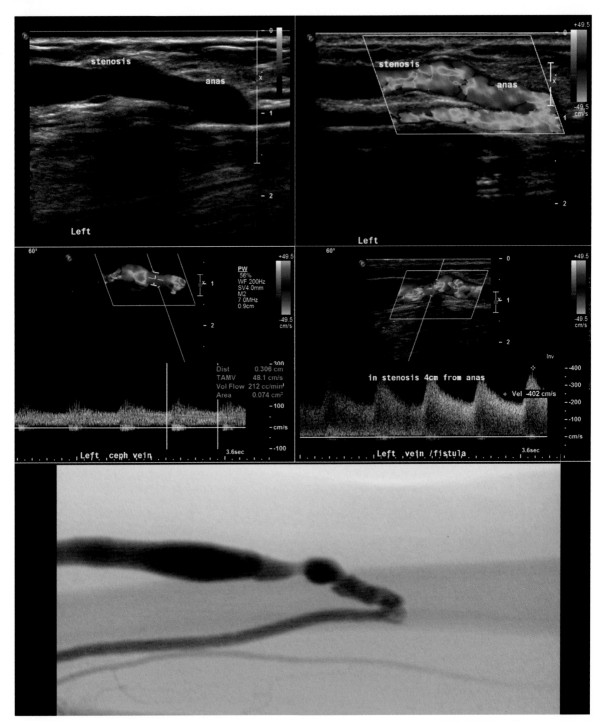

Figure 4-8. The images (*top left and right*) show narrowing of the outflow vein 4 cm proximal to the anastomosis. Middle left, Volume flow measurement of less than 500 mL/min is below normal (*middle left*). Spectral Doppler (*middle right*) and fistulogram (*bottom*) confirm the stenosis.

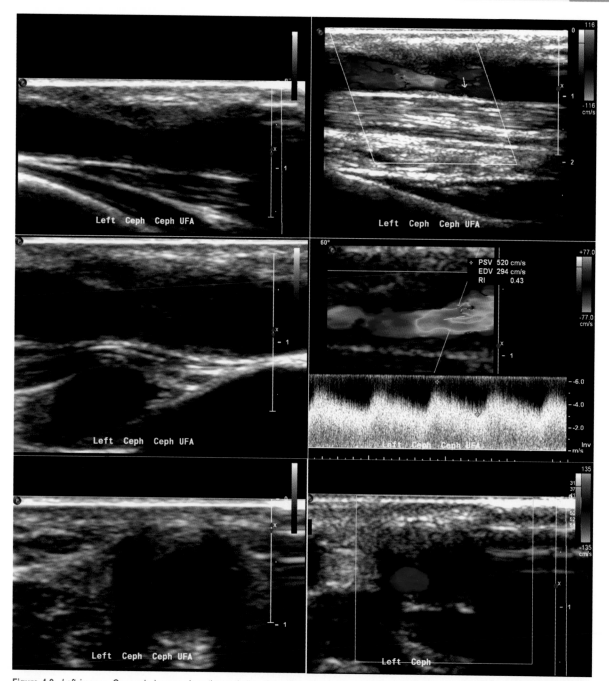

Figure 4-9. *Left images,* Grayscale images show the cephalic vein outflow of a forearm arteriovenous fistula with heterogeneous intraluminal echoes suggesting stenosis. *Right images,* Color and spectral Doppler images confirm this. The narrowing corresponds to the "buttonhole" site used for repeated puncture.

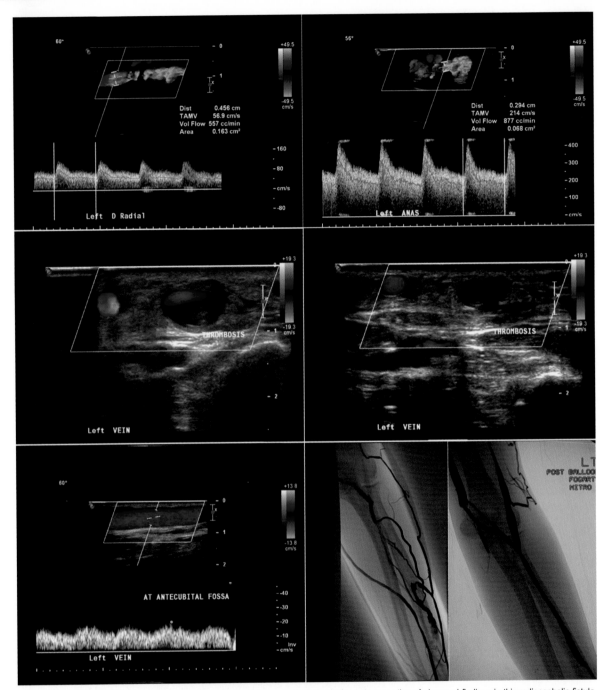

Figure 4-10. *Top left and right,* Long-axis views depict normal flow volume and velocity, not suggestive of abnormal findings in this radiocephalic fistula. *Middle left,* A short-axis view shows partial occlusion with thrombus of the main outflow vein. *Middle right,* The image taken further proximally shows complete occlusion and the presence of numerous collateral branches. *Bottom left,* Reduced velocity flow with a dampened waveform profile proximal to the occlusion in the upper forearm. *Bottom middle,* A fistulogram confirms segmental occlusion of the outflow vein with at least one large bridging collateral, the presence of which could explain why flow volume in the more distal segment appeared relatively unaffected by the occlusion. *Bottom right,* Patency of the outflow vein has been restored postangioplasty.

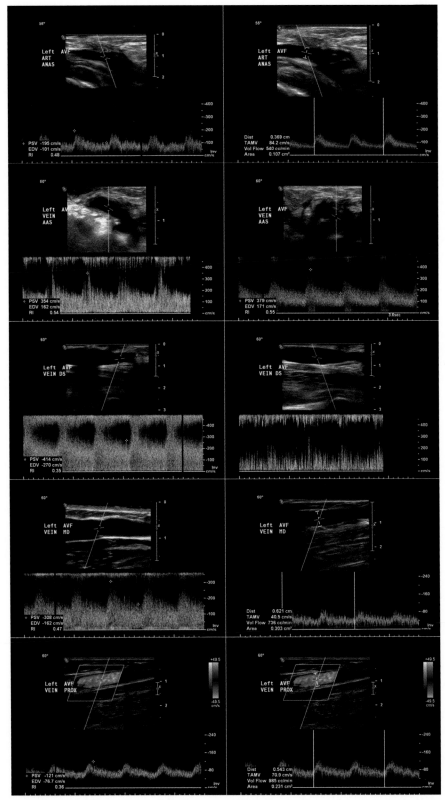

Figure 4-11. Baseline arteriovenous fistula: normal flow velocity and volume throughout the outflow vein from the anastomosis to the proximal segment and in the artery at the anastomosis. The third image on the right from the distal vein shows mild dilation and subsequent irregular flow pattern related to the variation (increase) in the luminal diameter.

5 Lower Extremity Arterial Disease

Key Points

■ Knowledge of normal and variant anatomy of the lower extremity arterial vasculature is critical.
■ A standardized and comprehensive duplex examination protocol is critical.
■ Knowledge of possible diseases/lesions potentially within the lower extremity arterial vasculature, and how to maximize their recognition, is critical.

This chapter is intended to review the ultrasound approach to assessment of arterial occlusive disease distal to the aorta. The arterial vasculature beyond the aorta has greater length than the aorta itself. As the arterial vasculature beyond the aorta involves progressively smaller and smaller vessels, it is more susceptible to occlusive disease than the aorta itself. Aneurysmal disease may occur at several levels in the lower extremity arterial vasculature. Duplex ultrasound of the lower extremity arterial vasculature is generally associated with noninvasive assessment of lower limb blood pressures, and may be associated as well with toe systolic blood pressure and transcutaneous oximetry.

ARTERIAL ANATOMY OF THE LOWER EXTREMITIES

The anatomy of the arterial vasculature (Figs. 5-1 to 5-3) of the lower abdomen, pelvis, and lower extremities is fairly consistent, with the level of branch origin being the most common type of variant. In 80% of cases, the aorta bifurcates within 1.25 cm of the iliac crest.

The right and left common iliac arteries are the continuation of the distal abdominal aorta at approximately the level of the fourth lumbar vertebra. The right and left common iliac arteries pass over the psoas muscle, run downward and laterally and themselves divide into internal (hypogastric) and external iliac arteries, the larger of the two branches, at a level between the last lumbar vertebra and the sacrum. The external iliac artery is larger than the internal iliac artery. The right common iliac artery is slightly longer than the left and passes over the fifth lumbar vertebra. There are small branches of the common iliac artery that supply the ureter, the peritoneum, and the psoas major muscle. Occasionally, accessory renal arteries arise from the common iliac artery.

Occlusion of the common iliac artery stimulates collaterals between branches of the abdominal aorta and the inferior mesenteric artery that bridge to the internal iliac artery and are thus one of the reasons that occlusive disease of the common iliac artery may be associated with bowel ischemia. Congenital atresia of one or both of the common iliac arteries is rare.

The external iliac artery has several small branches, which supply the psoas major muscle and lymph glands and two larger branches that arise from its distal segment. The first branch is the deep circumflex artery, which arises from the lateral surface of the external iliac artery and courses toward the anterior superior iliac spine, where it joins with branches of the lateral femoral circumflex artery. This connection is an important collateral source when common iliac artery occlusion extends into the internal iliac artery. The second branch of the external iliac artery is the inferior epigastric branch, which arises medially almost opposite the deep circumflex artery and courses superiorly beneath the rectus abdominis muscle.

In external iliac or common femoral artery occlusion, collateral vessels form between the gluteal branches of the internal iliac artery and the femoral circumflex branches of the profunda femoris artery.

The internal iliac artery, on average 4 cm long and with highly variable branching patterns, arises opposite the lumbosacral articulation and courses downward and medially with branches that supply the buttock, walls and viscera of the pelvis, reproductive organs, and medial side of the thigh.

The common femoral artery is a continuation of the external iliac artery. It originates at the inguinal ligament and is part of the femoral sheath, a downward continuation of the fascia lining the abdomen, which also contains the femoral nerve and vein. The common femoral artery extends approximately 3 to 4 cm below the inguinal ligament, where it then bifurcates into the superficial femoral and profunda femoris artery.

The profunda femoris artery, which lies lateral to the superficial femoral artery, gives rise to segmentally occurring circumflex and perforating branches which, when the superficial femoral artery is occluded, connect with the genicular branches of the popliteal artery to reconstitute the distal segment at the level of the adductus hiatus.

Clinical Pearls

- Even when the Doppler angle of insonation is inappropriate for acquisition of accurate velocity measurements, for example along the mid-external iliac artery where its course is parallel to pelvic floor, a suitably steered color box still reveals a focal narrowing by depicting turbulent flow and thereby gives some indication of the presence of stenosis.
- If a lower foreleg artery (such as the tibial artery) is subtotally occluded, its ongoing segments may be mistaken for the accompanying vein, as they may be easily compressible, due to low distending pressure, against shallowly underlying bone.
- A triphasic nonturbulent waveform at the common femoral level does not necessarily mean that there is no significant stenosis in either the common or external iliac arteries.
- At the femoral bifurcation, the profunda femoris artery may sometimes run in the usual position of the superficial femoral artery (i.e., more anteriorly for the first few centimeters) and the superficial femoral artery run more posteriorly. Hence, the vessels need to be followed along their length to identify them, and their courses may be atypical and engender confusion as to their identify. In a slim leg, this could result in the impression that the vessel is occluded by the time the mid thigh is reached and the profunda femoris artery had devolved into smaller branches.
- In a situation where the superficial femoral artery is chronically occluded and its ultrasonographic appearance blends into the surrounding tissues, it is possible to follow the profunda femoris artery until it divides into branches, giving the impression that the vessel is at least patent in the proximal thigh.
- A saphenous vein bypass graft typically lies closer to the skin surface than does the native vessel and is therefore more likely to be easily compressed by the probe during scanning, falsely suggesting narrowing. Hence when scanning, use very light pressure and lots of gel.
- Biphasic (increased diastolic) flow rather than the usual triphasic flow can be seen in the periphery of normal arteries when there is vasodilation and hyperemia as a result of infection, for example.

From the femoral bifurcation, the superficial femoral artery continues as the primary conduit between the common femoral and popliteal artery, giving off several small branches along its course and from the mid- to distal thigh, running under the sartorius muscle in the adductor canal along with the femoral vein and branches of the femoral nerve.

In the distal thigh, the superficial femoral artery courses deeply through the adductor hiatus and posteriorly into the popliteal fossa, to become the popliteal artery.

There are three groups of branches of the popliteal artery: (1) the genicular arteries, which form a collateral network around the knee; (2) the paired sural arteries, which arise from the posterior aspect and supply the gastrocnemius and soleal muscle; and (3) the anterior tibial artery, which crosses the upper edge of the interosseous membrane and extends down to the level of the medial malleolus.

The genicular branches connect with tibial branches to form a collateral network and bypass popliteal artery occlusions.

The tibioperoneal trunk extends approximately 2.5 cm from the takeoff of the anterior tibial artery to the bifurcation of posterior tibial and peroneal arteries, with the posterior tibial running distally to a point midway between the medial malleolus and the tip of the heel.

A common variant of anatomy is a small or absent posterior tibial artery, which is frequently diminished in size and absent in approximately 5% of limbs individuals (bilaterally). The peroneal artery is typically larger when the posterior tibial artery is small or absent.

There is generally a dearth of collateral availability and formation in the foreleg. Because there are few branch vessels present in the proximal foreleg to participate as collaterals, occlusion of the popliteal and proximal tibial arteries may result in severe distal ischemia.

The peroneal artery originates from the bifurcation of the tibioperoneal trunk and descends along the medial side of the fibula. The peroneal artery bifurcates behind the lateral malleolus into the lateral calcaneal arteries and may provide large collateral branches to the tibial arteries in the distal calf.

The dorsalis pedis artery is the continuation of the anterior tibial artery and runs lateral to the extensor tendon to the first toe. The line of demarcation of the two is held to be the level of the ankle. The artery is congenitally absent in approximately 4% to 5% of individuals but always bilaterally. In approximately 4% of individuals, the dorsalis pedis artery is a continuation of the perforating branch of the peroneal artery, and the anterior tibial artery does not extend to the ankle level or it is severely diminished in size. This variant artery may be detected by duplex scanning, and unless the anterior tibial artery is mapped, its continuation from the anterior tibial artery may be wrongfully assumed. As with the arteries within the hand, an arcade of vessels provides redundancy and digital branches.

The figures in this chapter represent numerous examples of ultrasound scanning of lower extremity arteries: common femoral artery (Figs. 5-4 to 5-7), superficial femoral artery (Figs. 5-8 to 5-15), profunda femoris artery (Figs. 5-16 and 5-17), common iliac artery (Figs. 5-18 to 5-28), external iliac artery (Figs. 5-29 to 5-33), internal iliac artery (Fig. 5-34), popliteal artery (Figs. 5-35 to 5-40), surgical cases (Figs. 5-41 to 5-48), and trifurcations (Figs. 5-49 to 5-52).

DUPLEX SCANNING

Purpose

The objective is to identify the presence or absence and location of occlusive or aneurysmal disease and subsequently to determine its extent and degree of severity.

Common Indications

❐ Patients with claudication
❐ Patients with ischemic rest pain/arterial ulcers
❐ Patients scheduled for invasive or surgical procedures in whom there is concern about arterial access and disease
❐ Follow-up post–peripheral angioplasty/stenting
❐ Follow-up bypass graft (see bypass graft protocol, page 99)
❐ Follow-up known peripheral vascular disease
❐ Evaluation prior to application of compression bandage therapy for venous ulceration
❐ Evaluation of arterial trauma
❐ Palpable mass/bruit/thrill post–vascular intervention
❐ Suspected popliteal entrapment
❐ Pulsatile mass in the lower abdomen or lower extremity
❐ Suspected Buerger disease (thromboangiitis obliterans)

Contraindications

❐ Ulceration
❐ Wound dressing

Equipment

❐ Color Duplex imaging system
❐ 5- to 12-MHz linear transducers
❐ 2- to 6-MHz sector/curved array transducers
❐ Coupling gel
❐ Digital recording system

Procedure

❐ Explain the procedure to the patient and answer any questions.
❐ Obtain and document applicable patient history on appropriate forms.
❐ Verify that the procedure requested correlates with patient's symptoms.
❐ Review pertinent medical history:
  • Determine if the patient has a history of recent deep vein thrombosis (ankle-brachial indices would not be performed in the presence of deep vein thrombosis).
  • Ascertain whether the patient is taking vasodilator medications because they may influence the observed peripheral arterial waveforms (rendering them low-resistance biphasic, whereas they are normally high-resistance biphasic/triphasic).
  • Ascertain whether there is a relevant cardiac history such as heart failure (which reduces flow velocity) or aortic valve stenosis or insufficiency (which alters waveforms).
❐ Perform a limited physical examination of the limbs in question.
❐ Review any previous duplex studies available.
❐ Select appropriate test settings.
❐ Select appropriate annotation throughout test.
❐ Record images.
❐ Complete sonographer's preliminary report when necessary.

Technique

❐ The patient lies supine for at least 10 minutes before scanning to avoid residual hemodynamic effects of exercise or muscular exertion.
❐ The sonographer stands or sits beside the patient.
❐ Gloves are worn by the sonographer where there is a threat of contamination by infected body fluids.

Scanning Protocol

❐ Ensure that both limbs are scanned.
❐ Ensure that the limb being scanned is externally rotated and the knee slightly bent.
❐ Using grayscale imaging and color Doppler flow mapping, identify all vessels (listed subsequently) in both their transverse and longitudinal planes and record flow velocities with pulsed-wave Doppler.
❐ Perform spectral Doppler using:
  • An angle of less than or equal to 60 degrees to the vessel wall where possible
  • A sample volume of 1.5 mm
❐ Sequentially image the:
  • Aorta
  • Common iliac arteries
  • External iliac arteries
  • Common femoral arteries
  • Femoral bifurcation
  • Profunda femoris arteries (proximal segment)
  • Superficial femoral arteries (proximal/mid/distal)
  • Popliteal arteries
  • Dorsalis pedis arteries (at the ankle level)
  • Posterior tibial arteries (at the ankle level)

Begin the scan at the level of the xiphisternum, slightly to the left of the midline (or above if the coeliac axis is more proximal) with the abdominal aorta. Use both transverse and longitudinal views to measure the maximal anteroposterior and transverse diameter of any aneurysmal dilatation. Document the location of aneurysmal disease with respect to the renal artery ostia. Turning the patient obliquely or into a decubitus position may be necessary to optimize arterial visualization in the presence of extensive bowel gas. Note, in passing, the splanchnic and renal branches of the aorta.

Continue to scan down the common and external iliac arteries, which can most easily be located by continuing to scan proximally from the common femoral artery (located at a point midway between the mid-symphysis pubis and the anterior superior iliac spine) just below the inguinal ligament and moving diagonally toward the umbilicus.

Then continue to scan following the common femoral artery through to its bifurcation. The profunda femoris artery dives deeply beyond its origin and can usually be followed only for several centimeters. Follow the superficial femoral artery along the medial aspect of the thigh to its distal segment, where it dives into the adductor hiatus. Scan the popliteal artery in the popliteal fossa from a posterior approach and then on, where possible, to the tibioperoneal trunk, noting the origins of the peroneal and posterior tibial arteries.

The posterior tibial artery is identified at the ankle level immediately posterior to the medial malleolus.

The dorsalis pedis artery is seen midway between lateral and medial malleoli.

If neither the posterior tibial nor the dorsalis pedis arteries are visualized, to scan the peroneal artery anterior or posterior to the lateral malleolus.

During the scan:

❏ Attempt to characterize the pathology (e.g., wall thickening/calcification [medial calcinosis]) and the appearance, length, location and extent of plaque.

❏ If aneurysmal dilation is identified in transverse scanning, measure the diameter, length, and the aneurysmal neck, as well as any endovascular treatment relevant details (see Chapter 7).

❏ Obtain representative peak systolic velocity (PSV) measurements along the vessels every 2 to 3 cm.

❏ When a lesion is detected with grayscale scanning and color Doppler flow mapping, record PSV measurements:
  • Immediately proximal to the site of stenosis
  • Within the stenosis
  • Immediately distal to it

❏ Note any obvious collateral vessel formation associated with a significant lesion.

❏ Document any identified retrograde flow.

Interpretation and Reporting
Normal Study
❏ Typical triphasic/biphasic Doppler waveform
❏ No evidence of plaque, calcification, or aneurysmal dilation on grayscale imaging
❏ Normal flow velocities

Abnormal Study
❏ Intraluminal echoes identified
❏ Abnormal waveforms
❏ Flow velocity changes

Classification of Stenosis
❏ Less than 50%
  • Plaque visualized on grayscale imaging
  • Triphasic/biphasic waveforms
  • 30% to 100% increase in PSV compared with that immediately proximal to the site of stenosis
❏ Between 50% and 99%
  • Plaque visualized
  • Loss of reverse flow component (variable)
  • More than 100% increase in peak systolic flow velocity compared with that immediately proximal to the site of stenosis
  • Evidence of poststenotic turbulent/disordered flow
  • Color flow representation of narrowed flow channel
❏ Complete occlusion
  • Intraluminal echoes observed throughout vessel
  • Absence of color and spectral Doppler signals

❏ Reconstitution postocclusion
  • Resumption of flow visualized by color Doppler
  • Spectral Doppler flow pattern usually contains both forward and reverse flow elements (influenced by reentry vessel flow)

Descriptions of Plaque/Stenosis
❏ Calcified: hyperechoic lesion causing acoustical shadowing
❏ Heterogeneous or complex: lesion of mixed echogenicity causing no acoustical shadowing
❏ Anechoic: hypoechoic, poorly delineated lesion but possibly causing flow disturbance
❏ Smooth: surface contour of lesion is smoothly defined
❏ Irregular: rough and irregular luminal surface

Other Lesions/Syndromes
❏ True aneurysm
  • Focal dilation of arterial wall
  • Pulsating mass seen on grayscale imaging
  • Possible visualization of an intimal flap if dissection is present
  • Turbulent flow in the aneurysmal sac
  • Intraluminal heterogeneous echoes suggestive of thrombus may be present
❏ False (or pseudo) aneurysm
  • Pulsating mass identified on grayscale and color Doppler imaging that is connected to the artery via a "tract"
  • Pattern of reciprocating high-velocity anterograde and retrograde ("to-and-fro") flow within the tract
  • Turbulent flow is present the body of the false aneurysm (apparent by color and spectral Doppler)
❏ Arterial compression syndrome (e.g., popliteal entrapment)
  • The artery may have normal appearance and show normal waveform contours at rest.
  • Even after exercise, although ankle-brachial values might diminish somewhat, there is often no dramatic change.
  • However, if the patient is asked to perform the provocative maneuvers that actually cause pain (e.g., plantar and dorsiflexion), high-velocity turbulent flow accompanied by visualization of a temporarily narrowed or obliterated flow channel by color Doppler can be readily seen.
❏ Arteriovenous fistula
  • Connection between artery and vein identified with color Doppler
  • Pulsatile flow identified in the vein distal to the fistula
  • Monophasic flow patterns possibly present in the artery proximal to fistula
  • High-velocity turbulent flow seen in arteriovenous connection
  • Observation of the following findings:

1. An increase in diastolic flow compared with proximal values
2. High-velocity flow within a persistent vein branch (rather than in the graft itself as in stenosis)
3. Mean velocities in proximal portions of the graft that are significantly higher than those obtained in normal or stenotic grafts
4. PSVs measured proximal to the fistula that are significantly greater than those measured distally

ANKLE-BRACHIAL INDEX

The ankle-brachial artery systolic blood pressure ratio is a venerable but still useful test in the assessment of peripheral arterial disease. It is not suitable as a stand-alone test to detect peripheral arterial disease because it may give false-negative results and does not localize or characterize disease suitability to revascularization. It is generally performed in conjunction with duplex assessment as a means to corroborate findings. Ankle-to-brachial pressures are listed in Table 5-1.

"False-Negatives" in Ankle-Brachial Testing for the Detection of Peripheral Arterial Disease
❐ Medial calcinosis rendering ankle arteries incompressible
❐ Extensive large collateral vessel formation
❐ Bilateral subclavian stenoses devalidating the brachial standard

Equipment
❐ Blood pressure cuffs: 13 × 85 cm, 11 × 85 cm
❐ Sphygmomanometer (manual/automatic)
❐ Continuous-wave probe 8 MHz/5 MHz
❐ Stethoscope
❐ Coupling gel

Resting Technique
❐ Ensure that the patient lies supine after having rested for at least 10 minutes.

TABLE 5-1 Ankle-Brachial Pressures

	NORMAL	ABNORMAL
Pre-exercise	>0.97	<0.97
Single segment disease		0.50–0.97
Multisegment disease		<0.50
Postexercise ankle pressure		Drop by 20%
Toe pressures	80 mm Hg	
Toe-to-brachial ratio	>0.65	

❐ If the room is cold, warm the patient with blankets.
❐ Wrap standard pneumatic blood pressure cuffs around the upper arms and the ankles.
❐ Place cuffs immediately proximal to the malleoli and attached to the sphygmomanometer.
❐ Using continuous-wave Doppler, auscultate the brachial artery, the dorsalis pedis artery, and the posterior tibial arteries at the ankle level distal to the cuff.
❐ Inflate the cuffs individually while continuing to listen to the pulse with Doppler.
❐ When the pulse disappears (must be at least 20 mm Hg of mercury above last sounds), slowly deflate until the pulse reappears.
❐ Look for the result displayed in mm Hg.
❐ Repeat the procedure on the contralateral limb.
❐ Calculate the ankle-brachial index by dividing the highest brachial pressure by each ankle pressure.
❐ If incompressible tibial arteries (medial calcinosis) are encountered (ankle-brachial index >1.3), proceed to perform toe pressure readings (see subsequent discussion), where possible.

Exercise Technique
Because there may be no obvious pressure gradient in the presence of early atherosclerotic disease, exercise stress (such as treadmill or toe raises) may be used to detect peripheral vascular disease. Exercise demands an increase in blood flow to the limbs and "reveals" a pressure drop where a hemodynamically significant lesion is present.

Toe Raises Technique
❐ Have the patient stand firmly on the ground while holding onto an immobile object in front of him or her and rising up on the toes and back down again, repeating a maximum of 50 times.
❐ Immediately after exercise, repeat the pressure test and compare it with the resting values.

TOE SYSTOLIC PRESSURES

Recording of toe systolic pressures is useful when ankle pressures cannot be recorded due to incompressibility.

Purpose
❐ As an indicator of the healing potential of lower extremity ulcers
❐ To obtain quantitative blood pressure data when ankle-brachial pressure measurements cannot be obtained

Common Indications
❐ When the tibial arteries are calcified, rigid, and incompressible (e.g., diabetes)
❐ When ankle cuff inflation is too painful
❐ When it is necessary to assess small vessel occlusive disease below the ankle

Equipment
- ❏ Digit cuffs of different sizes: 2.5 × 12 cm, 2.5 × 9 cm
- ❏ Photoplethysmograph sensors
- ❏ Chart recorder
- ❏ Double-sided adhesive tape

Technique
- ❏ If the feet are cold, warm them to room temperature.
- ❏ Wrap toe pneumatic cuffs around the proximal phalanx of each great toe.
- ❏ Attach photoplethysmographic (photosensor and infrared light-emitting diode that records signal proportional to the blood volume) sensors to the pad of each toe with double-sided adhesive tape/straps.
- ❏ Ensure that a pulsatile plethysmographic waveform is displayed on a chart recorder and amplitude adjusted where necessary (calibration is not required).
- ❏ Inflate the cuffs above arterial pressure until the waveform disappears.
- ❏ Look for the chart paper marked at 10-mm Hg increments while the cuffs are slowly deflated, until the waveform reappears.
- ❏ Document both waveform and pressure.

DUPLEX ULTRASOUND EXAMINATION OF BYPASS GRAFTS

Purpose
The goal is screening for early or late graft failure caused by any of the following:
- ❏ Retained valves (in situ)
- ❏ Myointimal hyperplasia
- ❏ Intimal flap
- ❏ Arteriovenous fistula
- ❏ Thrombosis/embolism
- ❏ Suture stenosis
- ❏ Infection
- ❏ Graft entrapment/torsion
- ❏ Atherosclerotic disease progression in graft or adjacent vessel

Common Indications
- ❏ Acute postoperative ischemia
- ❏ Return of preoperative symptoms
- ❏ Thrill/bruit over graft
- ❏ Pulsatile mass
- ❏ Follow-up as part of a surveillance program

Contraindications
- ❏ Wound dressings
- ❏ Open wound

Equipment
- ❏ Color duplex imaging system
- ❏ 5- to 12-MHz linear transducer
- ❏ 2- to 6-MHz sector/curved array transducer
- ❏ Coupling gel
- ❏ Digital reporting

Procedure
- ❏ Explain the procedure to the patient and answer any questions.
- ❏ Obtain and document applicable patient history on appropriate forms.
- ❏ Determine if the patient has a history of deep vein thrombosis (ankle-brachial indices would not be performed in the presence of deep vein thrombosis).
- ❏ Verify that the procedure requested correlates with patient's symptoms.
- ❏ Ascertain whether the patient is taking medication.
- ❏ Perform a limited physical examination of the limbs in question.
- ❏ Select appropriate test preset values.
- ❏ Select the appropriate annotation throughout test.
- ❏ Record images.
- ❏ Complete technologist's preliminary report when necessary.
- ❏ Auscultate for bruits along the length of the graft (bruits are usually significant, but the presence of a pulse can be misleading because the pulse can be felt often in the presence of a stenosis or even proximally to an occlusion).

Technique
The bypass study is always accompanied by a full lower extremity arterial study (see separate protocol) with particular attention being paid to the host vessels immediately proximal and distal to the graft anastomoses. Follow these guidelines:
- ❏ Have the patient lie supine.
- ❏ Perform the scan standing or sitting beside the patient.
- ❏ Wear gloves where there may be a threat of contamination by body fluids.
- ❏ Select appropriate transducer.
- ❏ Use grayscale imaging and pulsed Doppler.

Graft Types
- ❏ Saphenous vein in situ
- ❏ Saphenous vein reversed
- ❏ Axillofemoral (synthetic)
- ❏ Femoropopliteal (synthetic)
- ❏ Femorotibial (synthetic)
- ❏ Aortobifemoral
- ❏ Aortoiliac
- ❏ Femoral-femoral crossover
- ❏ Aortic tube

Views
Transverse
- ❏ Scan the graft in this mode first for identification of any abnormal dilatation.
- ❏ Measure the graft diameter at several sites and document.
- ❏ Utilize color flow mapping to identify any evidence of arteriovenous fistula.

❑ If an arteriovenous fistula is identified, perform spectral Doppler.

Sagittal
❑ Scan the entire graft from proximal to distal anastomoses.
❑ Perform spectral Doppler interrogation using an angle of less than or equal to 60 degrees where possible and a sample volume of 1.5 mm.
❑ Obtain representative PSVs throughout the length of the graft.
❑ Note areas of increased flow and obtain velocity measurements proximal to, within, and distal to the lesion.
❑ Measure the location of a stenosis with respect to a suitable landmark.
❑ Try to determine the nature of the lesion.

Interpretation and Reporting
❑ The normal Doppler velocity waveform should be triphasic or biphasic.
❑ In a normal graft, a bruit should not be heard during auscultation.
❑ The normal PSV is more than 40 cm/sec; this increases somewhat below the knee, as the graft narrows.
❑ The normal diameter of an in situ graft is 4 to 5 mm above the knee and 3 to 4 mm below it.
❑ A localized reddened area along or adjacent to the incision line (autologous grafts) may indicate the presence of an arteriovenous fistula.
❑ If a significant stenosis is present, the waveform distally will be dampened.
❑ An aneurysm suggested by palpation can be seen as a localized area of disturbed flow and a focal area of dilation visualized with grayscale imaging.
❑ A localized area of high-velocity flow indicates stenosis or arteriovenous fistula.
❑ Absence of a pulse and Doppler signal throughout accompanied by intraluminal echoes indicates complete occlusion.

Characteristics of Vein Graft Stenosis
The velocity characteristics of a significant (>50%) synthetic graft stenosis is similar to that of native vessel stenosis—a 100% increase in PSV compared with the segment immediately proximal to it.

Graft Stenosis: Less Than 20%
❑ Velocity ratio less than 2
❑ Mild turbulence in systole
❑ PSV less than 200 cm/sec

Graft Stenosis: 20% to 50%
❑ Velocity ratio greater than 2
❑ Turbulence throughout
❑ PSV less than 200 cm/sec

Graft Stenosis: 50% to 75%
❑ Velocity ratio greater than 2.5
❑ Severe turbulence with reversed flow components
❑ PSV greater than 200 cm/sec

Graft Stenosis: 75% to 99%
❑ Velocity ratio greater than 3.5
❑ End-diastolic velocity in flow jet greater than 100 cm/sec
❑ PSV greater than 300 cm/sec

Impending Graft Thrombosis
❑ Velocity ratio greater than 3.5
❑ PSV less than 50 cm/sec

PRACTICE GUIDELINES

The 2005 American College of Cardiology/American Heart Association (ACC/AHA) Practice Guidelines on Peripheral Artery Disease include indications for duplex ultrasonography of lower extremity arteries.[1]

ACCREDITATION

Intersocietal Commission for Accreditation of Vascular Laboratories (ICAVL) maintains the standards for testing and accreditation of vascular laboratories. Refer to Table 3-1 for a summary of standards for peripheral arterial testing.[2]

REFERENCES

1. Hirsch AT, Haskal ZJ, Hertzer NR, et al. ACC/AHA 2005 practice guidelines for the management of patients with peripheral arterial disease (lower extremity, renal, mesenteric, and abdominal aortic): executive summary. *J Am Coll Cardiol*. 2006;47:1239-1312.
2. Intersocietal Commission for Accreditation of Vascular Laboratories (ICAVL): The Complete ICAVL Standards for Accreditation in Noninvasive Vascular Testing. <http://www.icavl.org/icavl/Standards/2010_ICAVL_Standards.pdf.> Accessed April 20, 2010.

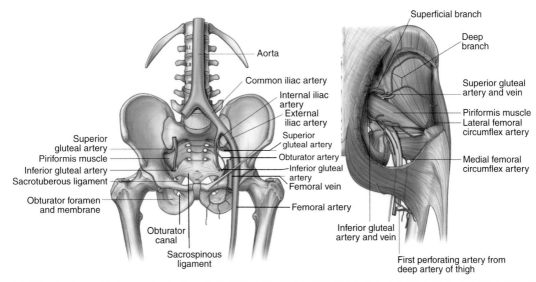

Figure 5-1. Arterial anatomy of the lower extremity. (From Drake R, Vogl AW, Mitchell AWM. *Gray's Anatomy for Students.* 2nd ed. Philadelphia: Elsevier; 2010; Figs. 6-36 and 6-48; used with permission.)

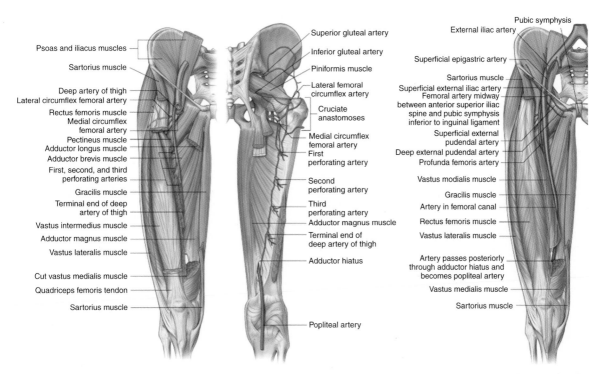

Figure 5-2. Arterial anatomy of the leg. (From Drake R, Vogl AW, Mitchell AWM. *Gray's Anatomy for Students.* 2nd ed. Philadelphia: Elsevier; 2010; Figs. 6-62 and 6-63; used with permission.)

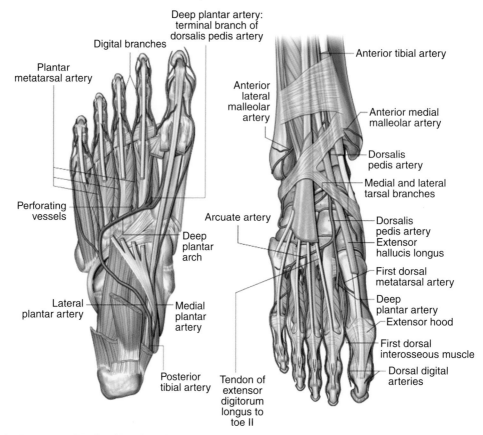

Figure 5-3. Arterial anatomy of the foot. (From Drake R, Vogl AW, Mitchell AWM. *Gray's Anatomy for Students*. 2nd ed. Philadelphia: Elsevier; 2010; Figs. 6-117 and 6-118; used with permission.)

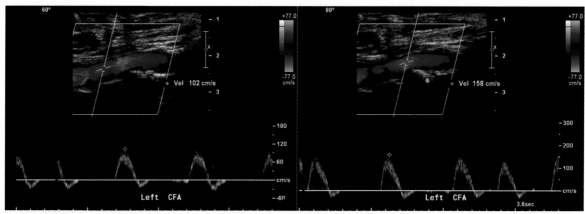

Figure 5-4. Stenosis of the common femoral artery by grayscale and color flow mapping is less than 50%. Spectral display of the flow before the plaque (*left*) and at the plaque (*right*) does not reveal an acceleration. The color Doppler flow pattern also does not show turbulence.

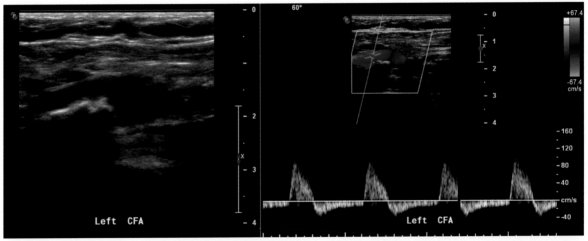

Figure 5-5. The grayscale image reveals the plaque in the common femoral artery. Spectral flow display reveals turbulence, but flow velocity is within the normal range. Without determining the flow velocity before the plaque, an acceleration of flow cannot be excluded.

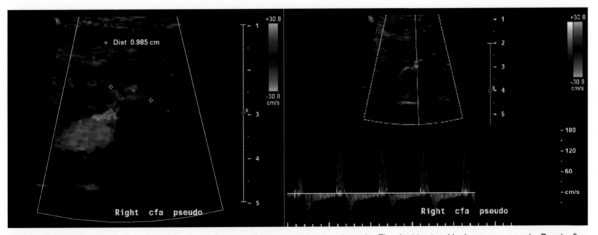

Figure 5-6. False aneurysm arising from the common femoral artery post–coronary angiography. The short tract and body are seen on color Doppler flow mapping. The reciprocating flow pattern is depicted by spectral display.

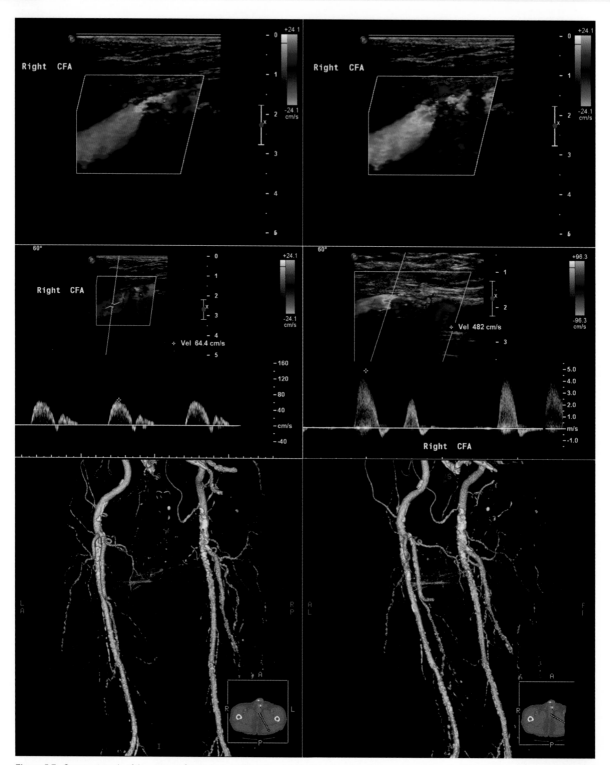

Figure 5-7. Severe stenosis of the common femoral artery. *Top left and right,* Color Doppler aliasing and reverberation into the tissues is seen. *Middle left and right,* Images confirm a systolic velocity ratio greater than 4 and considerable poststenotic turbulence consistent with stenosis. *Bottom left and right,* Computed tomography angiography images reveal heavy calcification of the common femoral arteries that on the right side obscures the underlying stenosis.

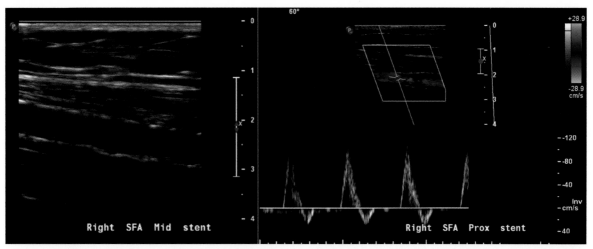

Figure 5-8. Stented superficial femoral artery. *Left,* On grayscale imaging, the stent is barely apparent. As the underlined atheromatous plaque is fairly homogenous, it is also barely visible. *Right,* The spectral flow pattern and velocities are normal.

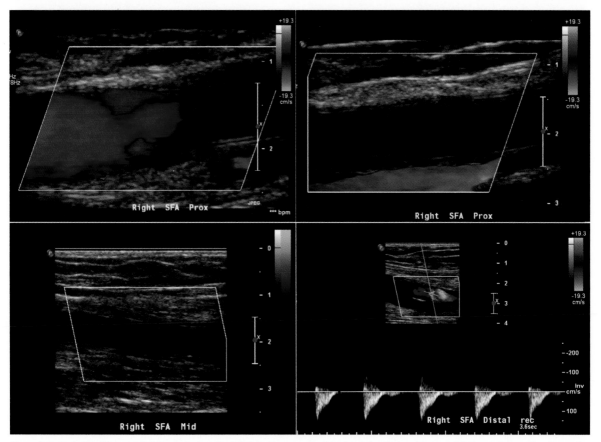

Figure 5-9. Occlusion of the superficial femoral artery. *Top left,* Color flow mapping at the level of occlusion of the superficial femoral artery. Abrupt cessation of flow is depicted with stem vessels, appearing blue by color Doppler flow mapping. *Top right,* A few centimeters more distally, no flow can be detected by color Doppler flow mapping. *Bottom left,* Flow cannot be detected by power angiography flow mapping. *Bottom right,* Further distally, color Doppler flow mapping at the far end of the occlusion demonstrates flow that seems to be reversed due to the inflow through reconstituting reentry vessels distally.

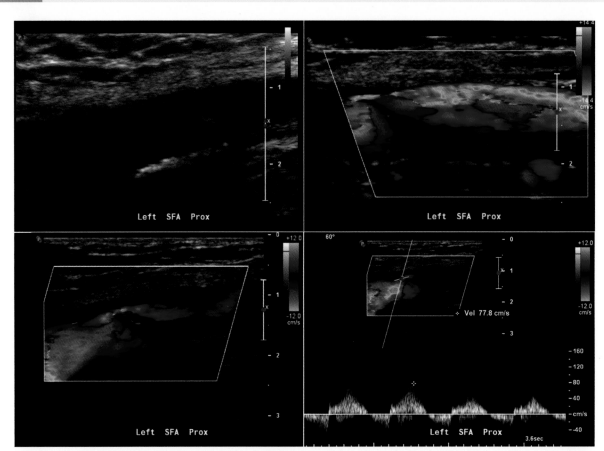

Figure 5-10. A greater than 50% stenosis of the superficial femoral artery. *Top left,* Grayscale imaging of the superficial femoral artery shows a tapering soft tissue linear lesion projecting into the lumen that was seen to have slight motion on real-time imaging. *Top right and bottom left,* Color Doppler flow mapping at this level more clearly shows the tapered shelflike lesion. This patient had a patent femoro-femoral bypass graft. *Bottom right,* The spectral Doppler waveform suggests that perhaps the graft is "stealing" flow from the artery here because the narrowed flow stream is not accompanied by high-velocity flow as would be expected and the flow pattern is tardus parvus and bidirectional (the shape of a "stealing" waveform).

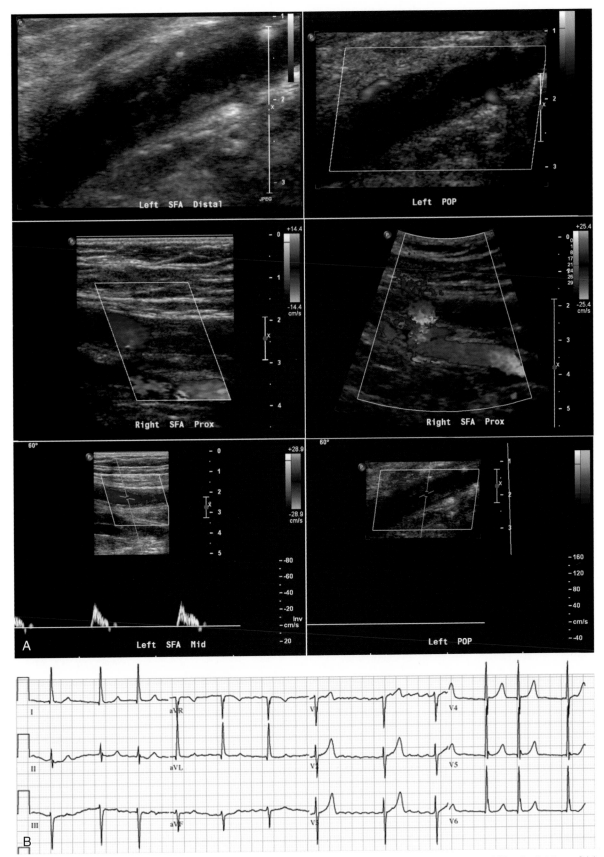

Figure 5-11. A, Embolic occlusion of the superficial femoral artery. *Top left,* Grayscale imaging reveals homogenous material filling the distal superficial femoral artery. *Top right,* Power angiography Doppler cannot delineate any flow within the popliteal artery. *Middle left,* There is abrupt termination of flow in the proximal superficial femoral artery. *Middle right,* Again, abrupt termination of flow seen in the proximal right superficial femoral artery with flow still in the profunda femoris artery. *Bottom left,* Blunted flow pattern proximal to the occlusion. *Bottom right,* No detectable flow by spectral display. **B,** Electrocardiogram revealing atrial fibrillation, the source of the occlusive embolus to the superficial femoral artery and popliteal arteries.

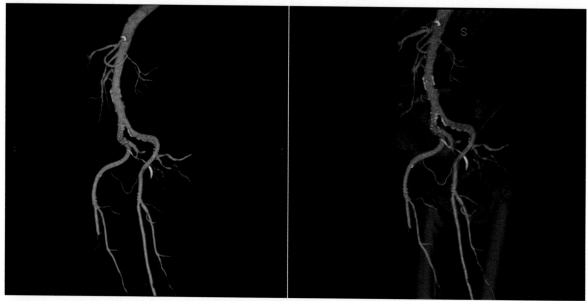

Figure 5-12. Three-dimensional reconstructions of a computed tomography aortogram. Abrupt occlusion of a right superficial femoral artery is seen due to embolization.

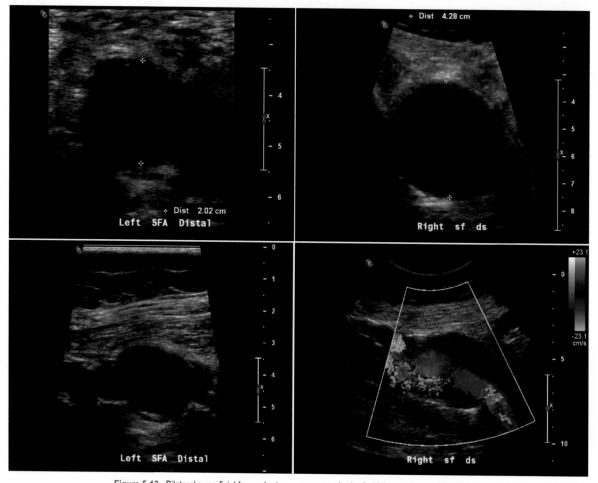

Figure 5-13. Bilateral superficial femoral artery aneurysms, both of which contain mural thrombus.

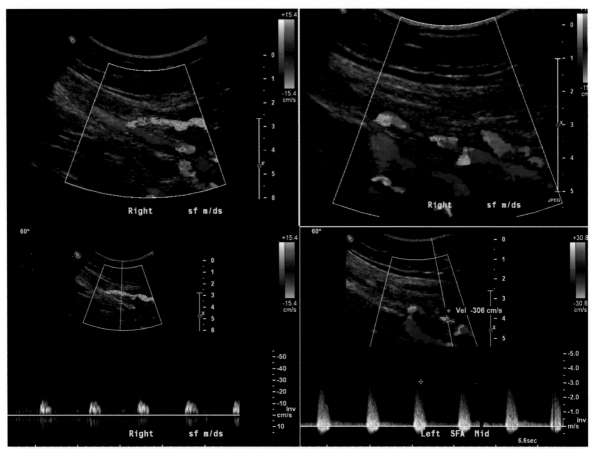

Figure 5-14. Long-standing stenosis of the superficial femoral artery (SFA) with large collaterals. *Top left,* A large collateral vessel arising from the SFA. *Top right,* Narrowing of the SFA after the collateral branch takeoff, turbulence at the site of narrowing, and other deeper collaterals. *Bottom left and right,* Spectral display of pulsed Doppler sampling before, and at the site of turbulence, with a significant velocity ratio consistent with stenosis.

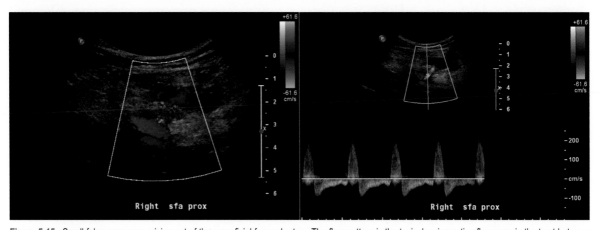

Figure 5-15. Small false aneurysm arising out of the superficial femoral artery. The flow pattern is the typical reciprocating flow seen in the tract between artery and pseudoaneurysm.

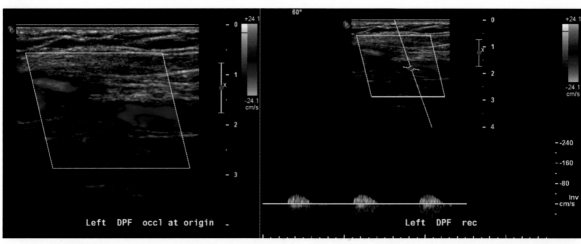

Figure 5-16. Occlusion of the profunda femoris artery. *Left,* The color Doppler flow mapping does not record flow at one level. *Right,* Immediately distal to the spectral flow recording is reconstitution via reentry vessels—hence the reversed flow component, which is also apparent on the color Doppler flow mapping.

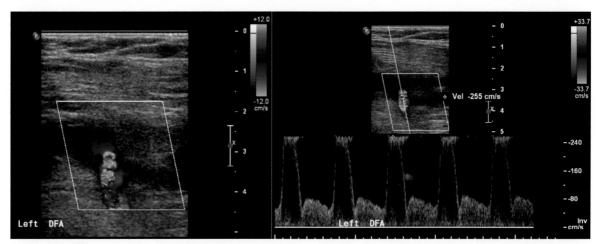

Figure 5-17. Significant stenosis at the ostium of the first branch profunda femoris artery. *Left,* Color Doppler flow mapping reveals turbulence at the ostium. The responsible plaque is not easily seen on the grayscale imaging. *Right,* The spectral display demonstrates significant increase in velocity consistent with greater than 50% stenosis.

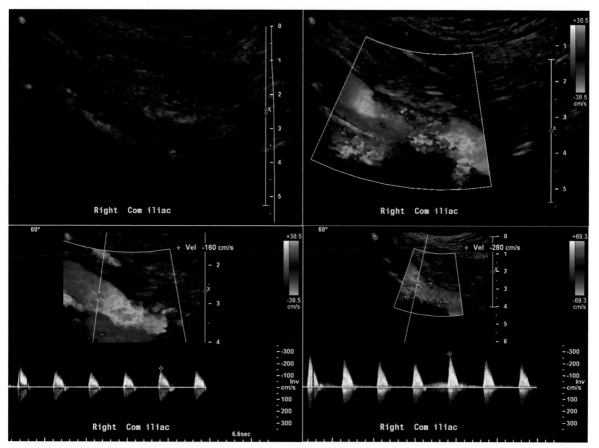

Figure 5-18. Less than 50% stenosis of the common iliac artery. *Top left,* Grayscale imaging reveals plaque that appears to be less than 50%. *Top right,* Color Doppler flow mapping depicts turbulence and acceleration of the site of the plaque. *Bottom left and right,* Spectral flow display before (*left*) and at the site of stenosis (*right*) reveals a less than 100% increase in velocity. Notably, there is variation for the peak systolic velocity in the samplings before and at the site of the stenosis, conferring some uncertainty as to the stenosis severity determination on the basis of the velocity ratio.

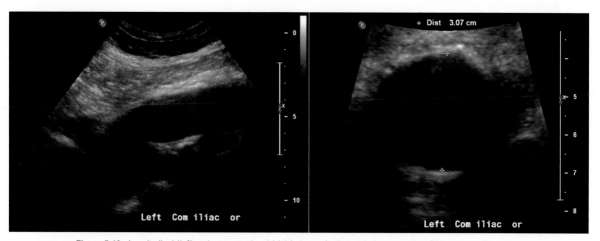

Figure 5-19. Longitudinal (*left*) and cross-sectional (*right*) views of a 3-cm tubular aneurysm of the common iliac artery.

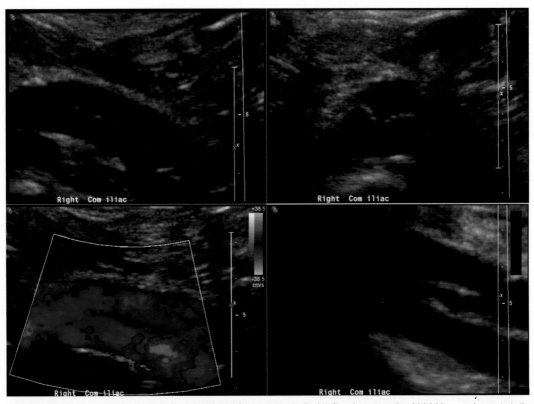

Figure 5-20. Dissection of the common iliac artery. *Top left and right,* Grayscale longitudinal (*left*) and cross-sectional (*right*) images demonstrate the intimal flap and resultant true and false lumen within the iliac artery. *Bottom left,* Color Doppler flow mapping reveals partitioning flow by the intimal flap and flow both in true and false lumens. *Bottom right,* There is notable complexity of the intimal flap at one portion along the artery.

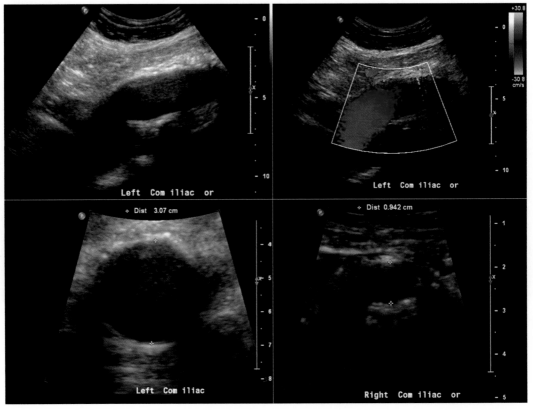

Figure 5-21. Bilateral aneurysms of the common iliac arteries.

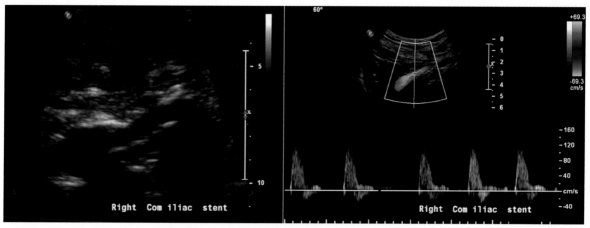

Figure 5-22. Views of the common iliac artery following stenting. In this case the stent is not visible, although the large volume of atherosclerotic plaque that has been responsible for the stenosis is apparent. Poststenting flow pattern and flow velocities are normal.

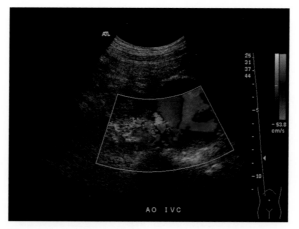

Figure 5-23. Iliac artery to vein fistula. An aneurysm of the iliac artery has ruptured into the adjacent vein.

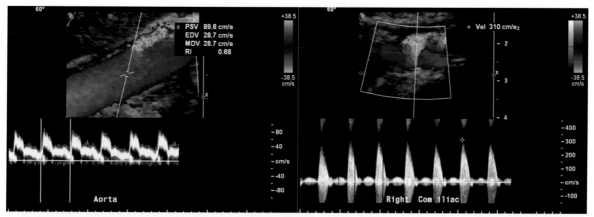

Figure 5-24. Ostial stenosis of the right common iliac artery. *Left,* Flow recorded in the distal abdominal aorta is of normal velocity and contour. *Right,* At he ostium of the right common iliac artery, color Doppler flow mapping depicts turbulence, and spectral display depicts velocities that are both elevated in the absolute sense and also elevated when compared with the upstream velocity within a distal aorta.

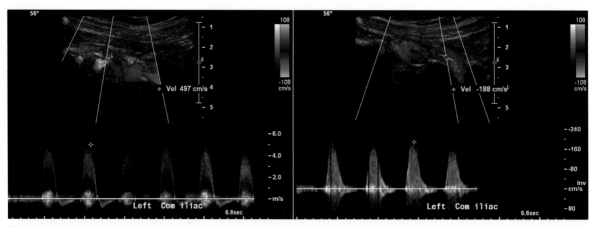

Figure 5-25. Greater than 50% stenosis of the common iliac artery. *Left,* Color flow mapping revealing acceleration and turbulence within the common iliac artery and spectral flow display revealing severely elevated systolic velocities. This is as well "color bruit" and "spectral bruit." *Right,* The velocity is almost normalized several centimeters downstream, but turbulence persists.

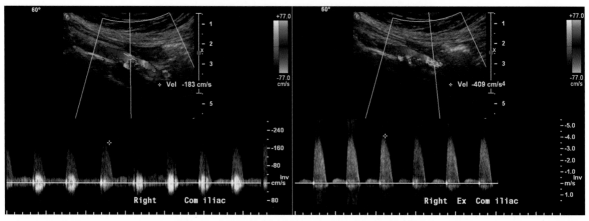

Figure 5-26. Fifty percent stenosis of the common iliac artery. Color Doppler flow mapping is consistent with acceleration and turbulence, and spectral display reveals significant increase (>100%) from before the site of stenosis (*left*) to the site of stenosis (*right*).

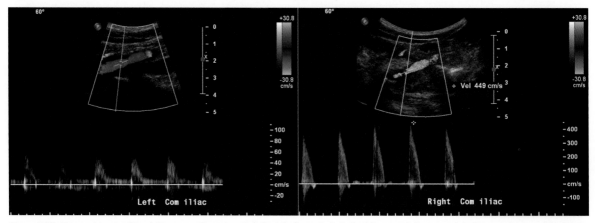

Figure 5-27. Severe stenosis of the right common iliac artery. *Left,* Systolic flow velocity in the left common iliac artery is in the normal range, although the early diastolic flow reversal component is absent. *Right,* Color flow aliasing is accompanied by severely elevated systolic flow velocity, although waveform morphology still suggests biphasicity.

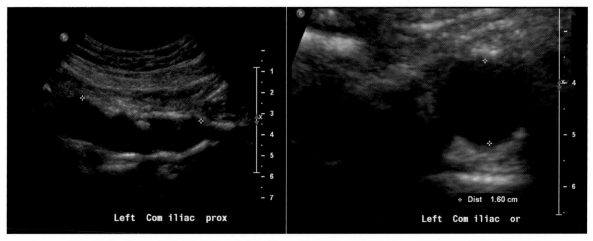

Figure 5-28. Atherosclerotic ectasia (irregularity and tortuosity, and also dilation in this case) of the common iliac artery.

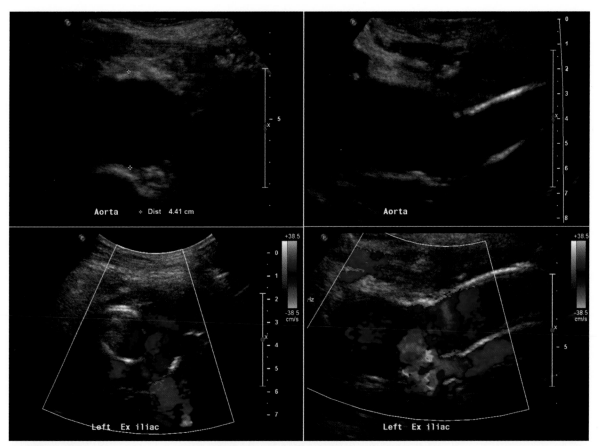

Figure 5-29. Type I endoleak following attempted endovascular repair of an iliac aneurysm. *Top left,* The infrarenal aorta is aneurysmal at 4.4 cm. *Top right,* The stent within the left common iliac is seen in long axis. *Bottom left,* Flow outside the stent is seen within the sack of the iliac aneurysm. *Bottom right,* Flow originating at the proximal end of the stent is responsible for the leak.

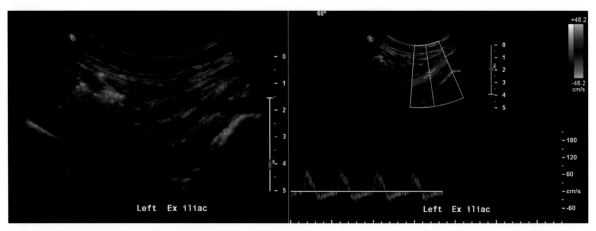

Figure 5-30. Less than 30% stenosis of the external iliac artery. *Left,* Some plaque is seen on grayscale imaging. *Right,* Spectral recording of flow does not reveal elevation of the velocities or turbulence, consistent with less than 50% stenosis.

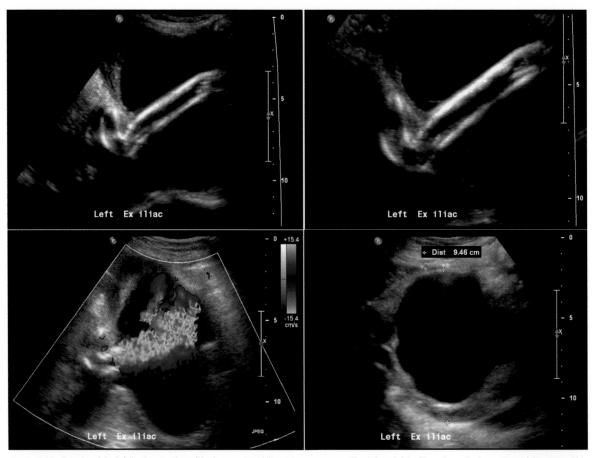

Figure 5-31. Type I endoleak following stenting of the large external iliac artery aneurysm. *Top left and right,* There is marked curvature of the stent within the body of the aneurysm. The body of the aneurysm has very little thrombus within it. *Bottom left,* Color Doppler flow mapping at the site of apposition of two of the stents reveals a large jet into the body of the aneurysm. *Bottom right,* The body of the iliac aneurysm measures 9.5 cm and has not thrombosed because of the large endoleak. There is only the same rind thrombus that has been present before the stenting.

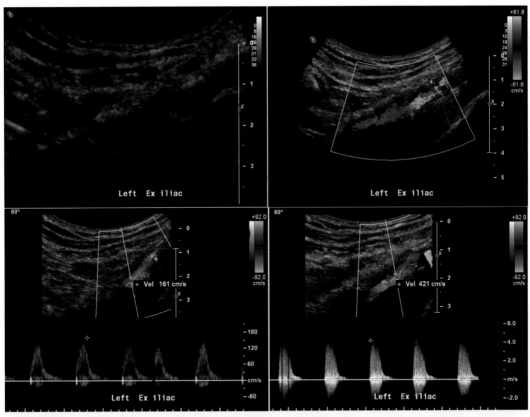

Figure 5-32. High-grade stenosis of the external iliac artery. *Top left,* Intraluminal echoes within the external iliac artery on grayscale imaging are suggestive of stenosis. *Top right,* Color Doppler flow mapping reveals a turbulent jet. *Bottom left and right,* Greater than 50% stenosis is confirmed by a marked (>100%) increase in velocity across the stenosis.

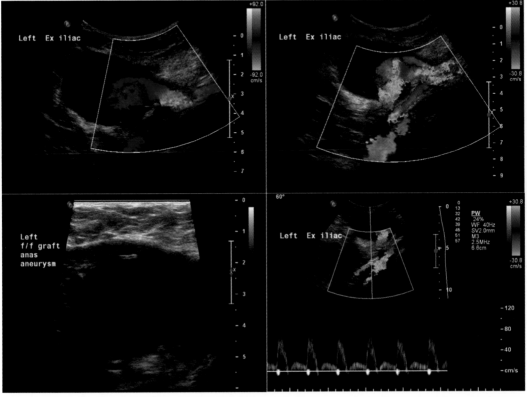

Figure 5-33. *Top left,* Long-axis view of a partially thrombosed pseudoaneurysm that has formed at the anastomosis of an occluded left-to-right femoro-femoral cross-over graft and left common femoral artery. *Top right,* Short-axis view reveals the pseudoaneurysm at 3 o'clock. *Bottom left,* Another view of the pseudoaneurysm. *Bottom right,* Patent external iliac artery proximal to the pseudoaneurysm.

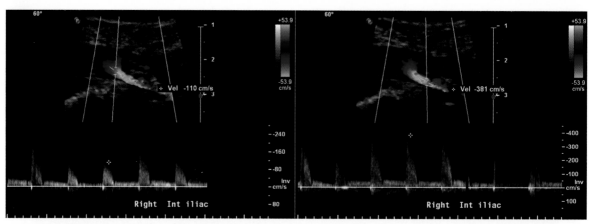

Figure 5-34. *Left,* Severe stenosis of the internal iliac artery. *Right,* Peak systolic velocity is high and color flow depicts poststenotic turbulence. Flow velocity just proximal to the stenosis is within the normal range, and the ratio of the two is well over the 100% increase required to place the stenosis in the greater than 50% category.

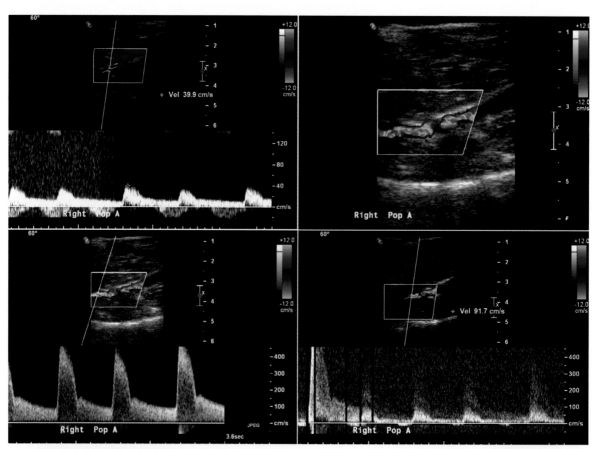

Figure 5-35. Greater than 50% stenosis at the popliteal artery. Grayscale and color Doppler flow mapping reveal plaque within the popliteal artery and more prominently, reveal turbulence. Flow measured before the turbulence (*top left*) and at the level of the turbulence (*bottom left*) demonstrate a significant increase in velocity. There is flow at the site of turbulence and what appears to be a small variation in the sampling position, which results in loss of the optimal sampling (*bottom right*).

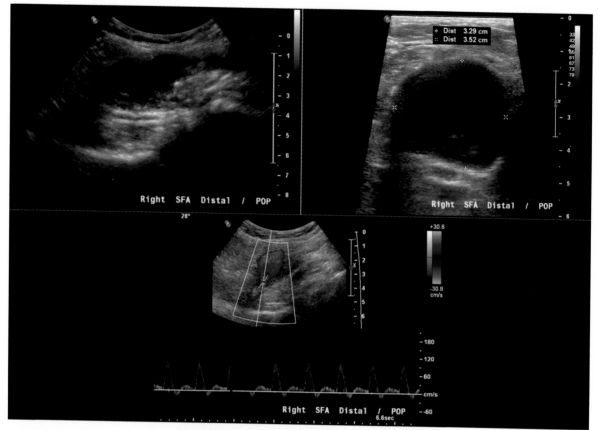

Figure 5-36. A 3.5-cm popliteal aneurysm with mural thrombus.

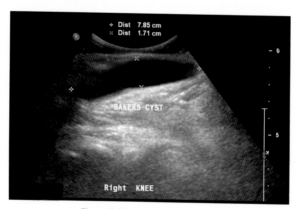

Figure 5-37. A popliteal Baker cyst.

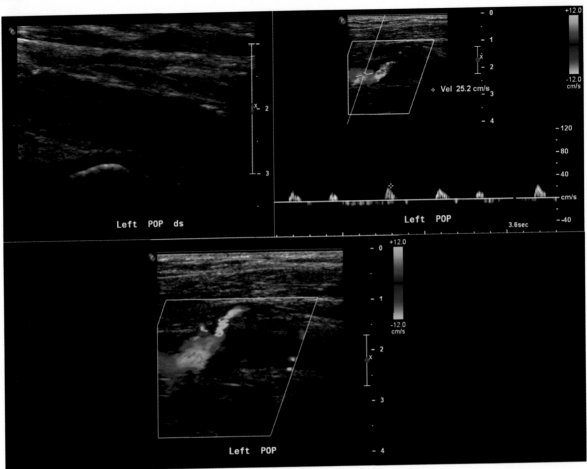

Figure 5-38. Popliteal occlusion from emboli. *Top left,* Grayscale imaging shows the typical appearance of a large bulk of thrombotic material within the artery. *Top right,* There is greatly blunted flow immediately proximal to a total cutoff of flow consistent with occlusion. *Bottom,* There is flow out of the popliteal artery into a branch artery immediately before the level of popliteal occlusion.

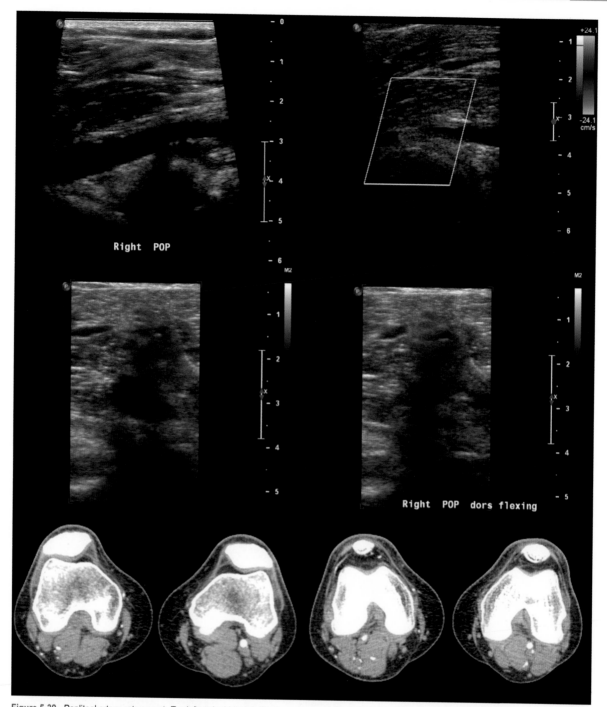

Figure 5-39. Popliteal artery entrapment. *Top left and middle left,* The knee is at rest. *Top left and middle right,* The knee is dorsiflexed. The popliteal artery becomes completely occluded when dorsiflexed (*upper and middle right*) when compared with the images of the artery on the left while the knee is at rest (*upper and middle left*). *Bottom left and right,* computed tomography scanning performed several months later shows the popliteal artery to be completely occluded. It was thought that a "slip" of soft tissue that is seen might represent fibromuscular insertion. During surgery, it was discovered that a very tight fascial band associated with a congenitally anomalous single gastrocnemius head was responsible for the entrapment.

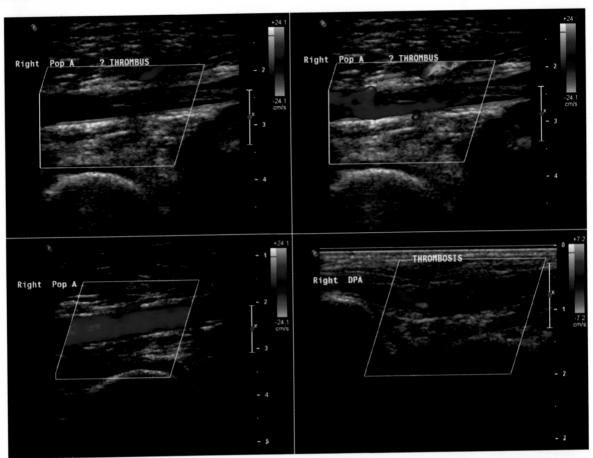

Figure 5-40. Acute thrombosis of the popliteal artery. *Top left,* Long-axis view. *Top right,* The thrombus is nonocclusive. *Bottom left,* Image taken after treatment a day later shows complete resolution of the popliteal thrombus. *Bottom right,* The occlusive thrombus remains in the dorsalis pedis artery.

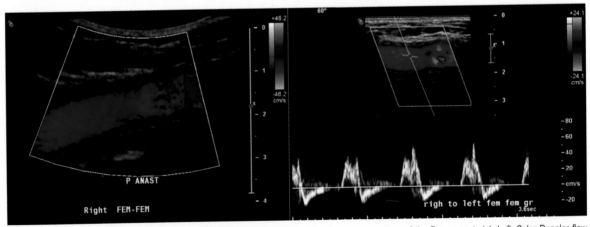

Figure 5-41. The right-to-left femoro-femoral bypass graft. Grayscale images reveal the woven pattern of the Dacron material. *Left,* Color Doppler flow mapping is unremarkable. The variable color of the flow mapping is an alignment phenomenon, not flow acceleration. *Right,* Spectral flow pattern is normal.

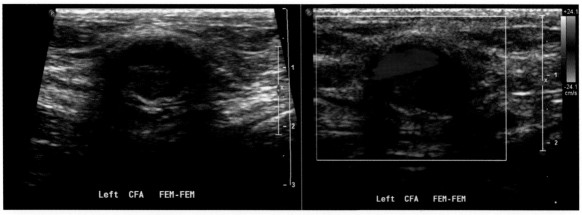

Figure 5-42. A femoro-femoral bypass graft seen in cross-section. There is a significant amount of soft tissue partially filling the lumen, and this is seen both on grayscale imaging (*left*) and color Doppler flow mapping (*right*).

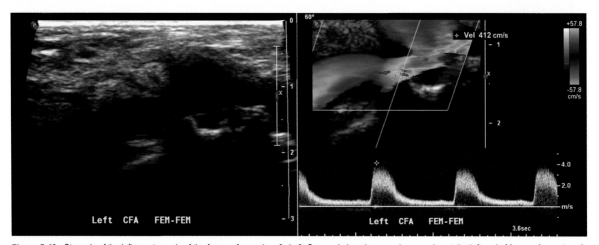

Figure 5-43. Stenosis of the left anastomosis of the femoro-femoral graft. *Left,* Grayscale imaging reveals narrowing at the left end of femoro-femoral graft. The slight bulge on the right corresponds to the graft seen in short-axis imaging. *Right,* Color Doppler flow mapping reveals flow acceleration and turbulence, and spectral display reveals severely elevated velocities and turbulence.

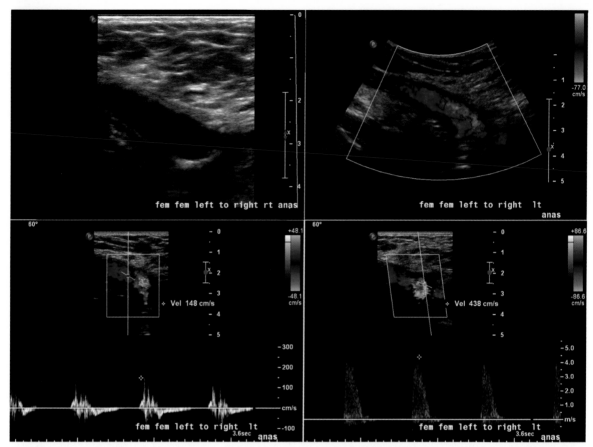

Figure 5-44. Distal anastomotic stenosis of the femoro-femoral graft. The right graft in long-axis anastomosis and its insertion into the common femoral artery (*top left*). Grayscale imaging of the graft is normal. Color Doppler flow mapping at the right anastomosis suggests stenosis and demonstrates turbulence (*top right*). There is significant flow acceleration from before (*bottom left*) to the site of greatest turbulence (*bottom right*).

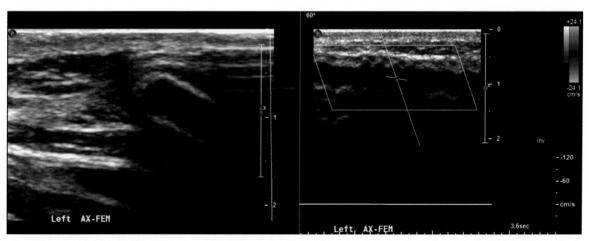

Figure 5-45. An occluded axillary-femoral bypass graft. *Left,* The woven texture of the graft walls is evident as is the intraluminal soft tissue on grayscale imaging and deformity of the graft material from its usual spherical shape. *Right,* Color Doppler flow mapping and pulsed Doppler sampling do not detect any flow.

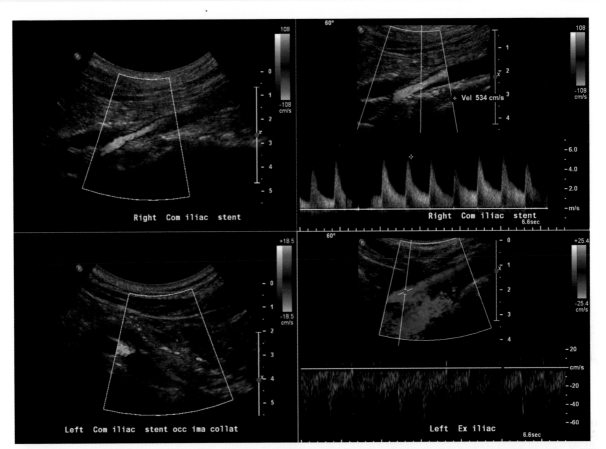

Figure 5-46. Previous bilateral common iliac stenting. *Top left and right,* Right common iliac stent with good grayscale and color Doppler depiction of narrowing (note the turbulence despite high pulse repetition frequency selection). Spectral display of pulsed-wave interrogation confirms stenosis with elevated systolic and diastolic velocities. *Bottom left and right,* Left common iliac stenting. Grayscale and color Doppler flow mapping reveal soft tissue throughout the stent and no flow within it. A collateral vessel is seen nearby.

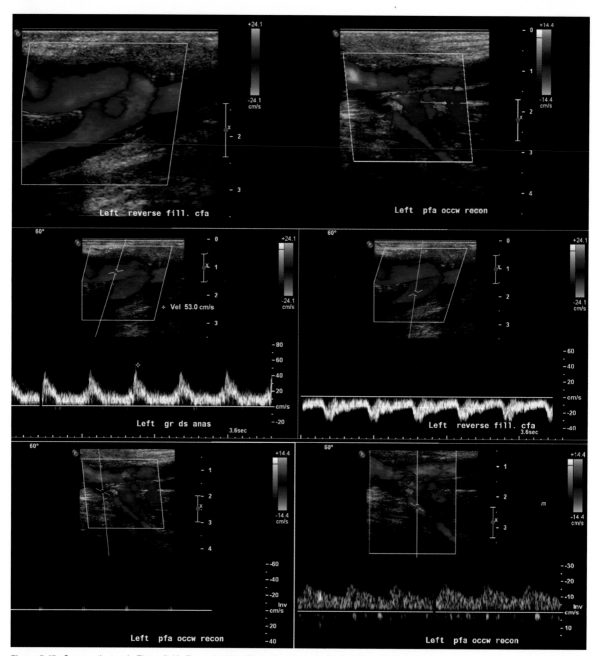

Figure 5-47. Same patient as in Figure 5-46. *Top and middle,* These four views depict the inflow of blood via a femoro-femoral graft into the left common femoral artery. The flow is without turbulence or other sign of stenosis. The runoff into the common femoral artery runs in opposite directions as the common iliac artery is occluded on this side. *Bottom left and right,* There is a complete occlusion of the ostium of the profunda femoris, with prompt reconstitution via collaterals, and ongoing pulsatile flow due to the adequacy of the collateral size.

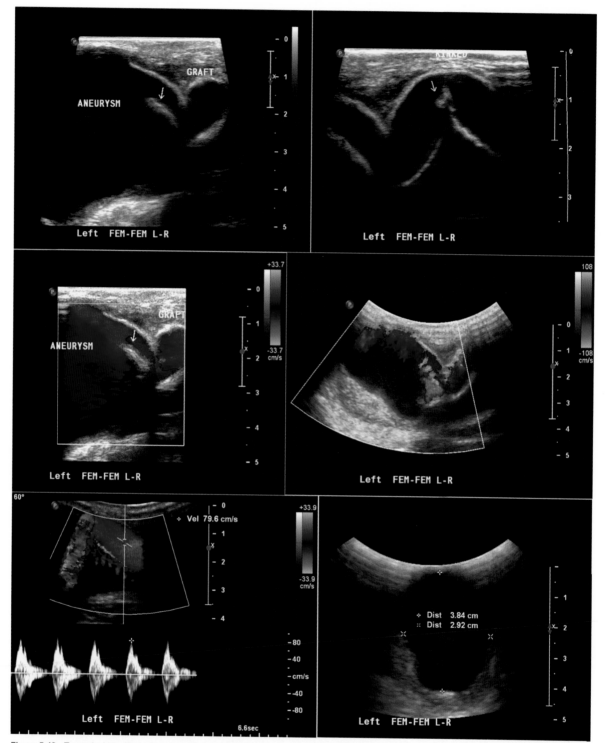

Figure 5-48. *Top and middle,* These four views depict a kinked femoro-femoral bypass graft. This patient, who had had this graft for several years, one day bent down to lift a heavy object and immediately experienced a large painful groin lump. Flow can be clearly seen to be entering a large pseudoaneurysm, which was the result of the graft tearing away from the anastomosis. *Bottom left and right,* The graft remains patent.

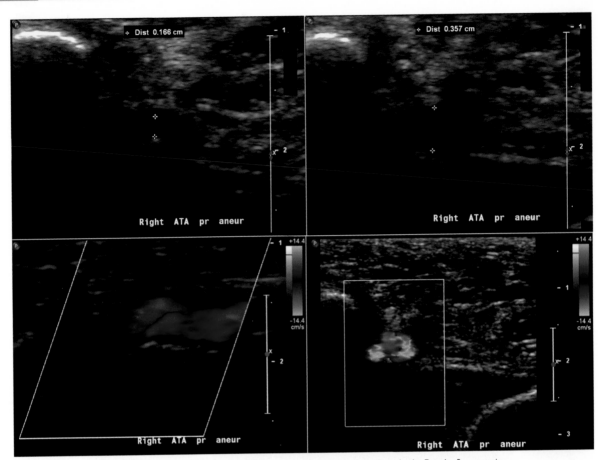

Figure 5-49. An aneurysm of the anterior tibial artery depicted on grayscale and color Doppler flow mapping.

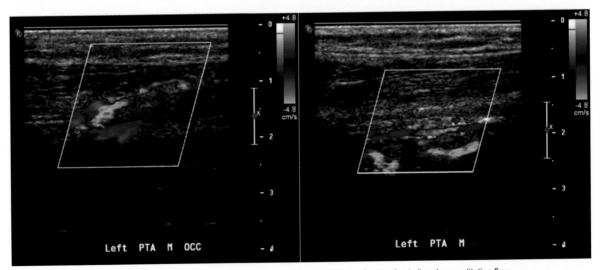

Figure 5-50. Occlusion of the posterior tibial artery, with collateral vessels returning to it and reconstituting flow.

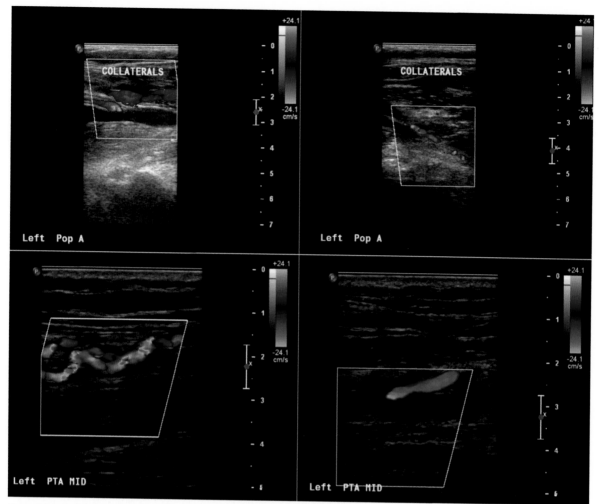

Figure 5-51. Occluded popliteal artery. *Top left,* Echo-filled lumen of an occluded popliteal artery is surrounded by large branching collaterals. *Top right,* There is a sliver of flow more distally and deep to the distal popliteal vein, representing another collateral branch, which is not to be confused with the still-occluded popliteal artery lying deep to that and suboptimally visualized. *Bottom left,* Ongoing collaterals. *Bottom right,* A collateral vessel returning to the tibial artery.

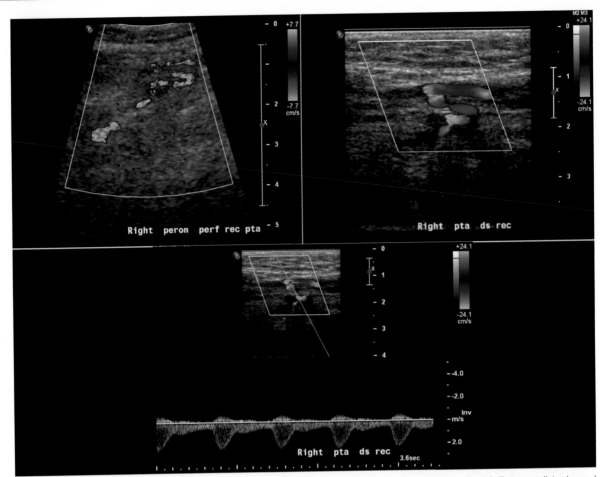

Figure 5-52. Occluded posterior tibial artery with reconstitution via perforating collaterals from the peroneal artery. *Top left,* Tortuous collateral vessel from the peroneal artery. *Top right,* Reconstitution of the occluded posterior tibial artery with flow reentering it via the collateral vessel. Note the lack of any flow and the material within the posterior tibial artery to the left side of the reconstitution. *Bottom,* Retrograde flow in the posterior tibial artery at the site of reconstitution.

6 Catheterization-Related Complications

Key Points

- Familiarity with the range of vascular complications that may be detected by ultrasound, and their respective findings, is critical.
- Patients may have more than one complication.

Catheterization-related complications detectable by ultrasound include hematomas (Figs. 6-1 to 6-3), false aneurysms (Figs. 6-4 to 6-10), arteriovenous fistulas (Figs. 6-11 to 6-17), bleeding tracts, thrombosis (Figs. 6-18 to 6-20), dissection, and malpositioned devices (Figs. 6-21 to 6-23). The incidence is variable and depends on the access site attempted/used, the urgency of the procedure, operator experience, degree of patient obesity, size of the catheters, and number of prior catheterizations at that site. Complications that are generally inapparent on duplex examination include embolization of small debris, such as atheroembolism.

Many catheter-related complications are due in part to puncture away from the intended site. The skin puncture site is a relatively poor marker of where a needle or catheter may have travelled internally because the obliquity and depth of introduction are unknown. Therefore, extensive scanning is needed to recognize the highest percentage of catheter-related complications. Some patients have more than one complication.

HEMATOMAS

Hematomas are the most common complication and may be either superficial or deep to the vessel. Leakage from puncture of the anterior aspect of the vessel typically generates a more superficial hematoma, and leakage from a posterior (e.g., transfixion) puncture generates a deep hematoma. Femoral puncture sites are the most common site of catheterization-related hematoma. Duplex examination of a patient with a large bulky hematoma confers discomfort to the patient (because the hematoma's tension renders it tender) and difficulty to the sonographer because of the increased depth to scan, patient discomfort, degradation of image quality of deeper structures, and distortion of underlying anatomy. A hematoma may be pulsatile if the pulsation of underlying artery is transmitted through it. If the hematoma distorts or compresses a nearby artery, turbulence in the artery may generate a bruit, commonly prompting consideration of the presence of a false aneurysm.

As with most duplex examinations at the level of the groin, the leg should be slightly externally rotated to optimize scanning. Duplex findings include:

- Lucent collection
- No evidence of flow by color flow mapping or spectral display within the hematoma

BLEEDING TRACT

Active bleeding, internally or externally, may occasionally be visualized at the time of scanning by color Doppler flow imaging. Duplex findings include flow within a needle or catheter tract depicted by color flow mapping or spectral display.

ARTERIOVENOUS FISTULAS

Arteriovenous fistulas may occur usually as the result of a needle or catheter tract into an artery that intersects a needle or catheter tract into a vein or a branch of a vein. Hence, most arteriovenous fistulas have length. Occasionally, an adjacent artery and vein have their adjacent walls lacerated or punctured, and flow is directed from the artery into the vein. Overlying arteries and veins are particularly likely to be rendered into a fistula by a single direct and deep puncture.

The flow pattern of an arteriovenous fistula is continuous/incessant and high velocity, differing from the reciprocating pattern of flow in a false aneurysm neck.

Auscultation typically reveals the continuous/incessant bruit, as long as the fistula is not too deep. Commonly, the arteriovenous fistula is tender. Many arteriovenous fistulas will close spontaneously, although some will not and may be closed by surgical repair. The volume of flow through catheter-related arteriovenous fistulas is usually not a significant hemodynamic burden, but on occasion it may be.

As with most duplex examination at the level of the groin, the leg should be slightly externally rotated to optimize scanning.

Duplex Scanning
Views, with grayscale and color Doppler flow mapping:
❑ Transverse
  • Common femoral artery/vein
  • Superficial femoral artery/vein
  • Profunda femoris artery/vein
❑ Longitudinal
  • External iliac artery/vein
  • Common femoral artery/vein
  • Superficial femoral artery/vein
  • Profunda femoris artery/vein
❑ Spectral recording of flow within the fistula

Duplex Findings
❑ Flow tract (fistulas)
❑ Continuous/incessant flow pattern, typically with high velocity of both the peak and diastolic components

PSEUDOANEURYSMS

Postcatheterization pseudoaneurysms (false aneurysms) are localized hematomas within tissue that are connected to the artery of origin by a tract. The pressurization of the tissue typically renders the false aneurysm tender. The reciprocating pulsatile flow into a false aneurysm, or an overlying an artery, may make it pulsate. A false aneurysm may be any size.

The flow pattern of a false aneurysm is reciprocating—into the body in systole and out of it in diastole ("to and fro"). The flow is typically high velocity. The most typical flow patterns are sampled from the tract, not the body.

As with most Duplex examinations at the level of the groin, the leg should be slightly externally rotated to optimize scanning.

Duplex Scanning
Views, with grayscale and color Doppler flow mapping:
❑ Transverse
  • Common femoral artery/vein
  • Superficial femoral artery/vein
  • Profunda femoris artery/vein
❑ Longitudinal
  • External iliac artery/vein
  • Common femoral artery/vein
  • Superficial femoral artery/vein
  • Profunda femoris artery/vein
❑ Spectral recording of flow within the tract and body of the false aneurysm
  • Measure the length of the tract.
  • Measure the size of the false aneurysm body.
  • Note the presence of thrombus within the false aneurysm.

Duplex Findings
❑ Mass extrinsic to an artery; may be pulsatile
❑ High velocity reciprocating ("to and fro") flow within the tract
❑ Turbulent flow within the mass, apparent by color Doppler flow mapping and spectral recording

CATHETER-RELATED DISSECTION

Catheters, wires, and introducer needles may result in dissection of either arteries or veins.

CATHETER-RELATED THROMBUS

Catheter-related thrombus is common in both veins and arteries. The thrombus may be attached to the catheter or arise from trauma to the vessel wall. Thrombosis of the vessel may also occur, particularly with large catheters, more trauma, and low-flow circulation.

PRACTICE GUIDELINES

The 2005 American College of Cardiology/American Heart Association (ACC/AHA) Practice Guidelines on Peripheral Artery Disease include indications for duplex ultrasonography for catheter-related femoral artery pseudoaneurysms.[1]

Catheter-Related Femoral Artery Pseudoaneurysms
Class I
1. Patients with suspected femoral pseudoaneurysms should be evaluated by duplex ultrasonography. *(Level of Evidence: B)*
2. Initial treatment with ultrasound-guided compression or thrombin injection is recommended in patients with large and/or symptomatic femoral artery pseudoaneurysms. *(Level of Evidence: B)*

Class IIa
1. Surgical repair is reasonable in patients with femoral artery pseudoaneurysms 2.0 cm in diameter or larger that persist or recur after ultrasound-guided compression or thrombin injection. *(Level of Evidence: B)*
2. Reevaluation by ultrasound 1 month after the original injury can be useful in patients with asymptomatic femoral artery pseudoaneurysms smaller than 2.0 cm in diameter. *(Level of Evidence: B)*

REFERENCES

1. Hirsch AT, Haskal ZJ, Hertzer NR, et al. ACC/AHA 2005 practice guidelines for the management of patients with peripheral arterial disease (lower extremity, renal, mesenteric, and abdominal aortic): executive summary. *J Am Coll Cardiol.* 2006;47:1239-1312.

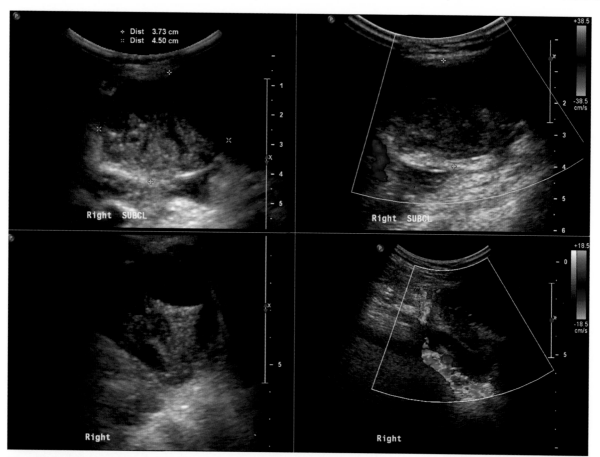

Figure 6-1. Hematoma at the site of subclavian catheter insertion. No flow can be demonstrated in the soft tissue collection, which has a marbled appearance. The subclavian vein, revealed by color Doppler flow mapping in the bottom right image, is displaced by the hematoma. The subclavian artery had been inadvertently punctured.

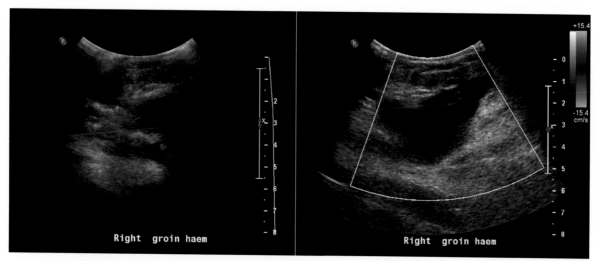

Figure 6-2. A large postcatheterization hematoma. Color Doppler flow mapping failed to detect flow within the mass.

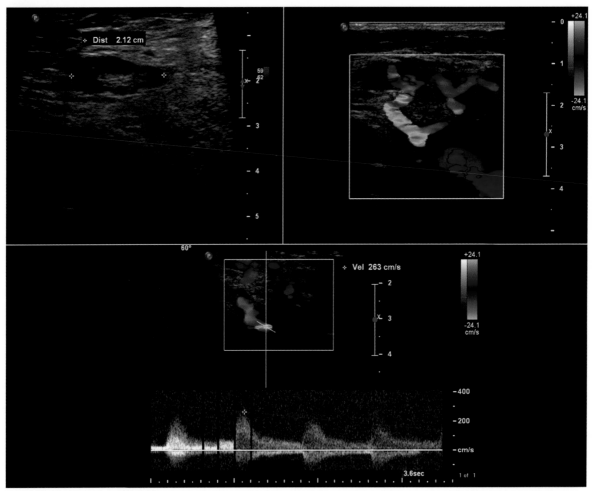

Figure 6-3. A small hematoma in the groin (*top left*). Color Doppler depicts tributaries extending superficially from the nearby femoral artery (*top right*), which might suggest tracks into a pseudoaneurysm, until the spectral Doppler sampling (*bottom*) fails to display the reciprocating flow pattern that would typically be seen within a pseudoaneurysm tract.

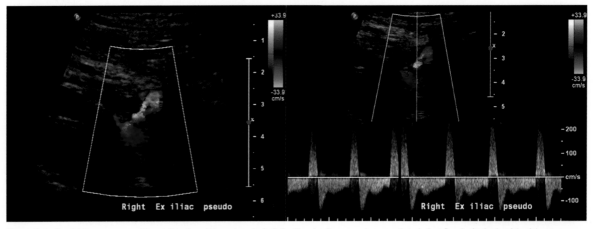

Figure 6-4. Small false aneurysm at the right external iliac artery. *Left,* Color Doppler flow mapping reveals turbulent flow in the body of the false aneurysm adjacent to the artery. *Right,* Spectral flow display reveals the reciprocating "to-and-fro" flow pattern characteristic of a false aneurysm.

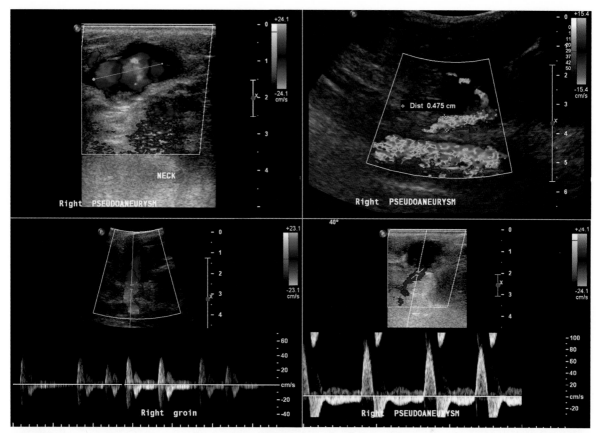

Figure 6-5. Common femoral artery false aneurysm post–coronary angiography. *Top left,* There is flow within a partially thrombosed lumen of the false aneurysm. *Top left,* The image depicts the serpiginous tract or neck of the false aneurysm. *Bottom left and right,* Spectral flow pattern is seen at different points along the tract joining the artery to the false aneurysm. Reciprocating flow is demonstrated.

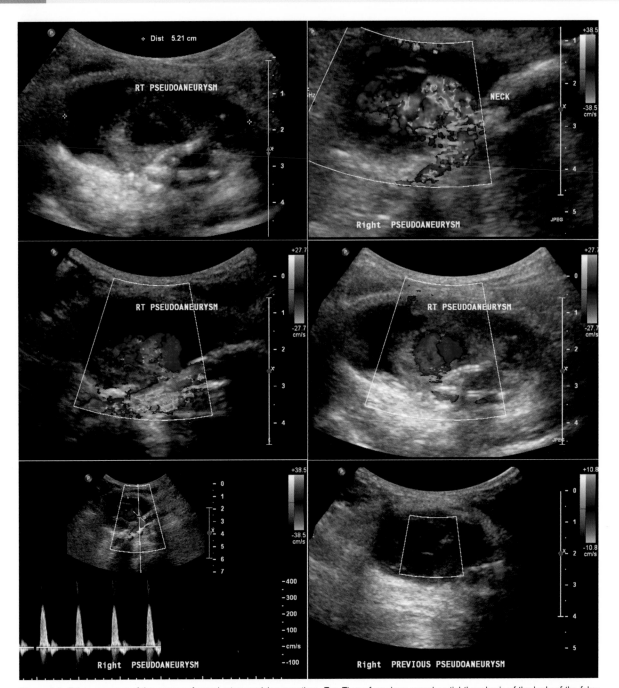

Figure 6-6. False aneurysm of the common femoral artery evolving over time. *Top,* These four views reveal partial thrombosis of the body of the false aneurysm. The flow pattern in the remaining body of the false aneurysm is typically turbulent. *Bottom left,* "To-and-fro" flow is depicted on the spectral display. *Bottom right,* The image taken 2 weeks later shows complete thrombosis of the body of the false lumen with no detectable flow, even with the reduced pulse repetition frequency selection.

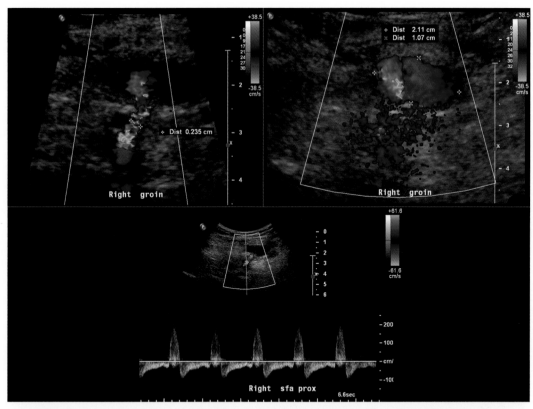

Figure 6-7. Small false aneurysm arising from the common femoral artery. The flow pattern is the typical reciprocating flow.

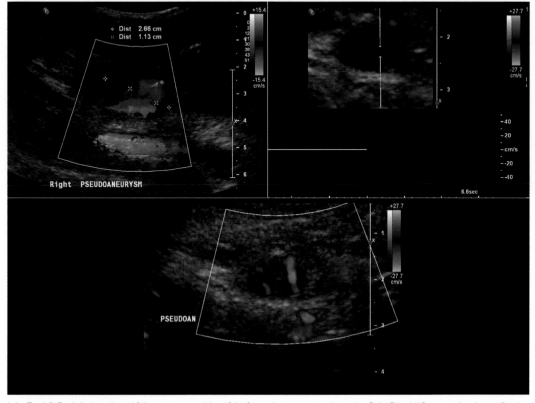

Figure 6-8. *Top left,* Partially thrombosed false aneurysm arising of the femoral artery postangiography. Color Doppler flow mapping detects flow in only half of the apparent body of the false aneurysm. *Top right,* The image taken 10 days later shows completion of thrombosis of the false lumen sac, without flow detected by color Doppler flow mapping or spectral Doppler. *Bottom,* Nearby branch vessels (as their course includes external to the sac) are detected by color Doppler flow mapping, falsely suggesting residual flow.

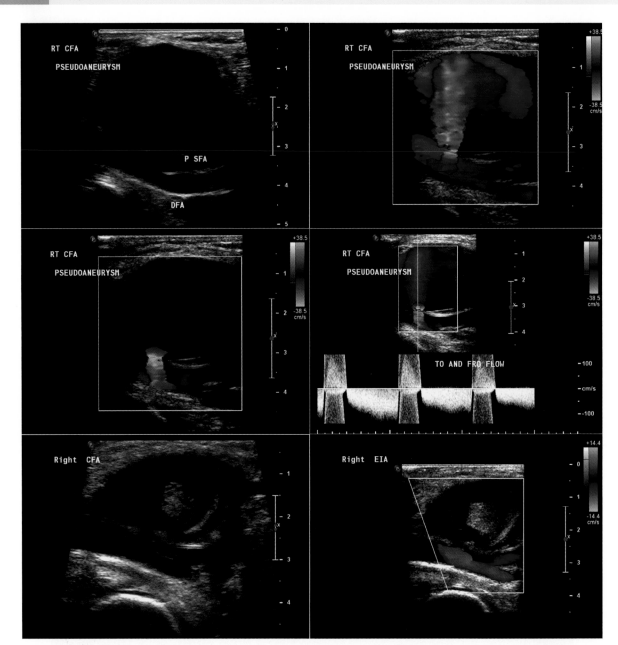

Figure 6-9. Postangiography false aneurysm of the common femoral artery. *Top four images,* The body and reciprocating flow into and out of it ("to and fro") are depicted. *Bottom left and right,* Following thrombin injection, the body has thrombosed, but a tail of thrombus that extended out of the body through the neck into the lumen of the femoral artery developed.

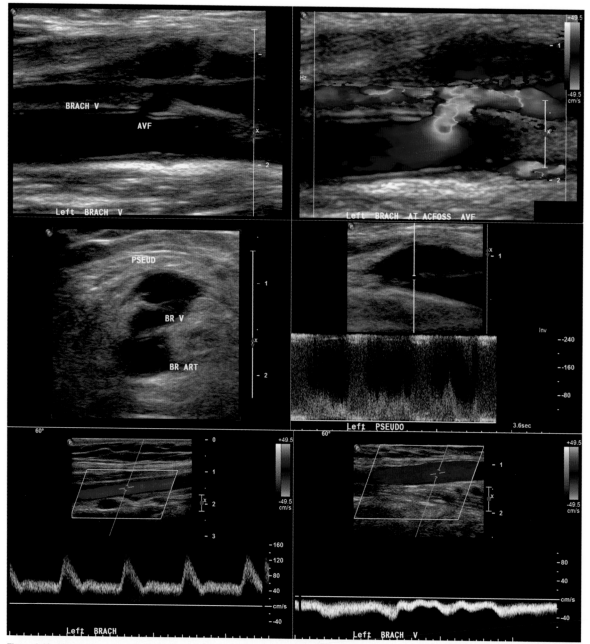

Figure 6-10. Brachial artery-to-vein arteriovenous fistula and false aneurysm arising from the vein following coronary angiography. The fact that the brachial vein overlies the brachial artery was likely responsible for this fistula as the needle tract transfixes the vein. *Top four images,* The tract of the fistula and the body of the false aneurysm are seen on grayscale imaging. Color Doppler flow mapping confirms the arteriovenous flow. Spectral depiction of the flow at the neck of the false aneurysm reveals an atypical pattern likely due to the fact that the false aneurysm arises from a venous structure that has been partially arterialized by the nearby arteriovenous fistula. The arteriovenous fistula and false aneurysm closed spontaneously over 2 months. *Bottom left and right,* Resolution of a brachial arteriovenous fistula and false aneurysm over 2 months, with normalization of the anatomy and of the flow patterns in the brachial artery and vein(s).

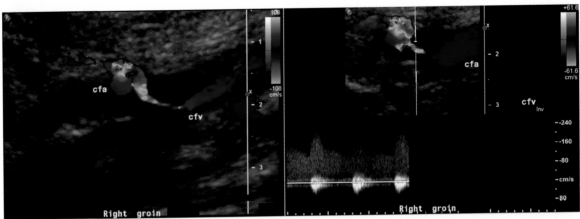

Figure 6-11. Right common femoral artery-to-vein arteriovenous fistula following coronary angiography. Color Doppler flow mapping reveals the tract and spectral flow display reveals the continuous and turbulent flow with increased velocity in the fistula.

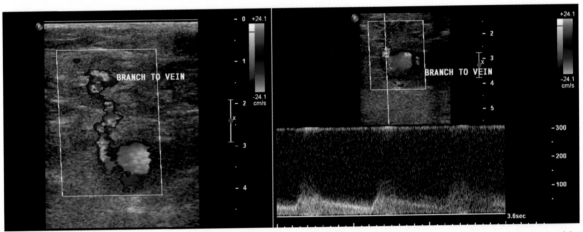

Figure 6-12. Common femoral artery-to-vein arteriovenous fistula following coronary angiography. Color Doppler flow mapping reveals the tract and the spectral flow display depicts the continuous-flow pattern typical of an arteriovenous fistula. The recorded velocities are less than usual, probably due to the fact that the sample volume is not cleanly within the tract but is more within the lumen of the femoral artery at the os of the tract.

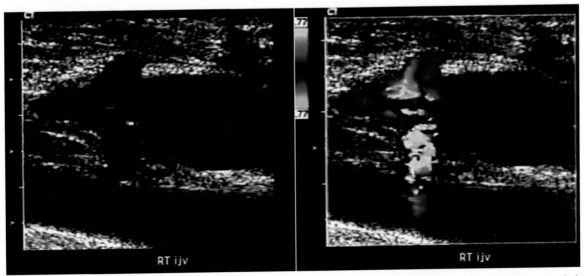

Figure 6-13. Common carotid artery-to-vein arteriovenous fistula following central venous catheter insertion. The wide body of the tract, apparent on both grayscale and color Doppler flow mapping, was due to the catheter having been inserted through the vein into the artery.

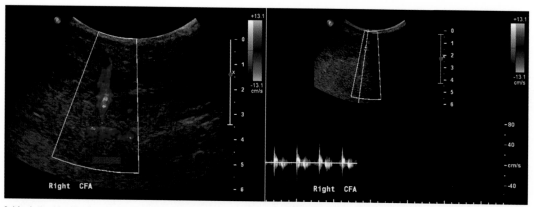

Figure 6-14. Active bleeding from the common femoral artery following coronary angiography. Flow is detected by color Doppler mapping and by postwave of sampling.

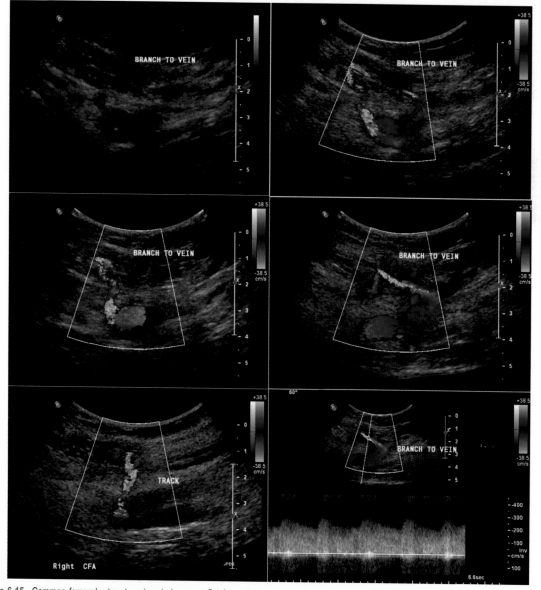

Figure 6-15. Common femoral artery-to-vein arteriovenous fistula post–coronary angiography. Two separate tracts, only apparent by color Doppler flow mapping, join the artery and vein. Spectral display reveals the typical continuous-flow and high-velocity flow of an arteriovenous fistula.

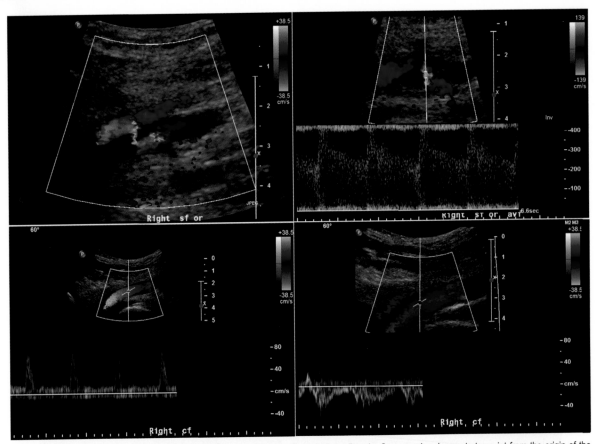

Figure 6-16. Arteriovenous fistula following catheterization via the groin. *Top left,* Color Doppler flow mapping demonstrates a jet from the origin of the superficial femoral artery, directly into the adjacent and deeper common femoral vein. *Top right,* Spectral display depicting the typical continuous flow pattern of the fistula. *Bottom left,* Spectral flow pattern in the common femoral artery reveals diastolic continuation due to runoff in the fistula. *Bottom right,* Spectral display of the flow velocity within the common femoral vein revealing systolic phasicity consistent with transmitted systolic flow from the fistula.

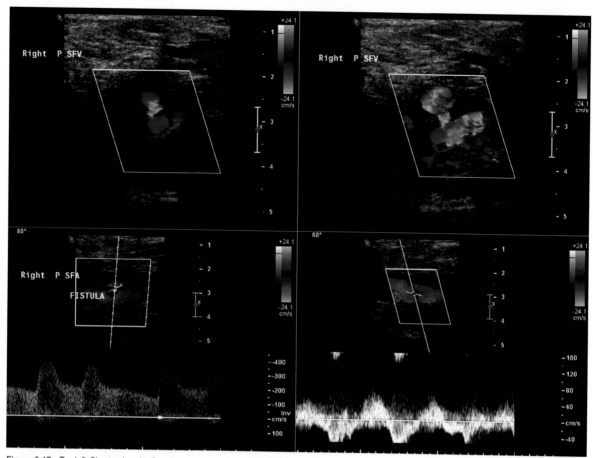

Figure 6-17. *Top left,* Short-axis color Doppler taken after catheterization demonstrates a tract running between the superficial femoral artery and vein consistent with an arteriovenous fistula. *Top right,* Another short-axis image depicts a color "bruit" deep to the vein, representing transmission of the high-velocity fistula flow into the tissues. *Bottom left,* Spectral Doppler shows the typical fistula flow pattern with low-resistance high peak and diastolic flow velocity. *Bottom right,* Long-axis color and spectral Doppler image of the more distal femoral artery showing both systolic forward and diastolic reverse flow (due to backward runoff into the fistula).

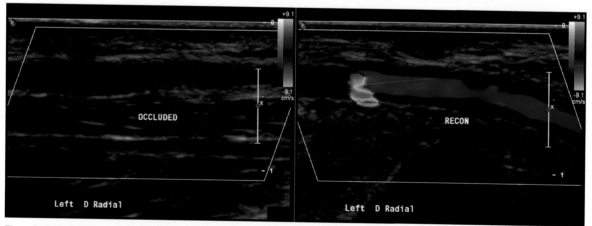

Figure 6-18. Radial artery occlusion following coronary angiography. *Left,* Grayscale findings suggest thrombosis. *Right,* Color Doppler flow mapping shows an absence of any flow over several centimeters, then reconstitution via a branch vessel.

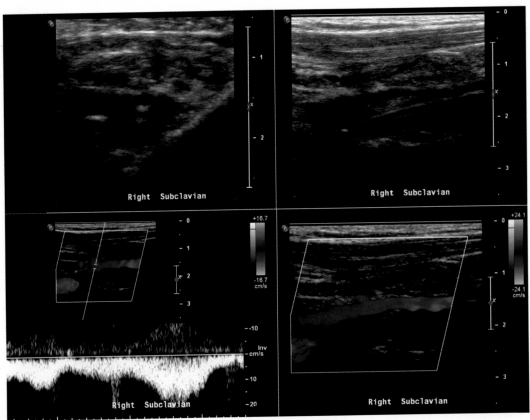

Figure 6-19. Left subclavian vein with a partially occlusive catheter-related thrombus. A peripherally inserted central catheter (PICC) had been present and inserted via the basilic vein. Clinically, the arm had developed edema, and the catheter was withdrawn. *Top left,* A cross-sectional view of the subclavian vein reveals a thrombus within the lumen and a cast of the catheter within the thrombus. *Top right,* A longitudinal view of the left subclavian artery depicting the large bulk of thrombus within the vein and a striking cast of the catheter. *Bottom left and right,* The images demonstrate flow within the remaining lumen.

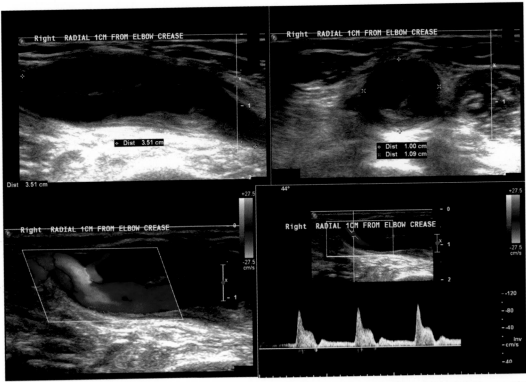

Figure 6-20. Proximal radial artery aneurysm following catheterization. *Top left,* A long-axis view shows heterogeneous intraluminal echoes consistent with thrombosis. *Top right,* A short-axis grayscale view shows the thrombus to be concentric within the aneurysm. *Bottom left,* A color long-axis view of the patent flow channel. *Bottom right,* Spectral Doppler flow signal shows a normal peripheral waveform shape.

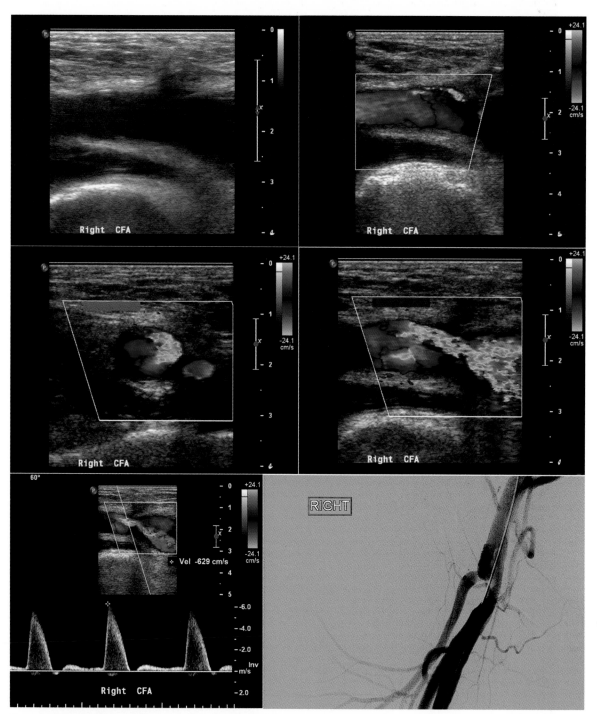

Figure 6-21. Views of the groin following coronary angiography using a percutaneous closure device. *Top left,* Grayscale long-axis view of the common femoral artery postcatheterization appears normal, without any obvious intraluminal echoes. *Top right,* Color Doppler shows color flow convergence anteriorly and reverse flow posteriorly, without obvious cause. *Middle left,* Color short-axis view again, showing color aliasing in the anterior part of the vessel. *Middle right,* Color Doppler taken at a different phase of the cardiac cycle, with turbulent flow extending further distally. *Bottom left,* Spectral Doppler taken at the site demonstrates high peak systolic flow consistent with significant narrowing, almost certainly caused by a malpositioned closure device. *Bottom right,* Femoral angiogram at the end of the angiogram, revealing the sideways displacement of the device into the lumen.

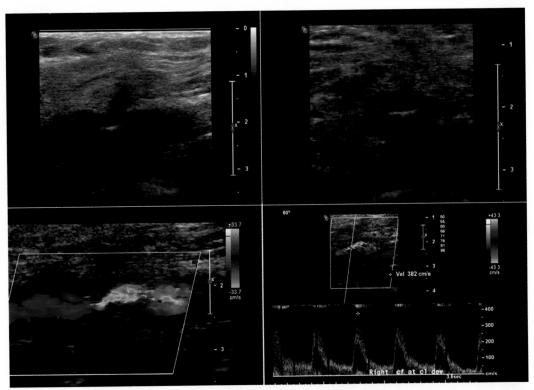

Figure 6-22. Long-axis grayscale imaging (*top left*) and short-axis grayscale imaging (*top right*) following catheterization of the common femoral artery, which demonstrates an intraluminal crescent-shaped echo, representing a closure device that has slipped out of position on the anterior wall to rest in mid-lumen. Color Doppler shows color flow convergence posterior to the device (*bottom left*); accompanying color aliasing suggests significant narrowing. Elevated peak systolic flow velocity demonstrated by spectral Doppler display (*bottom right*) corroborates the color Doppler findings.

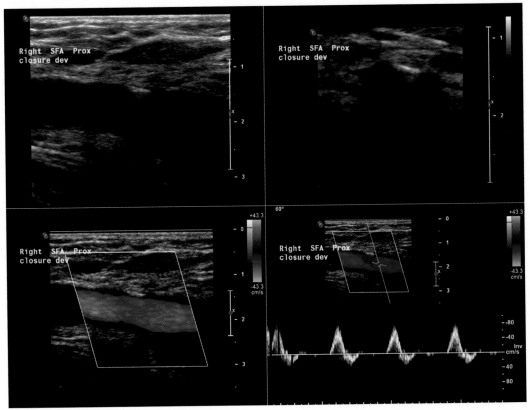

Figure 6-23. *Top left,* A long-axis grayscale image taken following catheterization and with a closure device in place, which clearly shows the device on the anterior wall of the superficial femoral artery. *Top right,* A short-axis view shows the device. *Bottom left,* Color flow filling is complete, with no evidence of flow disturbance. *Bottom right,* Spectral Doppler reveals normal multiphasic flow without turbulence beyond the device.

7 The Abdominal Aorta

Key Points

- The abdominal aorta is principally subject to aneurysmal disease in its infrarenal portion, to occlusive disease in its distal portion, and to dissection extending from thoracic aortic dissection.
- However, variations to these syndromes and other disorders such as aortitis, as well as concurrent branch vessel disease, confer a broad spectrum of abdominal aortic disease.

ANATOMY OF THE ABDOMINAL AORTA

The abdominal aorta begins at the level of the diaphragm and runs along the anterior longitudinal ligament in front of the vertebral column slightly to the left of both midline and inferior vena cava. As a result of the many branch vessels given off along its course, the aorta diminishes in size as it descends to the bifurcation. Because it lies in front of the convex-shaped vertebrae, it too is slightly curved, with the apex at the level of the third vertebra.

The branches of the aorta are divided into three sets:
- Visceral
  - Celiac
  - Superior mesenteric
  - Inferior mesenteric
  - Renal (paired)
  - Middle adrenal (paired)
  - Internal spermatic (male) (paired)
  - Ovarian (female) (paired)
- Parietal-inferior phrenic (paired)
  - Middle sacral
  - Lumbar (paired)
- Terminal—common iliac artery (paired)

The celiac artery (axis) is a 1.25-cm long stumpy artery arising from the anterior aspect of the aorta immediately below the diaphragm. The celiac artery divides into the left gastric, splenic, and common hepatic arteries, which supply the spleen, liver, stomach, duodenum, and pancreas.

The superior mesenteric artery, a large artery, arises from the aorta approximately 1.25 cm distal to the celiac artery, supplies the whole of the small intestine, cecum, head of the pancreas, ascending colon, and half of the transverse colon. The superior mesenteric artery lies behind the pancreas where the splenic vein crosses over its proximal segment and then courses downward and forward, crossing in front of the inferior vena cava, diminishing in size to its terminus and anastomosis with one of its own branches, the ileal branch of the ileocolic artery. There are 12 to 15 branches that run down the left side of the superior mesenteric artery, divide, and then anastomose with adjacent branches to form a series of arches supplying the small intestine.

The middle, right, and ileocolic arteries arise from the right side of the superior mesenteric artery. Of particular note is the middle colic artery, which forms an anastomosis with the left colic branch of the inferior mesenteric artery to create the marginal artery, an important collateral in the presence of celiac artery occlusive disease.

The inferior mesenteric artery is smaller than the superior mesenteric artery, arising from the anterior aspect of the aorta approximately 3 cm proximal to the aortic bifurcation at the level of the third lumbar vertebra. This artery supplies the left half of the transverse colon, a greater part of the rectum, and the descending colon.

The inferior mesenteric artery lies anterior to the aorta and then runs downward on the left side, eventually crossing the left common iliac artery. After this point it continues as the superior rectal hemorrhoidal artery, an important stem artery that joins with other hemorrhoidal branches to provide a collateral network in cases of aortic obstruction.

The suprarenal arteries arise from either side of the aorta at the level of the superior mesenteric artery. They run laterally and proximally where they pass over the crura of the diaphragm to join with suprarenal branches of the renal and inferior phrenic arteries.

The lumbar arteries are a series of four paired vessels that arise from the back of the spine, passing behind the quadratus lumborum and psoas muscles. There they join with other arteries in the area and can provide collaterals as far away as the inguinal ligament.

Similarly, the subcostal arteries (intercostal arteries of the twelfth rib) can supply important collaterals in the presence of aortoiliac artery occlusion. The third lumbar artery is the most common source of collateral blood supply in the presence of renal artery stenosis or occlusion.

Clinical Pearls

- A bowel "prep" is recommended before performing abdominal (vascular) ultrasound for patients who do not have diabetes:
  - Low-fat meal night before
  - Plenty of clear fluids throughout with medications, if necessary
  - No gum chewing, caffeine, or carbonated beverages
  - Bowl of flavored gelatin the morning of the test (helps abate the appetite and reduces excessive aerophagia)
- The waveforms in the aorta vary in shape between the proximal and distal segments:
  - Relatively low resistance proximal flow patterns are influenced by the low-resistance end bed of the renal and celiac arteries.
  - In contrast, flow patterns in the higher resistance infrarenal segment are shaped by the high resistance of the lumbar, peripheral arteries, and (non-postprandial) superior and inferior mesenteric arteries.
- Use a small color box when imaging for endoleaks.
- Optimize settings so that the color gain is set just below speckle, then circle the circumference of the sac carefully to search for any evidence of flow within the sac or connecting channel of flow.

TABLE 7-1 Protocol for Aortoiliac Duplex Scanning

ANATOMIC SEGMENT	TECHNIQUE	DUPLEX MODALITY
Aorta	SAX sweep Proximal Mid Distal	Grayscale, color Doppler
	LAX Proximal Mid Distal	Grayscale, color/ spectral Doppler
Common iliac artery	SAX sweep Proximal Mid Distal	Grayscale
	LAX sweep Proximal Mid Distal	Grayscale, color/ spectral Doppler
Internal iliac artery	SAX	Grayscale, color Doppler
	LAX	Grayscale, color/ spectral Doppler
External iliac artery	SAX	Grayscale
	LAX sweep Proximal Mid Distal	Grayscale, color/ spectral Doppler

LAX, long-axis imaging; SAX, short-axis imaging.

The internal spermatic arteries arising from the anterior aorta just below the renal arteries are small. In contrast, the paired ovarian arteries are large and join in an arcade with the uterine arteries, which are part of the internal iliac artery system.

The renal arteries arise from the aorta at approximately the level of the second lumbar vertebra immediately below the superior mesenteric artery, although some variation is known. Major accessory renal arteries are usually fewer than two or three in number and most commonly arise from the aorta, but smaller arteries can originate from vessels such as the suprarenal artery. Approximately 50% of these accessory arteries extend to the hilum and the other 50% to either the upper or lower poles of the kidney.

As both renal arteries cross the crura of the diaphragm, they almost form a right angle with the aorta. The left renal artery extends superior and posterior to the left renal vein and inferior and posterior to the pancreas and splenic vein. The right renal artery is longer than the left renal artery and passes behind the inferior vena cava, right renal vein, head of the pancreas, and descending segment of the duodenum.

Before entering the hilum of the kidney, each renal artery gives off four or five branches, which extend to the adrenal gland, ureter, muscle, and neighboring tissue. Closer still to the hilum, the anterior and posterior segmental, or lobar, arteries arise and supply the various segments of the kidney.

The segmental arteries further divide into the interlobar arteries, which run alongside the renal pyramids and then divide again into the arcuate arteries at the corticomedullary junction. The arcuate arteries then divide into the interlobular arteries, which become the afferent glomerular arteries supplying the glomerular body, a capillary tuft that is part of the main filtration system of the kidney.

Besides the third lumbar artery previously mentioned, the collateral circulation for the kidney is usually provided by the internal iliac, testicular, ovarian, intercostal, and inferior adrenal arteries, and the first three lumbar arteries are the main supply for an ischemic kidney.

ANEURYSMAL DISEASE OF THE ABDOMINAL AORTA

Abdominal aortic aneurysms (AAAs) are common in the older population, in 3.5% of males older than 65 years of age (although most of these are small), and the incidence increases with increasing age. Unfortunately, the same is true with obesity, which is increasingly common and severe with aging. AAAs occurring within the context of familial/ genetic syndromes are seen at much earlier ages.

TABLE 7-2   Aortic Aneurysm Terminology

Normal artery	<3 cm*
Aneurysmal	≥3 cm*
Fusiform	Spindle-shaped
Saccular	Rounded or bag-shaped

*With some intent to index to the body size of the patient.

Most aneurysms are small, but all enlarge over time and, if the patient lives long enough, eventually rupture. The risk of rupture of AAAs relates to size, which is generally expressed as the maximal transverse diameter. At diameters of more than 4.5 cm, the risk increases.

Physical diagnosis detection of AAA is at best modestly successful; in the presence of abdominal obesity, it is frankly poor. Screening for AAAs is most commonly performed by ultrasound because it is widely available, accurate, and without risk. Computed tomography aortography better and more extensively delineates aortic (and branch vessel) anatomy and pathology than ultrasound but with the potential of contrast nephropathy. Although ultrasound may image some cases of rupture or leak of an AAA, computed tomography is a far more reliable test to recognize leak.

In the era of endovascular aneurysm repair (EVAR), determination of the anatomy of the AAA relevant to EVAR repair requires the delineation of details relevant to EVAR technique such as the suitability of proximal and distal "landing zones."

DUPLEX PROTOCOL FOR EVALUATION OF ABDOMINAL AORTIC ANEURYSMS

Purpose
The objective is to evaluate and calculate pertinent measurements of the aneurysm.

Technique
The patient lies supine initially, but an oblique or decubitus position may be necessary.

Views
Transverse
❏ Scan the abdominal aorta from the xiphisternum to the bifurcation.
❏ Identify the superior mesenteric, celiac, renal, and inferior mesenteric arteries where possible and image them with color Doppler flow mapping.
❏ Measure the anteroposterior diameter of the aorta (outside to outside wall) at the following locations:
  • Suprarenal
  • Infrarenal
  • Aneurysmal neck
  • Aneurysm itself

❏ In addition, measure the:
  • Distance of neck from the ostium of the left renal artery (when possible)
  • Diameter of the common iliac artery bilaterally

Sagittal
❏ Scan the proximal, middle, and distal abdominal aorta, and common iliac arteries bilaterally using color and spectral Doppler.
❏ Measure the length of the aneurysm.
❏ Determine if the aneurysm is saccular or fusiform:
  • Saccular: saclike
  • Fusiform: spindle-shaped

Interpretation and Reporting
❏ Notable criteria include: aneurysm: focal dilation of arterial wall
❏ True aneurysm (vs. pseudoaneurysm)
  • Pulsating mass seen on grayscale imaging
  • Turbulent flow, which may be present in the aneurysmal sac
  • Heterogeneous intraluminal echoes suggestive of mural thrombus. These are commonly present.
  • Intimal flap, which may develop within an AAA

Post–Endovascular Aneurysm Repair/Postsurgical Repair
Ultrasound is useful post-EVAR to check for the presence of endoleaks, which are apparent on Doppler flow mapping. Care to scan all levels of the aneurysm sac for endoleak is required to avoid failing to detect a leak in any one part. The EVAR-covered stent is commonly seen to lie at an angle in the aneurysm sac. Development of thrombus in the aneurysm sac is apparent by ultrasound, when the body of the aneurysm is excluded (partially or completely) by the stent. The size/diameter of the body of the aneurysm may remain stable following successful EVAR but more commonly diminishes partially. Increase in the size of the aneurysm sac is a worrisome finding. Follow-up of patients who previously underwent EVAR repair is usually performed with either computed tomography aortography or ultrasound, with the choice of test depending on the imageability of the patient by ultrasound, the degree of renal dysfunction, the age of the patient and the consideration of long-term radiation risks, and the availability of the tests.

DUPLEX PROTOCOL FOR THE EVALUATION OF ENDOVASCULAR STENT GRAFTS

Purpose
❏ To establish patency and search for possible endoleak
❏ To measure the size of the aneurysmal sac and compare with baseline study (if possible)

Limitations

- Excessive bowel gas
- Obesity
- Abdominal tenderness

Patient and Study Preparation

Patient preparation is as with full arterial duplex scanning.

For study preparation, follow these guidelines:

- Establish preoperative aneurysm size.
- As different complications may arise with different graft and disease configurations, review:
  - EVAR procedure documentation
  - Other pertinent ancillary procedure information
  - Previous scan data (where applicable)
  - Possible ancillary procedures
- Effect precoiling of inferior mesenteric or hypogastric arteries, if "chimney" iliac grafts were placed due to small or diseased iliac arteries, to insert the endovascular device for other procedures such as angioplasty/stenting

Possible Stent Types

- Tube graft
- Bifurcated graft
- Aortoiliac grafts (involve exclusion or occlusion of the contralateral iliac artery to prevent retrograde flow from entering the aneurysmal sac and usually a femoral-femoral bypass to restore flow to the limb)
- Aorto-uni-iliac graft, with a femoral-to-femoral cross-over (left-right) graft

Note that some stents are totally supported and some are unsupported, except for the attachment ends.

Views

Transverse

- Identify and measure the maximal anteroposterior and transverse diameter of the aneurysmal sac.
- Identify superior and inferior attachment sites—look for linear reflective metal struts used as anchors.

Transverse and Long-Axis

- Optimize color settings and scan the entire graft in grayscale, color Doppler, and spectral Doppler.
- Record any flow entering the aneurysm and annotate location and direction.
- Attempt to determine the extent of the leak (i.e., whether the leak extends through the entire length of the AAA sac or is confined only to the immediate area of the suspected origin of the leak).
- Answer this question—what is the direction of flow and source of the leak?

Potential Leak Sites

More than one type of leak can occur at the same time. Assess for graft deformities such as "telescoping," kinking, or twisting, which may lead to stenosis or thrombosis.

- Record flow velocity throughout.
- Attempt to identify:
  - Inferior mesenteric artery origin (flow direction) (might be occluded at origin but reconstituted distally)
  - Aorta: anterior-middle
  - Renal arteries
- With native iliac arteries, look for intimal flaps, hematoma, arteriovenous fistulas, or atherosclerotic disease.

Types of Leaks

- Type I: attachment endoleak; seen at either the superior attachment or the inferior attachment
- Type II: branch leak (these originate from native vessels such as the inferior mesenteric artery or the lumbar arteries of the aorta through which retrograde flow returns into the residual aneurysmal sac outside the endograft)
- Type III: modular connect endoleak; seen where stent connection sites do not provide a seal.
- Type IV: transgraft leaks, which can occur from tiny tears in the fabric or exudates from thin-walled fabric

Complications

Apparent by Ultrasound

- Endoleak
- Graft stenosis
- Thrombosis
- Dissection
- Perforation (some)
- Graft migration (some)
- Remodeling of the aneurysm sac
- Graft infection (few)
- Delayed rupture (some)
- Pseudoaneurysm

Not Apparent by Ultrasound

- Perforation
- Graft migration
- Lower extremity ischemia due to embolization
- Graft infection
- Delayed rupture
- Bleeding
- Hematoma
- Bowel ischemia

Postsurgical Tube Graft Repair of an Abdominal Aortic Aneurysm or Aortobifemoral Graft

Ultrasound is useful to assess status and complications of surgical repair of the abdominal aorta, including tube graft repair and aortobifemoral repair. Ultrasound is able to detect obstruction of grafts and anastomotic false aneurysms. Ultrasound is less useful to recognize leak or infection of surgical grafts.

DUPLEX PROTOCOL FOR THE EVALUATION OF AORTOBIFEMORAL BYPASS FOR ABDOMINAL AORTIC ANEURYSM REPAIR

Purpose
The objective is to assess patency of the graft, and anastomotic integrity, as part of a surveillance regimen post-AAA aneurysm repair.

Equipment
The equipment needed is the same as for lower extremity imaging.

Technique
The patient lies supine.

Views
Transverse
❑ Identify the body of the graft and the anastomoses.
❑ Measure and record the largest anteroposterior diameter.

Long-Axis
❑ Use flow map with color Doppler and record flow by pulsed-wave Doppler.
❑ When recording with pulsed-wave Doppler, when possible, use:
  • An angle of 60 degrees to the vessel wall where possible
  • A sample volume of 1.5 mm

Interpretation
Normal
There is no evidence of intraluminal echoes or peak systolic velocity elevation.

Abnormal
This involves classification of stenosis.
❑ Less than 50%
  • Plaque visualized on B-mode
  • Triphasic/biphasic waveforms

  • From a 30% to 100% increase in peak systolic velocity compared with that immediately proximal
❑ Between 50% and 99%
  • Plaque visualized
  • Loss of reverse flow component (variable)
  • Greater than 100% increase in peak systolic flow velocity compared with that immediately proximal
  • Evidence of true poststenotic disordered flow on color flow representation of narrowed flow channel
❑ Occlusion: intraluminal echoes and no flow identified
❑ Anastomotic pseudoaneurysm:
  • Pulsating mass identified on grayscale and color Doppler imaging and color and connected to the main lumen by a narrow "neck"
  • High-velocity antegrade and retrograde ("to and fro") flow within the track
  • Turbulent flow in body of the false aneurysm (apparent by spectral and color Doppler)

PRACTICE GUIDELINES

The 2005 American College of Cardiology/American Heart Association (ACC/AHA) Practice Guidelines on Peripheral Artery Disease include indications for duplex ultrasonography of the abdominal aorta.[1]

ACCREDITATION

The Intersocietal Commission for Accreditation of Vascular Laboratories (ICAVL) maintains the standards for testing and accreditation of vascular laboratories. The standards for duplex ultrasonography of the abdominal aorta are summarized in Table 7-3.[2]

TABLE 7-3 ICAVL* Standards for Accreditation: Abdominal Aortic Duplex Testing Summary Points

- A range of imaging frequencies appropriate for the vessels and structures evaluated must be available.
- The indication for testing must be documented.
- Generally accepted indications vary depending on clinical considerations provided by the referring health care provider and in some instances can only be assessed at the time of examination. Appropriate indications for peripheral arterial examination include, but are not limited to, exercise-related limb symptoms, limb pain at rest, extremity ulcer/gangrene, assessment of healing potential, follow-up of limb revascularization, absent peripheral pulses, digital cyanosis, cold sensitivity, arterial trauma, aneurysms/pseudoaneurysms, follow-up of arterial reconstruction, and endovascular procedures or surgical intervention.
- The laboratory must have a written protocol to determine the anatomic extent of the study. Bilateral testing is considered an integral part of a complete examination.
- Limited examinations may be performed for an appropriate or recurring indication. The reasons for a limited examination must be documented.
- A written protocol must be in place for all supplemental testing examinations that defines the components and documentation of the complete examination.
- Abdominal aortic duplex: grayscale—representative grayscale images of the aorta must be documented as required by the protocol with additional documentation of any abnormalities and must include at a minimum:
  - Transverse views with diameter measurements proximal, middle, and distal
  - Longitudinal views proximal, middle, and distal
  - Transverse view of common iliac arteries at aortic bifurcation
- Documentation of aneurysms, if present, must include the widest size of the aorta measured outer wall to outer wall. Additional images proximal and distal to the aneurysm must be recorded.
- Representative spectral Doppler waveforms of the aorta must be documented as required by the protocol and must include at a minimum waveforms taken from each specified artery.
- One site in the aorta as described in the laboratory protocol
- Other aortoiliac sites as appropriate
- Representative color-coded Doppler images must be documented as required by the laboratory protocol.
- There must be criteria for interpretation of aortic duplex examination (i.e., aneurysm and stenotic disease).

*IACVL, Intersocietal Commission for Accreditation of Vascular Laboratories.
Adapted from Intersocietal Commission for Accreditation of Vascular Laboratories (ICAVL): The Complete ICAVL Standards for Accreditation in Noninvasive Vascular Testing. <http://www.icavl.org/icavl/Standards/2010_ICAVL_Standards.pdf>.

REFERENCES

1. Hirsch AT, Haskal ZJ, Hertzer NR, et al. ACC/AHA 2005 practice guidelines for the management of patients with peripheral arterial disease (lower extremity, renal, mesenteric, and abdominal aortic): executive summary. *J Am Coll Cardiol*. 2006;47:1239-1312.

2. Intersocietal Commission for Accreditation of Vascular Laboratories (ICAVL): The Complete ICAVL Standards for Accreditation in Noninvasive Vascular Testing. <http://www.icavl.org/icavl/Standards/2010_ICAVL_Standards.pdf>; Accessed April 20, 2010.

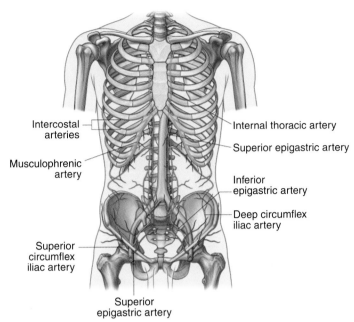

Figure 7-1. Arterial supply to the anterolateral abdominal wall. (From Drake R, Vogl AW, Mitchell AWM. *Gray's Anatomy for Students.* 2nd ed. Philadelphia: Elsevier; 2010; Fig. 4-39; used with permission.)

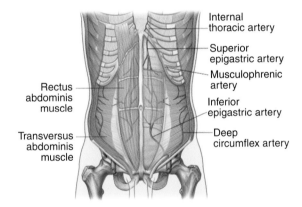

Figure 7-2. Superior and inferior epigastric arteries. (From Drake R, Vogl AW, Mitchell AWM. *Gray's Anatomy for Students.* 2nd ed. Philadelphia: Elsevier; 2010; Fig. 4-40; used with permission.)

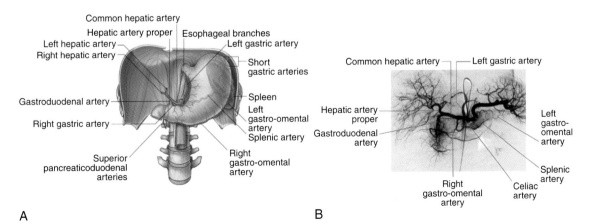

A

B

Figure 7-3. Celiac trunk. **A,** Distribution of the celiac trunk. **B,** Digital subtraction angiography of the celiac trunk and its branches. (From Drake R, Vogl AW, Mitchell AWM. *Gray's Anatomy for Students.* 2nd ed. Philadelphia: Elsevier; 2010; Fig. 4-111; used with permission.)

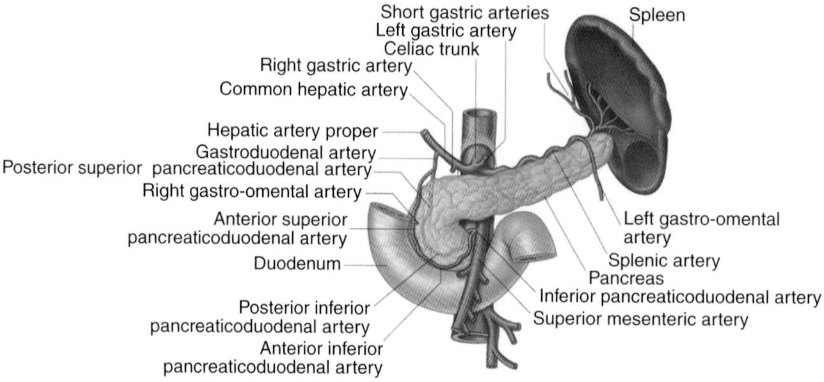

Short gastric arteries
Left gastric artery
Celiac trunk
Spleen
Right gastric artery
Common hepatic artery

Hepatic artery proper
Gastroduodenal artery
Posterior superior pancreaticoduodenal artery
Right gastro-omental artery
Anterior superior pancreaticoduodenal artery
Duodenum

Left gastro-omental artery
Splenic artery
Pancreas
Inferior pancreaticoduodenal artery
Superior mesenteric artery

Posterior inferior pancreaticoduodenal artery
Anterior inferior pancreaticoduodenal artery

Figure 7-4. Arterial supply to the pancreas. (From Drake R, Vogl AW, Mitchell AWM. *Gray's Anatomy for Students.* 2nd ed. Philadelphia: Elsevier; 2010; Fig. 4-112; used with permission.)

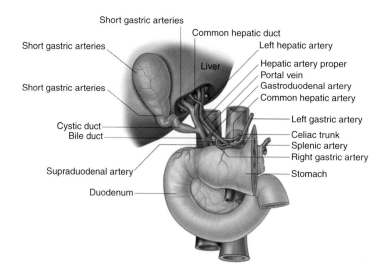

Short gastric arteries

Common hepatic duct
Short gastric arteries
Left hepatic artery

Liver
Hepatic artery proper
Portal vein
Gastroduodenal artery
Common hepatic artery

Short gastric arteries

Cystic duct
Bile duct
Left gastric artery
Celiac trunk
Splenic artery
Right gastric artery

Supraduodenal artery
Stomach

Duodenum

Figure 7-5. Distribution of the common hepatic artery. (From Drake R, Vogl AW, Mitchell AWM. *Gray's Anatomy for Students.* 2nd ed. Philadelphia: Elsevier; 2010; Fig. 4-113; used with permission.)

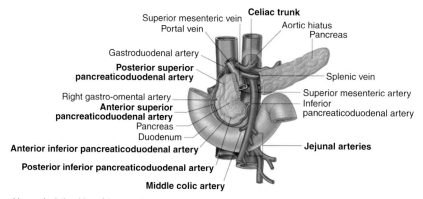

Superior mesenteric vein
Portal vein
Celiac trunk
Aortic hiatus
Pancreas

Gastroduodenal artery
Posterior superior pancreaticoduodenal artery

Splenic vein

Right gastro-omental artery
Anterior superior pancreaticoduodenal artery
Pancreas
Duodenum
Superior mesenteric artery
Inferior pancreaticoduodenal artery

Anterior inferior pancreaticoduodenal artery
Jejunal arteries

Posterior inferior pancreaticoduodenal artery

Middle colic artery

Figure 7-6. Initial branching and relationships of the superior mesenteric artery. (From Drake R, Vogl AW, Mitchell AWM. *Gray's Anatomy for Students.* 2nd ed. Philadelphia: Elsevier; 2010; Fig. 4-114; used with permission.)

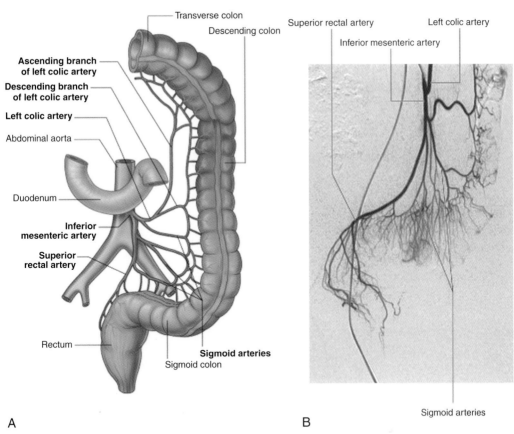

Figure 7-7. Inferior mesenteric artery. **A**, Distribution of the inferior mesenteric artery. **B**, Digital subtraction angiography of the inferior mesenteric artery and its branches. (From Drake R, Vogl AW, Mitchell AWM. *Gray's Anatomy for Students.* 2nd ed. Philadelphia: Elsevier; 2010; Figure 4-116; used with permission.)

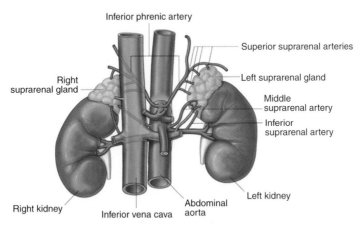

Figure 7-8. Arterial supply to the suprarenal glands. (From Drake R, Vogl AW, Mitchell AWM. *Gray's Anatomy for Students.* 2nd ed. Philadelphia: Elsevier; 2010; Fig. 4-147; used with permission.)

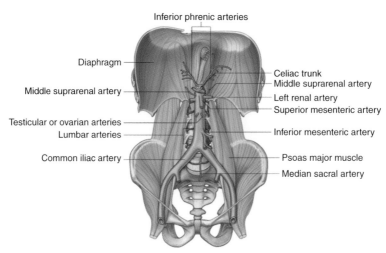

Figure 7-9. Abdominal aorta. (From Drake R, Vogl AW, Mitchell AWM. *Gray's Anatomy for Students*. 2nd ed. Philadelphia: Elsevier; 2010; Fig. 4-148; used with permission.)

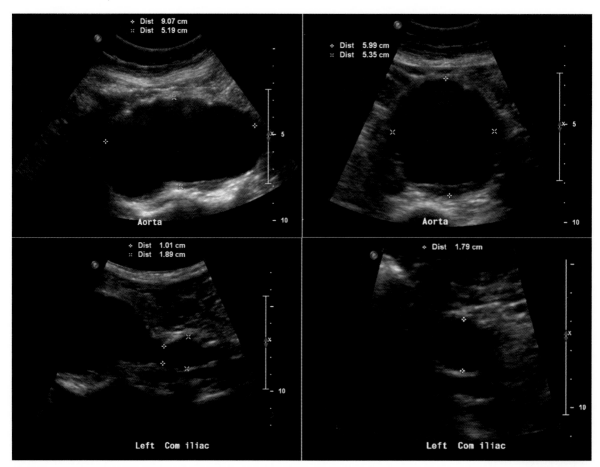

Figure 7-10. A 6.0-cm large infrarenal abdominal aortic aneurysm with a small amount of mural thrombus and an associated small, and separate, left common iliac aneurysm.

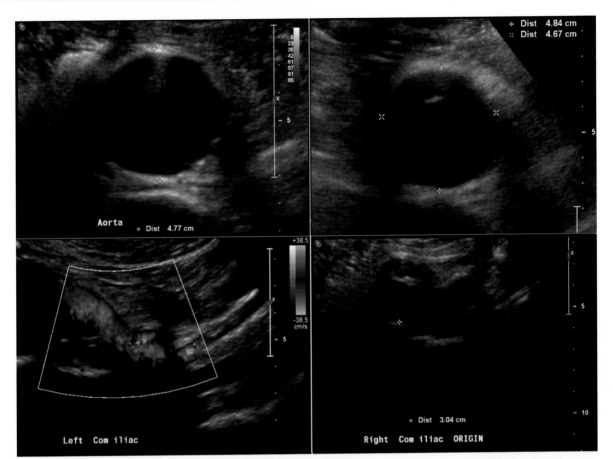

Figure 7-11. *Top left and right,* A 4.8-cm infrarenal abdominal aortic aneurysm with little mural thrombus. *Bottom left,* Mild enlargement of the left common iliac artery. *Bottom right,* A separate aneurysm of the right common iliac artery.

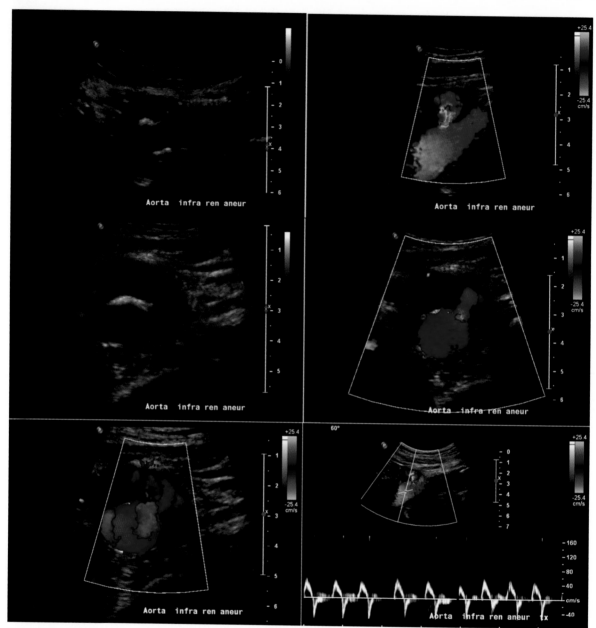

Figure 7-12. Infrarenal abdominal aortic aneurysm with dissection. *Top left,* Longitudinal view of the abdominal aorta revealing the abdominal aortic aneurysm and intimal flap resulting in true and false lumens. *Top right,* Color flow mapping reveals a jet into the false lumen through the intimal flap. *Middle left,* Abdominal aortic aneurysm with dissection in cross-section. The intimal flap and the intimal tear through the flap are depicted. *Middle right,* Color flow mapping revealing flow across the intimal flap through the intimal tear. *Bottom left,* Same. *Bottom right,* Spectral flow recording at the intimal tear. Reciprocating flow into and out of the false lumen, which is acting as a false aneurysm, through the single tear is demonstrated.

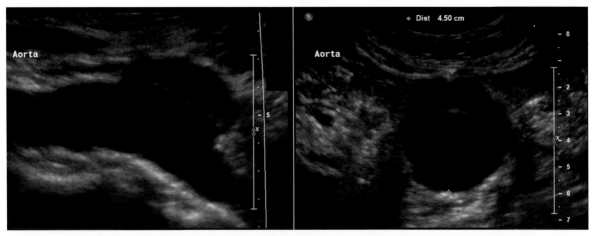

Figure 7-13. A 4.5-cm infrarenal saccular abdominal aortic aneurysm. There is a moderate amount of anterior mural thrombus.

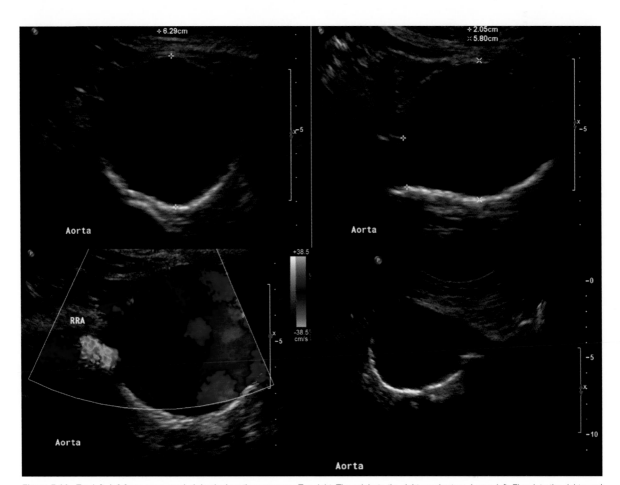

Figure 7-14. *Top left,* A 6.3-cm suprarenal abdominal aortic aneurysm. *Top right,* The origin to the right renal artery. *Lower left,* Flow into the right renal artery as seen by color Doppler flow mapping. *Lower right,* The origin to the left renal artery. Abdominal aortic aneurysm extending above the level of the renal arteries.

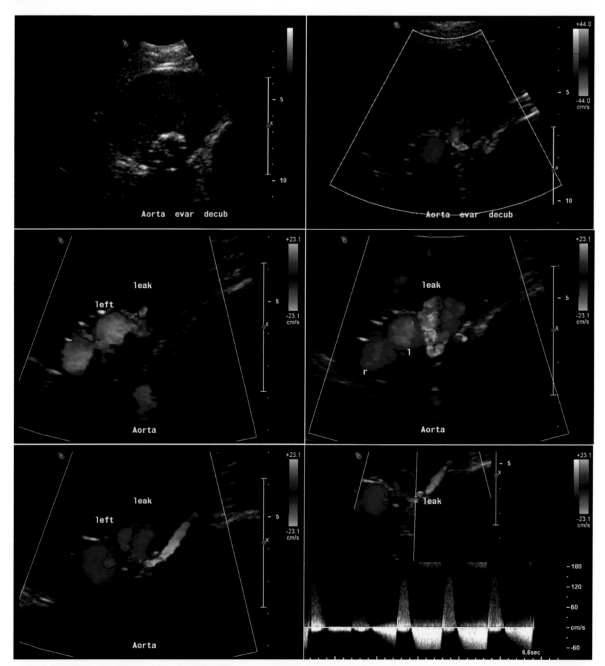

Figure 7-15. Type I endoleak post–endovascular aneurysm repair (EVAR) of an abdominal aortic aneurysm. *Top left,* The sac of the abdominal aortic aneurysm is largely thrombosed, and the EVAR is apparent. *Top right, middle left and right, and bottom left,* Color flow mapping revealing a leak from the site of the overlap with the left iliac stent leg with that of the EVAR. *Bottom right,* Spectral display of the reciprocating "to and fro" flow into and out of the sac through the leak.

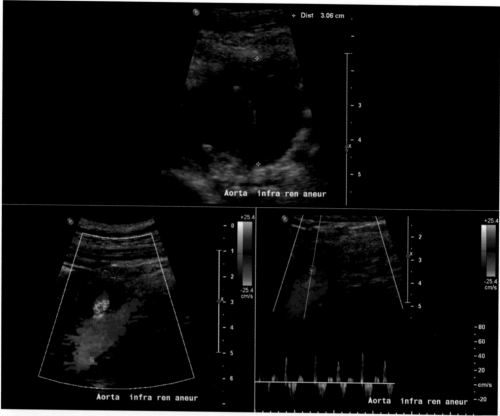

Figure 7-16. Infrarenal abdominal aortic aneurysm with dissection. *Top,* Short-axis view of the abdominal aorta revealing the abdominal aortic aneurysm and an intimal flap resulting in true and false lumens. *Bottom left,* Color flow mapping reveals a jet into the false lumen through the intimal flap. *Bottom right,* Spectral flow recording at the intimal tear. There is reciprocating flow into and out of the false lumen, which is acting as a false aneurysm, through the single tear.

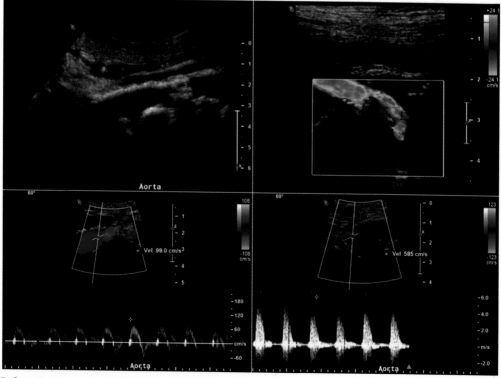

Figure 7-17. Stenosis of the distal aorta. *Top left,* Grayscale imaging revealing a large plaque more than 50% compromising the lumen of the distal aorta. *Top right,* Color flow mapping revealing the same. *Bottom,* Spectral display of flow before (*left*) and at the site of (*right*) the plaque. There is a nearly sixfold increase in systolic velocity.

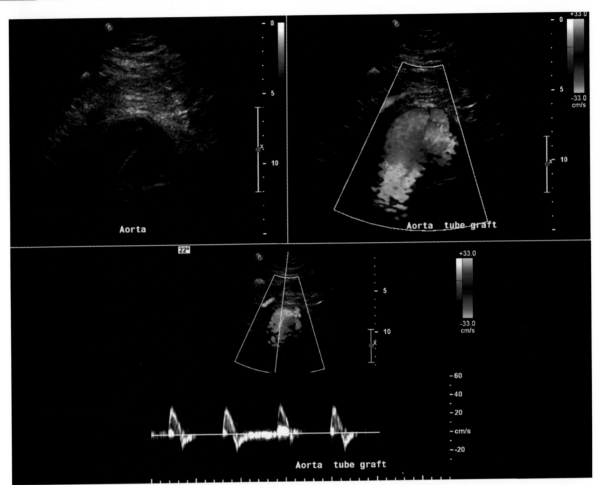

Figure 7-18. Folded aortic tube graft. *Top left and right,* Images revealing extensive thrombus formation within the sac of the abdominal aortic aneurysm and the tube graft deep to this, which is folded almost 90 degrees as seen on the grayscale and color Doppler flow mapping. *Lower image,* The flow, as depicted on the spectral display, is within the normal velocity range and phasic pattern, and there is no effective narrowing of the lumen of the graft.

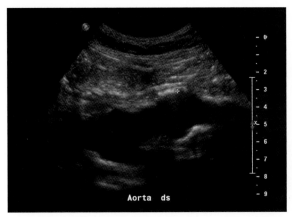

Figure 7-19. Dumbbell-shaped infrarenal abdominal aortic aneurysm.

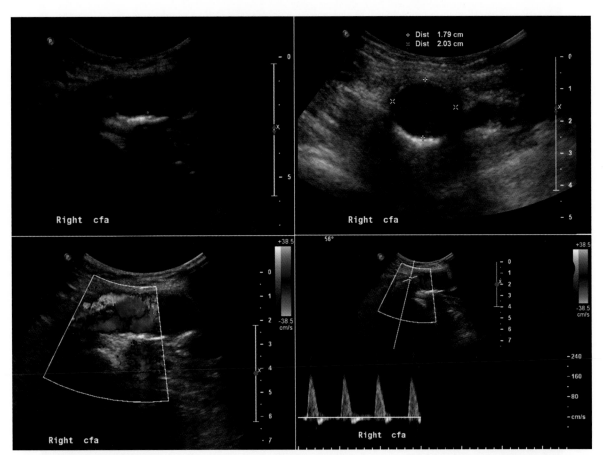

Figure 7-20. Distal anastomosis of an aortobifemoral graft. Grayscale long-axis (*top left*) and short-axis (*top right*) images of an aortobifemoral graft entering a tubularly aneurysmal common femoral artery, approximately 2 cm in diameter. Color Doppler (*bottom left*) and spectral Doppler (*bottom right*) spectral depiction of the normal flow pattern at the distal end of the graft. Bilaterally, the common femoral arteries had developed aneurysms, without flow disturbances.

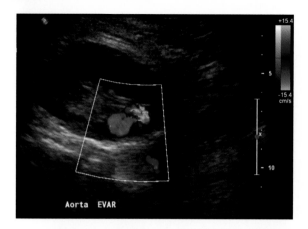

Figure 7-21. Type I endovascular aneurysm repair (EVAR) endoleak. Turbulent flow extending outside/beside the lumen of the EVAR is depicted by Doppler flow mapping.

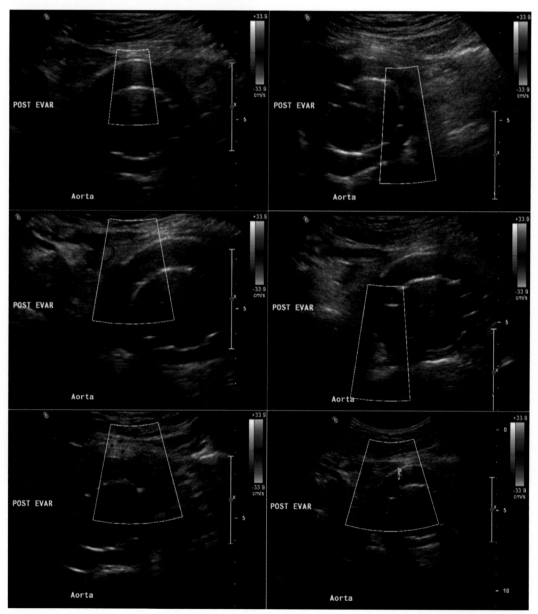

Figure 7-22. Methodical and meticulous flow mapping is needed to interrogate all around and the full length of the endovascular aneurysm repair (EVAR). In the bottom right image, there is a transducer color Doppler speckle artifact at 11 o'clock, not an endoleak. The selection of pulse repetition frequency is higher than ideal (18 cm/sec is ideal).

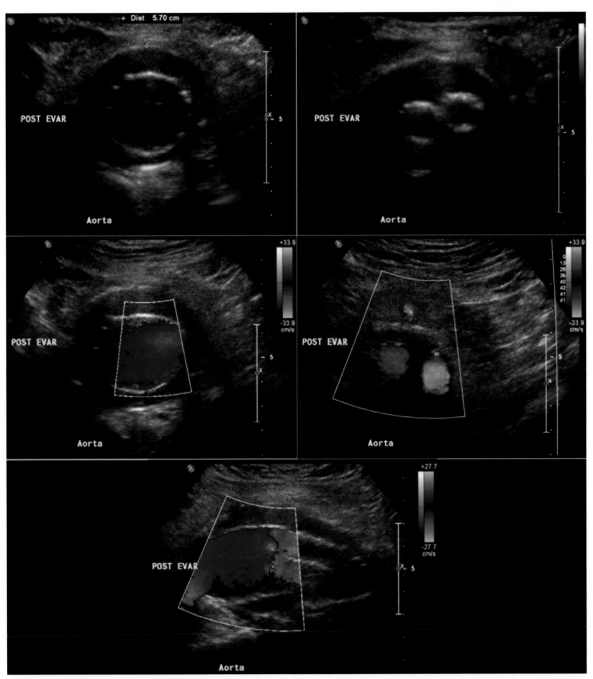

Figure 7-23. Grayscale and color Doppler flow imaging post–endovascular aneurysm repair (EVAR). No endoleak is seen. Flow is seen in a vessel *outside* the aneurysm sac (*middle right*); hence, the flow is not an endoleak.

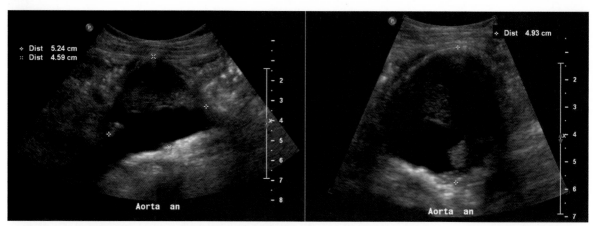

Figure 7-24. An approximately 5-cm saccular infrarenal abdominal aortic aneurysm largely filled by mural thrombus. Such a case reveals the limitations of angiography alone in determining dimensions of an abdominal aortic aneurysm.

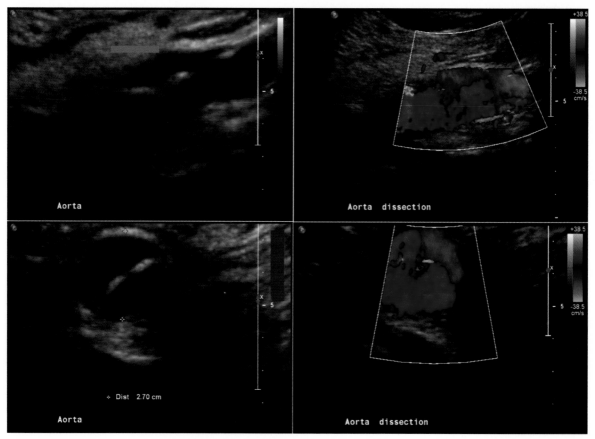

Figure 7-25. A localized dissection of the abdominal aorta.

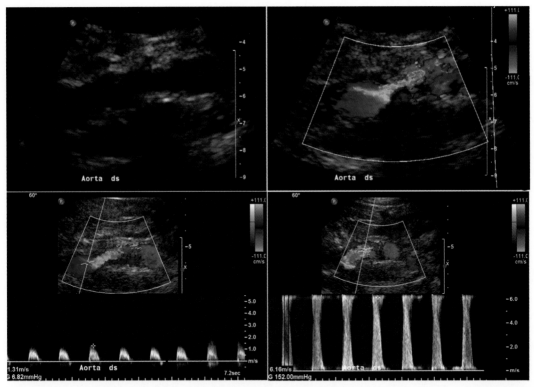

Figure 7-26. Stenosis of the distal aorta. *Top left,* Grayscale imaging of a large mass of plaque in the distal aorta. *Top right,* Color Doppler flow mapping reveals convergence of flow and turbulence at the site of greatest narrowing. *Bottom left and right,* Spectral display of the flow before (*left*) and after (*right*) revealing a high ratio of velocity increase, consistent with severe stenosis of the distal aorta.

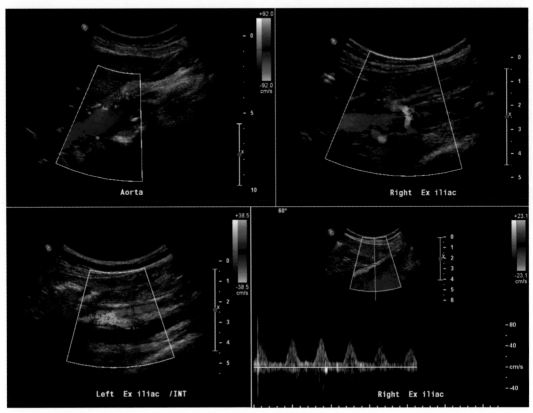

Figure 7-27. Occlusion of the distal aorta. Grayscale and color Doppler flow mapping reveal an abrupt termination of the lumen of the aorta (*top left and right*). Following the aorta past its termination is difficult because there is so much plaque and no residual lumen. Flow is converging into and flowing within the inferior mesenteric artery (IMA), which is anterior to the aorta. *Top right,* Flow returning to the right external iliac artery via a collateral vessel. *Bottom left,* Flow returning retrograde up the internal iliac artery to the iliac bifurcation, and then running down the external iliac artery. The IMA collateralized to the external iliac artery beyond the aortic obstruction. *Bottom right,* The flow in the external iliac artery is pulsatile, due to the size of the feeding collateral vessel.

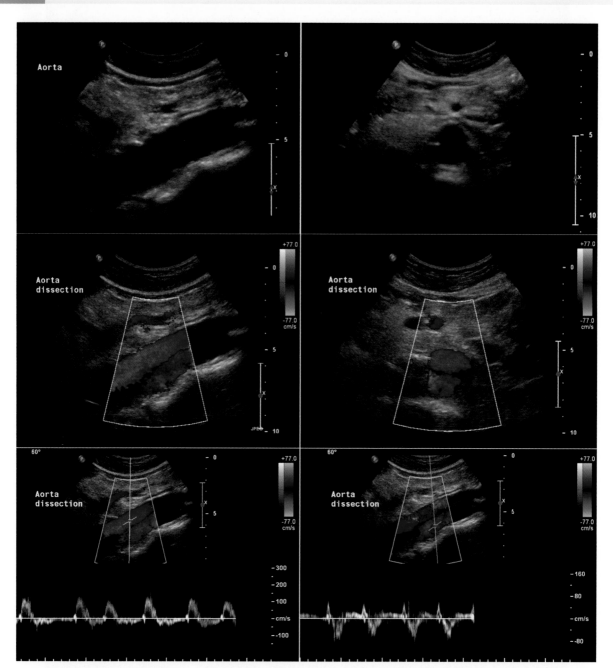

Figure 7-28. Long-axis views (*left*) and short-axis views (*right*) of a dissection of the abdominal aorta, residual after a type A dissection repair. The intimal flap can be seen as well as flow in both the true and false lumens. Notably, at this level, the flow in the false lumen is ascending in the false lumen, rather than running off distally. This is due to a more distal entry tear.

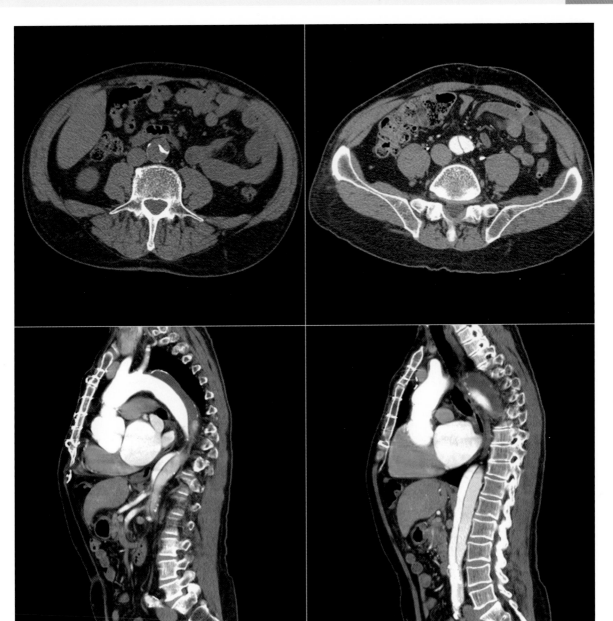

Figure 7-29. Computed tomography scans with contrast enhancement of the same case as in Figure 7-28. *Top left,* The intimal flap, now chronic, is seen to be calcified on the noncontrast images. *Top right,* The patency of the false lumen at the level image is demonstrated. *Bottom left and right,* Sagittal views revealing the sternal wires of the ascending aortic repair, with complete thrombosis of the proximal descending aortic false lumen proximally, then patency of the false lumen by the level of the retrocardiac aorta with a patent false lumen.

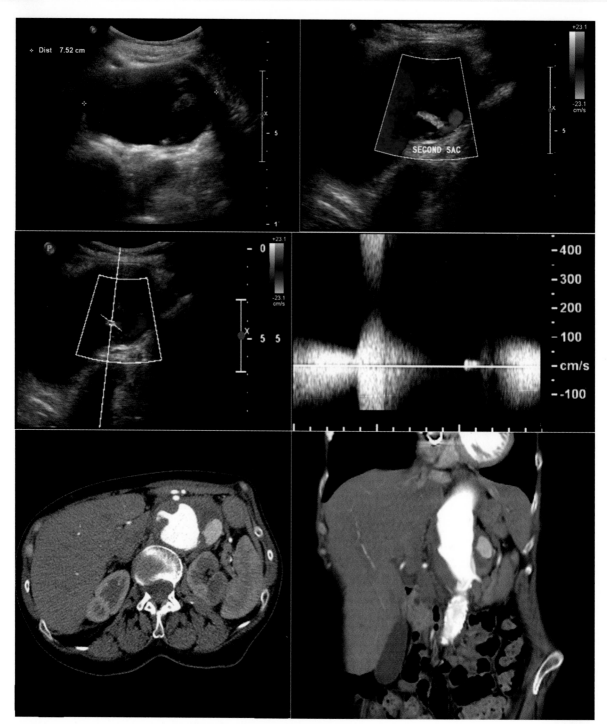

Figure 7-30. Abdominal aortic aneurysm with a small saccular false aneurysm within (presumably) its mural thrombus. The flow into and out of the second sac is through a small orifice and at high velocity. The computed tomography images confirm the same.

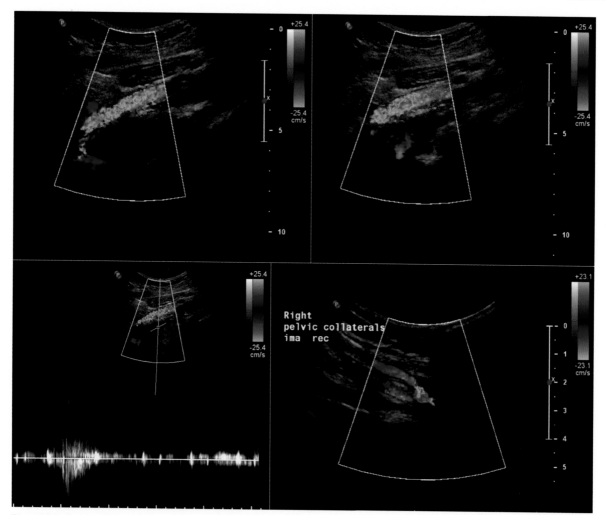

Figure 7-31. Chronic occlusion of the distal aorta with IMA to right external iliac artery collaterals. *Top left and right,* The aliasing color Doppler flow pattern is in a substantially dilated IMA, serving as a collateral. Deep to the enlarged IMA is the abdominal aorta with specular echoes in it and no color Doppler representation of flow. *Bottom left,* Spectral flow display from sampling within the aorta reveals no flow, only noise. *Bottom right,* A branch of the IMA (orange flow mapping) is reconstituting flow in the right external iliac artery (blue flow mapping).

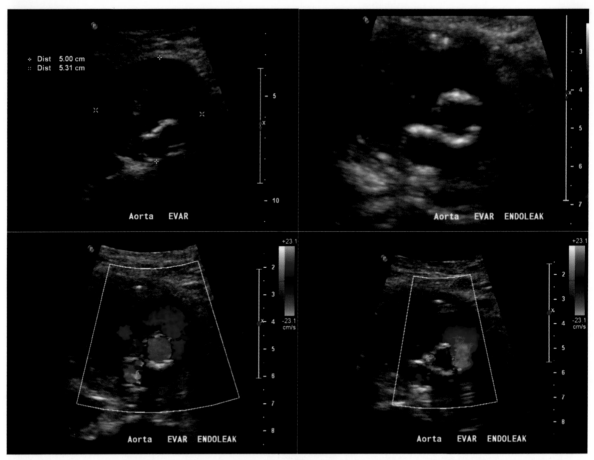

Figure 7-32. Post–endovascular aneurysm repair (EVAR) endoleak with partial thrombosis of the aneurysm sac. Partial thrombosis is revealed by both the visible presence of thrombus in some areas of the aneurysm sac and by lucency and color Doppler flow mapping in (other) areas.

8 Renal Artery Disease

ANATOMY OF THE RENAL ARTERY

The renal arteries arise from the aorta at approximately the level of the second lumbar vertebra immediately below the superior mesenteric artery, although some variation is known (Fig. 8-1). Major accessory renal arteries are usually fewer than two or three in number. They most commonly arise from the aorta, but smaller arteries can originate from vessels such as the suprarenal artery. Approximately 50% of these accessory arteries extend to the hilum and the other 50% to either the upper or lower poles of the kidney (Fig. 8-2).

Both renal arteries cross the crus of the diaphragm, and as a result, they almost form a right angle with the aorta. The left renal artery extends superior and posterior to the left renal vein and inferior and posterior to the pancreas and splenic vein. The right renal artery is longer than the left renal artery and passes behind the inferior vena cava, right renal vein, head of the pancreas, and descending segment of the duodenum.

Before entering the hilum of the kidney, each renal artery gives off four or five branches that extend to the adrenal gland, ureter, muscle, and neighboring tissue. Closer still to the hilum, the anterior and posterior segmental, or lobar, arteries arise and supply the various segments of the kidney.

The segmental arteries further divide into the interlobar arteries, which run alongside the renal pyramids and then divide again into the arcuate arteries at the corticomedullary junction. The arcuate arteries then divide into the interlobular arteries, which become the afferent glomerular arteries supplying the glomerular body, a capillary tuft that is part of the main filtration system of the kidney.

RENAL ARTERY STENOSIS

Renal artery stenosis (RAS) may be caused by atherosclerosis, fibromuscular dysplasia, or aortitis. RAS may be clinically silent, or it may result in hypertension, ischemic nephropathy, or recurrent pulmonary edema. The quest for accurate noninvasive tests to detect RAS evolves, as does the quest for accurate noninvasive tests to predict clinical response to renal artery revascularization. Although percutaneous intervention of stenotic renal arteries is technically successful in a high percentage of cases,[1] the debate continues as to whether atherosclerotic RAS hypertension benefits more from renal revascularization than from antihypertensive medications.[2-4]

Criteria for the Presence of Renal Artery Stenosis

Renal artery duplex findings predict the presence or absence of significant RAS. The peak systolic velocity (PSV) correlates with the severity of angiographic stenosis and the translesional pressure gradient.[5] Stenosis PSV greater than 1.8 to 2.0 at an angle of 45 to 60 degrees or a renal artery PSV–to–aortic PSV ratio of more than 3.5 predicts the presence of significant RAS (Table 8-1).[5-8]

Criteria Purported to Be Predictive of Response to Renal Artery Revascularization

Pulsed-wave Doppler recordings of intrarenal (interlobar) arterial flow are used to calculate the resistance index (RI): the ratio of PSV to end diastolic velocity (EDV). The RI affords some predictiveness of response to revascularization. As stenosis of the renal artery worsens, the early systolic peak diminishes, resulting in a "tardus et parvus" contour. As well, as stenosis worsens, the diastolic velocities increase. The RI is influenced by the severity of the stenosis but also its extent, the distensibility of the vessel, nonrenal/cardiac factors (e.g., tachycardia and aortic valve insufficiency), and the location of Doppler sampling (as the RI decreases from the hilum to the cortex).[8]

Radermacher and colleagues demonstrated that the RI, calculated as $(1 - EDV/ESV) \times 100$ (where ESV is end systolic velocity), of less than 80 was highly predictive of blood pressure response to renal artery angioplasty or stenting, and that the relative risk of worsening of renal function was over 100 times higher with a RI of greater than or equal to 80.[9] However this study did not clearly describe whether the RI was calculated from the stenotic or the contralateral kidney. The stenosis influences the poststenotic RI; therefore, the RI should not be determined on the

Clinical Pearls

- A bowel "prep" is recommended before performing abdominal (vascular) ultrasound for patients who do not have diabetes:
  - Low-fat meal night before
  - Plenty of clear fluids throughout with medications, if necessary
  - No gum chewing, caffeine, or carbonated beverages
  - Bowl of flavored gelatin the morning of the test (helps abate the appetite and reduces excessive aerophagia)
- Often, the best windows are achieved from lateral decubitus positions:
  - The right kidney is best imaged through the liver.
  - The left kidney is best imaged through the spleen.
- Place the patient in the lateral decubitus position and raise the upper arm over his or her head, to raise the diaphragm and provide better imaging of the upper kidney.
- It is helpful as well to place the lower extremities in optimal position, with the upper leg crossed over the lower leg and straight, and the lower leg placed behind and bent at the knee (if possible).
- Choose an approach where possible that is the shortest distance from skin to vessel.
- Keep the frame rate low by maintaining a narrow color box.
- Better color enhancement may be achieved with a phased array transducer rather than a curved linear transducer. Grayscale images are generally better with a curved linear transducer.
- Scan the most important (e.g., renal, if that is the main goal of study) vessels first and with limited breath holding, because continual transducer compression and breath holding can cause excessive gas formation, compromising the latter part of a study.
- The left renal vein is normally a useful landmark for the ostium/proximal right renal artery because the left renal vein crosses rightward over the abdominal aorta to the left side of the inferior vena cava. Rarely, the left renal vein can run posterior to the aorta.
- For flow sampling of the renal parenchyma, be sure to sample both the upper and lower poles of the kidney because there might be more than one renal artery supplying each pole.
- Disease parameter findings (such as the peak systolic velocity and renal-aortic ratio) should yield congruent findings; if they do not, then the basis of the disagreement needs to be resolved. For example, stenosis of the aorta proximal to the renal arteries may confound use of the renal-aortic ratio such that it is inapplicable, whereas the peak systolic velocity is more applicable.

affected kidney. Furthermore, the presence of bilaterality of RAS confounds as well the utility of RI as a descriptor of renal parenchymal damage. The inclusion of RAS of greater than 50% in the study also included some cases of borderline hemodynamic consequences that would not achieve treatment benefit.[8]

Subsequently, some authors described utility to RI, and others did not. Voiculescu and associates did not establish the utility of contralateral kidney RI greater than or equal to 80 in predicting blood pressure response, although poststenotic RI less than 55 was somewhat predictive of response.[10] Similarly, in a small series of 36 cases, Garcia-Criado and coworkers did not observe predictiveness of blood pressure response or renal function according to RI less than or greater than 80.[11] Among a larger series of (241) patients treated with stenting for RAS (>70%), RI greater than 80 (39 cases) was associated with improvement in blood pressure and renal function.[12]

Limitations of using intrarenal measurements to diagnose renal artery stenosis are:
- Inability to distinguish between occlusion and stenosis
- Inability to distinguish between renal artery stenosis and other factors that may alter the waveform (e.g., aortic stenosis or coarctation)
- Inability to localize site of the lesion
- Inability to identify less than 60% stenosis
- Insensitivity to lesions in accessory or segmental arteries

DUPLEX PROTOCOL FOR EVALUATION OF RENAL ARTERY STENOSIS

Purpose
The objective is to identify the presence or absence of occlusive disease or aneurysmal disease and, subsequently, determine its extent and degree of severity.

Common Indications
- Upper abdominal bruit
- Follow-up renal artery stent, bypass, or angioplasty procedure
- Suspected renovascular hypertension

Equipment
- Color duplex imaging system
- 5- to 7-MHz linear transducers
- 2- to 5-MHz sector/curved array transducers
- 2- to 4-MHZ vector transducer
- Coupling gel
- Digital image acquisition

Procedure
- Explain procedure to patient and answer any questions.
- Obtain and document applicable patient history on appropriate forms.
- Verify that the procedure requested correlates with patient's symptoms.
- Ascertain whether or not the patient is taking medication.
- Review any previous duplex studies available.
- Select appropriate test preset values.

TABLE 8-1 Ultrasound Criteria for the Presence of Renal Artery Stenosis

PARAMETER	REFERENCE	ANGIOGRAPHIC STANDARD	SENSITIVITY	SPECIFICITY	PPV	NPV
PSV > 200 cm/sec	Staub[5]	>50%	92%	81%		
RAR > 2.5	Staub[5]	>50%	92%	79%		
PSV < 200 cm/sec and RAR < 2.5		>70%				100%
PSV > 219 cm/sec	Kawarada[6]		89%	89%	83%	93%
PSV ≥ 200 cm/sec	Hua[7]	>60%	91%	75%	60%	95%
RAR ≥ 3.5		>60%	72%	92%	79%	88%

NPV, negative predictive value; PPV, positive predictive value; PSV, peak systolic velocity; RAR, renal-to-aortic ratio.

❐ Select appropriate annotation throughout test.
❐ Acquire and store digital images.
❐ Complete technologist's preliminary report when necessary.

Technique
❐ The patient lies supine for at least ten minutes before testing.
❐ The technologist stands/sits beside the patient.
❐ Gloves are worn by the technologist where there is a threat of contamination by infected body fluids.

Views
❐ Origin
❐ Middle
❐ Distal
❐ Stenotic sites: prestenotic, stenotic, and poststenotic peak systolic velocity readings plus post-stenotic turbulence

Sites to Survey
❐ Aorta (assess for significant stenosis, aneurysm, or anatomic variant)
❐ Celiac axis
❐ Superior mesenteric artery origin
❐ Renal artery (proximal, middle, and distal)
❐ Accessory arteries; these occur up to 20% of the time and are more commonly unilateral
❐ Kidneys
❐ Arcuate arteries in the renal cortex
❐ Interlobar arteries in the renal parenchyma
❐ Segmental arteries in the renal pelvis

Imaging of the Aorta
Take sagittal and transverse views to look for aneurysm, plaque, thrombus, tortuosity, and anomalies.

Grayscale and Color Imaging
❐ Identify origins of the superior mesenteric and celiac arteries.
❐ Record the normal aorta in maximal anteroposterior diameter from outside to outside diameter, at the level of the renal arteries.

❐ If an aneurysm is identified, record it in the sagittal plane.

Doppler Imaging (Sagittal)
❐ Image at the bifurcation in sagittal view to confirm the grayscale findings and to ensure there are no hidden areas of stenosis.
❐ Record an aorta velocity at a point just inferior to the superior mesenteric artery to be used in the renal-to-aortic PSV ratio (RAR).
❐ If abdominal aortic disease is suspected (based on image or velocity criteria), or if PSV in the proximal aorta is less than 40 cm/sec, the RAR may not be reliable.
❐ A delay in systolic upstroke of the spectral waveform in the proximal renal artery or its orifice suggests disease in the aorta proximal to the origin of the renal artery.

Imaging of Renal Vessels
Right Renal Artery
❐ Identify the superior mesenteric artery and left renal vein and locate the renal artery as it lies on the right anterior side of the aorta directly beneath the left renal vein.
❐ Find an optimal window to display the kidney and aorta in the same plane (i.e., spleen; it may be necessary to use an intercostal approach).
❐ Activate color and spectral Doppler to follow the artery from the ostium into the kidney, measuring PSV along the way.

Left Lateral Decubitus (Right Kidney)
❐ Turn the patient onto his or her left side on a small pillow and repeat steps.

Left Renal Artery
❐ Appreciate that the left renal artery lies directly across from the right but is quite variable in position, ranging from anterolateral to posterolateral.
❐ Document flow from the ostium to the proximal renal artery with spectral Doppler and record flow

---

TABLE 8-2 ICAVL* Standards for Accreditation: Visceral Vascular/Renal Vasculature Summary Points

- Visceral vascular testing is performed for appropriate clinical indications.
- The indication for testing must be documented.
- The entire course of the accessible portions of each visceral vessel should be examined.
- The laboratory must have a written protocol to determine the extent of the study and the appropriate documentation of normal and abnormal studies.
- Limited examinations may occur for an appropriate or recurring indication. The reason for a limited examination must be documented.
- A written protocol must be in place that defines the components and documentation of the complete examination. The protocol should also describe how color-coded Doppler is utilized to supplement grayscale imaging and spectral Doppler. If other flow imaging modes (e.g., power Doppler) are used, the protocol should describe how they are utilized.
- Representative grayscale spectral Doppler and/or color Doppler images from the following vessel groups must be documented as required by the protocol. Abnormalities require additional images that demonstrate the type and severity of the abnormality present.
- Renal system:
  - Adjacent aorta
  - Renal arteries
  - Renal veins
  - Grayscale pole-to-pole renal length measurement
- A complete renal vasculature examination includes bilateral evaluation.
- Interpretation of the renal vascular duplex examination must use validated diagnostic criteria to assess the presence of disease and to document its location, etiology, extent, and severity.
- Diagnostic criteria must be laboratory specific and documented.
- These criteria can be based on published reports or internally generated and internally validated as outlined.
- There must be criteria for interpretation of grayscale images; spectral Doppler; and when utilized, plaque morphology and color-coded Doppler images specific for each examination performed.
- The findings generate an interpretation and report that indicates the absence or presence of abnormalities in the vessels that were investigated. Disease, if present, must be characterized according to its location, etiology, extent, and severity.
- The laboratory must have a written procedure for regular correlation of visceral vascular examinations with angiographic findings produced by digital subtraction arteriography, contrast-enhanced computed tomography, or magnetic resonance angiography. The correlation must be reported using the categories of stenosis and/or disease defined by the diagnostic criteria utilized by the laboratory. Surgical correlations may be used when angiographic correlation is not available.
- A minimum of 15 patient examinations are to be correlated. These correlations must reflect a mix of all vessel groups performed by the laboratory and have been completed within the 3 years preceding submission of the application.
- The correlation matrix should demonstrate greater than 70% agreement.
- Documentation of correlation must be maintained.

*ICAVL, Intersocietal Commission for Accreditation of Vascular Laboratories.
Adapted from Intersocietal Commission for Accreditation of Vascular Laboratories (ICAVL): The Complete ICAVL Standards for Accreditation in Noninvasive Vascular Testing. < http://www.icavl.org/icavl/Standards/2010_ICAVL_Standards.pdf>.

---

velocity if possible at an angle of less than or equal to 60 degrees.
- ❏ Use three sampling locations around each stenosis: prestenotic, stenotic, and poststenotic (turbulence increases with severity of disease and may be easily missed due to autoregulation of blood flow).

Right Lateral Decubitus (Left Kidney)
- ❏ Turn the patient onto his or her right side on a small pillow and repeat steps.

Kidney
- ❏ Image the kidney in long-axis view without color to measure length, thickness, and anomalies (e.g., cysts).

- ❏ Take three separate measurements and document the most reproducible figures. If there is greater than 1-cm difference, remeasure to rule out a technical cause of size disparity.
- ❏ Document the RIs in the arcuate and segmental arteries.

Interpretation and Reporting
Normal Study
- ❏ PSV: 0.80 ± 0.20
- ❏ Renal-to-aortic PSV ratio (RAR): less than 3.5
- ❏ Normal waveform: biphasic
- ❏ No focal velocity increase
- ❏ Low resistance waveform

Less Than 60% Diameter Reduction

☐ Low resistance waveform
☐ RAR: less than 3.5
☐ PSV: less than 1.8 m/sec
☐ Focal velocity increase

Greater Than 60% Diameter Reduction

☐ RAR: greater than 3.5
☐ True poststenotic turbulence
☐ Focal PSV increase greater than 1.8 m/sec

Normal Kidney

☐ Length: 9 to 13 cm
☐ Width: 4 to 6 cm
☐ Reasonable difference in length: 1 cm
☐ Length difference greater than 1 cm: suggests smaller kidney is abnormal
☐ Texture: similar to liver except for echogenic renal sinus fat (normal)

Spectral Velocity Criteria

☐ Biphasic: normal (similar to internal carotid artery)
☐ Triphasic flow: highly abnormal
☐ Monophasic flow: also highly abnormal, consistent with distal occlusion or significant renal malfunction

Renovascular Resistance

RI is measured in the body of the kidney vasculature to assess renal resistance and suggest perfusion. An RI less than 0.70 is considered normal, one between 0.70 and 0.80 is questionably elevated, and one greater than 0.80 is abnormally elevated.

PRACTICE GUIDELINES

The 2005 American College of Cardiology/American Heart Association (ACC/AHA) Practice Guidelines on Peripheral Artery Disease include indications for duplex ultrasonography of renal arteries.[13]

ACCREDITATION

The Intersocietal Commission for Accreditation of Vascular Laboratories (ICAVL) maintains the standards for testing and accreditation of vascular laboratories. The standards for peripheral arterial testing are summarized in Table 8-2.[14]

REFERENCES

1. Morellato C, Bergelin RO, Cantwell-Gab K, et al. Clinical and duplex ultrasound follow-up after balloon angioplasty for atherosclerotic renal artery stenosis. *Vasc Surg.* 2001;35:85-93.

2. van Jaarsveld BC, Krijnen P, Pieterman H, et al. The effect of balloon angioplasty on hypertension in atherosclerotic renal-artery stenosis: Dutch Renal Artery Stenosis Intervention Cooperative Study Group. *N Engl J Med.* 2000;342:1007-1014.

3. Roussos L, Christensson A, Thompson O. A study on the outcome of percutaneous transluminal renal angioplasty in patients with renal failure. *Nephrol Clin Pract.* 2006;104:c132-c142.

4. Wong JM, Hansen KJ, Oskin TC, et al. Surgery after failed percutaneous renal artery angioplasty. *J Vasc Surg.* 1999;30:468-482.

5. Staub D, Canevascini R, Huegli RW, et al. Best duplex-sonographic criteria for the assessment of renal artery stenosis: correlation with intra-arterial pressure gradient. *Ultraschall Med.* 2007;28:45-51.

6. Kawarada O, Yokoi Y, Takemoto K, et al. The performance of renal duplex ultrasonography for the detection of hemodynamically significant renal artery stenosis. *Catheter Cardiovasc Interv.* 2006;68:311-318.

7. Hua HT, Hood DB, Jensen CC, et al. The use of color flow duplex scanning to detect significant renal artery stenosis. *Ann Vasc Surg.* 2000;14:118-124.

8. Krumme B, Hollenbeck M. Doppler sonography in renal artery stenosis: does the resistive index predict the success of intervention? *Nephrol Dial Transplant.* 2007; 22:692-696.

9. Radermacher J, Chavan A, Bleck J, et al. Use of Doppler ultrasonography to predict the outcome of therapy for renal artery stenosis. *N Engl J Med.* 2001; 344:410-417.

10. Voiculescu A, Schmitz M, Plum J, et al. Duplex ultrasound and renin ratio predict treatment failure after revascularization for renal artery stenosis. *Am J Hypertens.* 2006;19:756-763.

11. Garcia-Criado A, Gilabert R, Nicolau C, et al. Value of Doppler sonography for predicting clinical outcome after renal artery revascularization in atherosclerotic renal artery stenosis. *J Ultrasound Med.* 2005;24: 1641-1647.

12. Zeller T, Muller C, Frank U, et al. Stent angioplasty of severe atherosclerotic ostial renal artery stenosis in patients with diabetes mellitus and nephrosclerosis. *Catheter Cardiovasc Interv.* 2003;58:510-515.

13. Hirsch AT, Haskal ZJ, Hertzer NR, et al. ACC/AHA 2005 practice guidelines for the management of patients with peripheral arterial disease (lower extremity, renal, mesenteric, and abdominal aortic): executive summary. *J Am Coll Cardiol.* 2006;47:1239-1312.

14. Intersocietal Commission for Accreditation of Vascular Laboratories (ICAVL). The Complete ICAVL Standards for Accreditation in Noninvasive Vascular Testing. <http://www.icavl.org/icavl/Standards/2010_ICAVL_Standards.pdf>:Accessed April 20, 2010.

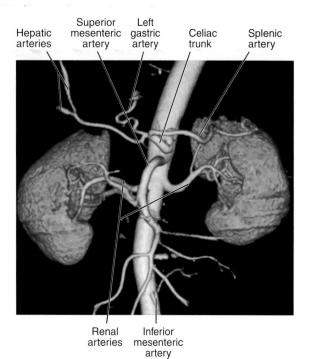

Hepatic arteries | Superior mesenteric artery | Left gastric artery | Celiac trunk | Splenic artery

Renal arteries | Inferior mesenteric artery

Figure 8-1. Volume-rendered surface-shaded computed tomography angiogram of the major branches of the abdominal aorta: renal, celiac, and superior mesenteric arteries. (Courtesy of Dr Nasir Khan, Chelsea & Westminster Hospital, London.)

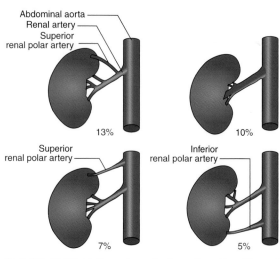

Abdominal aorta
Renal artery
Superior renal polar artery

13%

10%

Superior renal polar artery

Inferior renal polar artery

7%

5%

Figure 8-2. Variations in the number and patterns of branching of the renal artery (percentages are approximate). (From Standring S, ed. *Gray's Anatomy*. 40th ed. London: Elsevier; 2009; Fig. 74-10B; used with permission.)

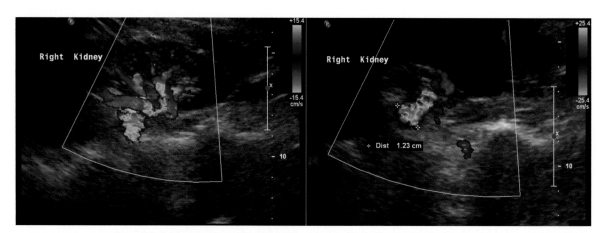

Figure 8-3. A 1.2-cm aneurysm of the distal right renal artery detected by color Doppler flow mapping.

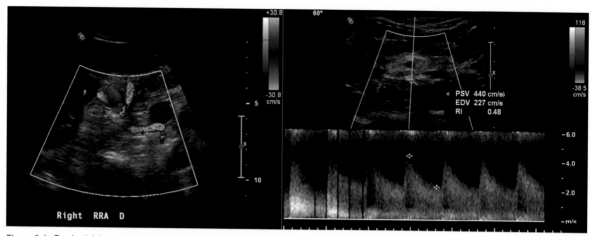

Figure 8-4. Proximal right renal artery stenosis. *Left,* Color Doppler flow mapping (patient in the decubitus position) depicts aliasing. *Right,* Spectral recording (patient in a supine position and aorta seen in short-axis view) reveals severely elevated systolic and diastolic velocities.

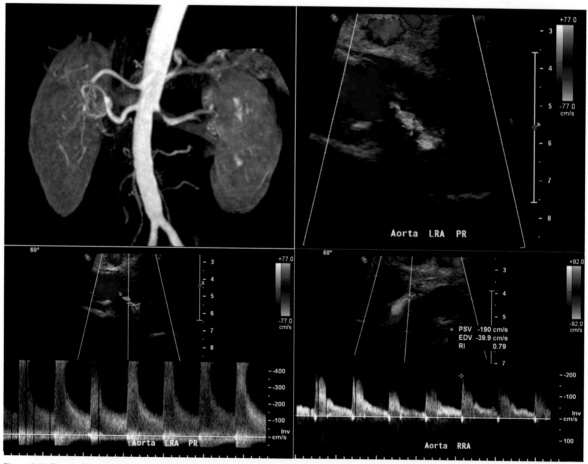

Figure 8-5. Renal artery stenosis resulting in secondary hypertension. *Top left,* The initial investigation, a magnetic resonance angiogram (MRA), is consistent with either a severe, a subtotal, or a short occlusion of the left renal artery. *Top right,* Color Doppler flow mapping depicts turbulent flow in the proximal left renal artery at the site of narrowing. *Bottom left,* Spectral display of flow in the proximal left renal artery, revealing severely elevated velocities. *Bottom right,* Spectral display of the proximal (lower) right renal artery, revealing normal flow velocities consistent with the normal appearance of color Doppler flow mapping and as well of the MRA. Note the superior right renal artery as seen on the MRA.

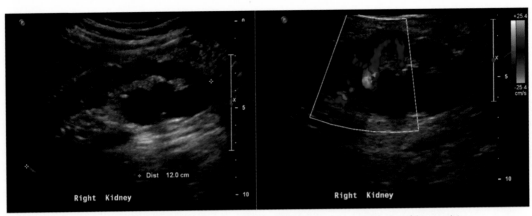

Figure 8-6. Polycystic kidney disease with enlargement of the kidney, cysts, and distortion of the vasculature.

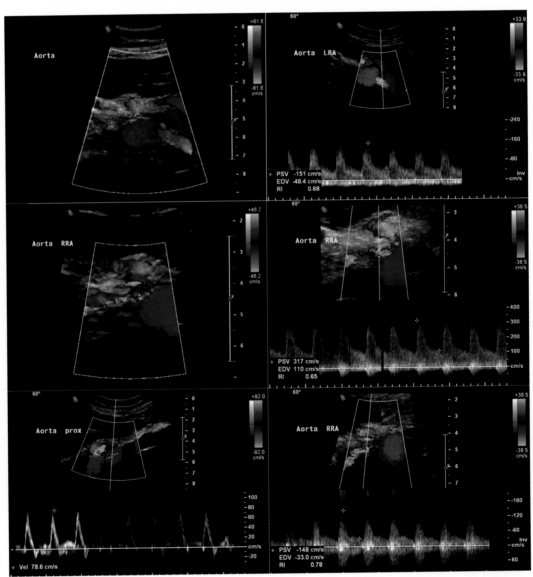

Figure 8-7. *Top left and right,* Normal color Doppler flow mapping of the left renal artery, and normal spectral Doppler flow velocity recordings. *Middle left,* Aliased flow in the proximal right renal artery. *Middle right,* Elevated systolic and diastolic flow velocities consistent with stenosis. *Bottom left and right,* Aortic reference flow yielding a renal-to-aortic ratio of 4.1 (with 3.5 the cutoff for greater than 60% stenosis).

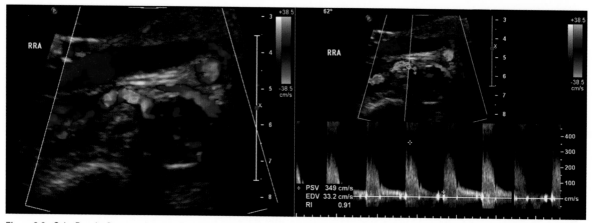

Figure 8-8. Color Doppler flow mapping revealing aliasing within the proximal right renal artery and spectral Doppler recording of elevated systolic velocities. The diastolic velocities are not proportionately elevated, consistent with elevated distal resistance (parenchymal/small vessel disease).

9

Splanchnic/Visceral Arteries

Key Points

■ Duplex ultrasound assessment of the splanchnic/visceral arteries, with careful technique and adherence to a comprehensive duplex protocol, is feasible and accurate in the majority of patients.

A therosclerotic aortic disease may result in stenosis of the origins to the celiac or to either of the mesenteric arteries. Most atherosclerotic disease of the splanchnic/mesenteric arteries occurs at the ostium and in the proximal segment. Disease, when present, commonly involves more than one vessel.

Anatomic variants of the splanchnic/mesenteric vessels occur. Anomalies such as a right hepatic artery arising from the superior mesenteric artery (SMA), a common hepatic artery arising from the SMA, or a common celiac-mesenteric trunk may be correctly recognized by ultrasound.[1]

Many patients with disease involving the splanchnic vessels are hypertensive because their aortas are extensively and severely diseased (resulting in noncompliance systolic hypertension). Concurrent, if not adjacent, renal artery stenosis may further incite hypertension. The greater the hypertension, the higher the PSV needed to establish severity of the splanchnic (or other) vessel stenosis by use of that criterion alone.

Use of PSV appears more useful than does end-diastolic velocity, which provides little additional information.[2] The use of both fasting and postprandial scanning offers little incremental information if the SMA PSV is greater than or equal to 275 cm/sec. Patients with symptoms of chronic visceral ischemia and positive duplex studies should be considered for confirmatory angiographic testing.[3] Duplex imaging also appears useful to follow surgical revascularization procedures (Figs. 9-1 to 9-6).[3]

ANATOMY OF THE SPLANCHNIC ARTERIES: THE CELIAC, SMA, AND IMA

The celiac artery (axis) is a 1.25-cm long stumpy artery arising from the anterior aspect of the aorta immediately below the diaphragm. It divides into the left gastric, splenic, and common hepatic arteries, which supply the spleen, liver, stomach, duodenum, and pancreas.

The SMA, a large artery, arises from the aorta approximately 1.25 cm distal to the celiac artery. This artery supplies the whole of the small intestine, cecum, the head of the pancreas, the ascending colon, and half of the transverse colon. The SMA lies behind the pancreas where the splenic vein crosses over its proximal segment and then courses downward and forward, crossing in front of the inferior vena cava, then diminishing in size to its terminus and anastomosis with one of its own branches, the ileal branch of the ileocolic artery. There are 12 to 15 branches that originate from the left side of the SMA; these divide and then anastomose with adjacent branches to form a series of arches supplying the small intestine.

The middle, right, and ileocolic arteries arise from the right side of the SMA. Of particular note is the middle colic artery, which forms an anastomosis with the left colic branch of the inferior mesenteric artery to create the marginal artery, an important collateral in the presence of celiac artery occlusive disease.

The inferior mesenteric artery is smaller than the SMA, arising from the anterior aspect of the aorta approximately 3 cm proximal to the aortic bifurcation at the level of the third lumbar vertebra. The inferior mesenteric artery supples the left half of the transverse colon, a greater part of the rectum, and the descending colon.

The inferior mesenteric artery lies anterior to the aorta and then runs downward on the left side, eventually crossing the left common iliac artery, after which it continues as the superior rectal hemorrhoidal artery. This important stem artery joins with other hemorrhoidal branches to provide a collateral network in cases of aortic obstruction.

Celiac Stenosis

Duplex scans are technically adequate in a very high percentage of celiac artery studies (96%); angiograms have a slightly higher technical adequacy rate (98%).[4] A less than 50% stenosis of the celiac artery is not readily detected by ultrasound scanning, and fortunately, is not likely directly a (flow-limiting) lesion (Table 9-1).[2,4-6]

Clinical Pearls

- It is important to note that portal venous flow is toward the probe, whereas that of the inferior vena cava and away from the liver.
- In the case of a high takeoff of the celiac axis, it is often possible to image/scan through the xiphisternum.
- To identify the celiac axis, look for the classic "seagull" sign, reminiscent of the body (axis) and wings (common hepatic arching to the right and then to the liver and the splenic artery arching left and onto the spleen). The axis itself can vary in its takeoff from the aorta (i.e., more lateral than anterior).
- If the superior mesenteric or celiac artery is severely diseased, there may be a compensatory increase in flow velocity in the other, and this could lead one to infer stenosis. Therefore, it is important to assess whether the identified flow velocity increase is focal or occurs throughout the vessel.
- Postprandial flow:
  - In the celiac artery, there is little variation postprandially because the metabolic needs of the liver and/or spleen are relatively stable.
  - The superior and inferior mesenteric artery flows change prominently postprandially; there can be a doubling of the peak systolic velocity (PSV) and a tripling of the diastolic flow in the celiac artery.
- In the abdomen, it can be relatively easy to inadvertently compress the veins being interrogated.
- The hepatic artery normally arises from the celiac axis, but it can occasionally arise from the proximal superior mesenteric artery, resulting in turbulent flow at the confluence of the two vessels. This can possibly lead to an erroneous diagnosis of narrowing.
- Median arcuate ligament compression: where a band of this ligament (that connects the two sides of the diaphragmatic crura) is caught around the celiac axis and can cause its compression, narrowing and increasing the flow velocity at that point. This occurs in 0% to 24% of people.[1] Because median arcuate ligament compression is most noticeable at the end of expiration, it is useful to instruct the patient to inspire deeply; this will temporarily release the band, and in doing so decrease the velocity, thus indicating that the process is not atherosclerotic.

Superior Mesenteric Artery Stenosis

Duplex scans are technically adequate in a very high percentage of SMA studies (98%). Angiograms have an 100% technical adequacy rate.[4]

A specific PSV cutoff for the determination of the presence of a significant stenosis of the SMA has been elusive, because hypertension is common in this patient population (Table 9-2).[2,4]

A positive determination of SMA stenosis by ultrasound is usually verified by another modality. A negative determination by ultrasound is unlikely to be disproven by other modalities (Figs. 9-7 to 9-12).

DUPLEX PROTOCOL FOR EVALUATION OF THE SPLANCHNIC/VISCERAL ARTERIES

Purpose

The objective is to identify the presence or absence of occlusive or aneurysmal disease of the celiac, superior mesenteric, and inferior mesenteric arteries.

Common Indications

- ❒ Upper abdominal bruit
- ❒ Stent surveillance
- ❒ Postprandial upper abdominal pain
- ❒ Suspected bowel ischemia

Equipment

- ❒ Color Duplex imaging system
- ❒ 1- to 5-MHz curved array transducer
- ❒ 2- to 4-MHz vector transducer
- ❒ Coupling gel
- ❒ Digital image acquisition

Procedure

- ❒ There is no preparation for patients with type 1 diabetes.
- ❒ Ensure that the patient has followed a bowel preparation regimen of:
  - A low-fat meal the night before
  - No carbonated drinks
  - No smoking the morning of the test
  - Clear fluids throughout with medication, where necessary
  - A bowl of clear flavored gelatin the morning of the test
- ❒ Explain the procedure to the patient and answer any questions.
- ❒ Obtain and document an applicable patient history.
- ❒ Verify that the procedure requested correlates with the patient's symptoms.
- ❒ Ascertain whether the patient is taking medication.
- ❒ Review any previous duplex studies available.
- ❒ Select appropriate test preset values.
- ❒ Select appropriate on-screen annotation throughout the test.
- ❒ Record images.
- ❒ Complete the technologist's preliminary report.

Technique

- ❒ The patient lies supine.
- ❒ The technologist stands or sits beside the patient.
- ❒ Gloves are worn by the technologist where there is a threat of contamination by infected body fluids.

Views

Standard recording sites are the aorta, celiac, superior mesenteric artery, and inferior mesenteric artery—to assess for significant stenosis, aneurysm, or anatomic

TABLE 9-1 Ultrasound Assessment of Celiac Stenosis

PARAMETER	REFERENCE	ANGIOGRAPHIC STANDARD	SENSITIVITY	SPECIFICITY	PPV	NPV
PSV ≥ 275 cm/sec	Mitchell[5]	≥70% Stenosis	92%		80%	99%
PSV ≥ 275 cm/sec or no flow	Moneta[2]		89%	92%	80%	
PSV ≥ 275 cm/sec	Gentile[6]	70%–99%				
Fasting			89%	97%	80%	99%
Postprandial			67%	94%	60%	91%
Fasting and postprandial			67%	100%	100	96%
PSV ≥ 275 cm/sec	Zwolak[4]	≥50%–100%	60%	100%		
EDV ≥ 275 cm/sec	Zwolak[4]		90%	91%	90%	91%

EDV, end diastolic velocity; NPV, negative predictive value; PPV, positive predictive value; PSV, peak systolic velocity.

TABLE 9-2 Ultrasound Assessment of Superior Mesenteric Artery Stenosis

PARAMETER	REFERENCE	ANGIOGRAPHIC STANDARD	SENSITIVITY	SPECIFICITY	PPV
PSV > 200 cm/sec or no flow	Moneta[2]	≥70%	75%	89%	85%
Retrograde common hepatic flow	Zwolak[4]	50%–100%	100%		
EDV ≥ 55 cm/sec or no flow	Zwolak[4]		93%	100%	
PSV ≥ 200 cm/sec or no flow	Zwolak[4]		93%	94%	

EDV, end diastolic velocity; PPV, positive predictive value; PSV, peak systolic velocity.

variant axis (e.g., median arcuate ligament, compression of the celiac artery). For the aorta, take short-axis and long-axis views, with grayscale and color Doppler, and spectral Doppler, looking for aneurysms, atherosclerotic plaque, thrombus, dissection, tortuosity, and anomalies. If necessary, turn the patient to the decubitus position for improved visualization of the aorta.

In addition, identify the celiac axis, and superior and inferior mesenteric arteries in grayscale, color Doppler, and spectral Doppler. Measure the PSV throughout using an angle of insonation of less than or equal to 60 degrees. Identify the splenic and common hepatic arteries.

Interpretation and Reporting
Celiac Axis

Normal
- ❏ No plaque visualized
- ❏ Laminar and forward flow throughout diastole
- ❏ PSV: 100 to 180 cm/sec (approximately)

Less Than 70% Stenosis
- ❏ Plaque visualized; variable and dependent on image quality

- ❏ PSV: less than 200 cm/sec
- ❏ Color Doppler evidence of focal and poststenotic turbulence

Greater Than 70% Stenosis
- ❏ Plaque visualized
- ❏ PSV: greater than 200 cm/sec
- ❏ Color Doppler evidence of focal and poststenotic turbulence

Occlusion
There is no flow.

Superior Mesenteric Artery

Normal
- ❏ No plaque visualized
- ❏ Laminar and forward flow throughout diastole
- ❏ PSV: 125 to 180 cm/sec (approximately)

Less Than 70% Stenosis
- ❏ Plaque visualized
- ❏ PSV: less than 275 cm/sec
- ❏ Color Doppler evidence of focal and poststenotic turbulence

TABLE 9-3   Ultrasound Criteria for the Detection of Severe IMA Stenosis

	SENSITIVITY	SPECIFICITY	PPV	NPV	ACCURACY
EDV >25 cm/sec	40%	91%	57%	83%	79%
Mesenteric-to-aortic PSV ratio	80%	88%	67%	93%	86%
PSV >200 cm/sec	90%	97%	90%	97%	95%

EDV, end diastolic velocity; NPV, negative predictive value; PPV, positive predictive value; PSV, peak systolic velocity.
From Pellerito JS, Revzin MV, Tsang JC, Greben CR, Naidich JB. Doppler sonographic criteria for the diagnosis of inferior mesenteric artery stenosis. *J Ultrasound Med.* 2009;28(5):641-650.

Greater Than 70% Stenosis
❑ PSV: greater than 275 cm/sec
❑ Color Doppler evidence of focal and poststenotic turbulence

Occlusion
No flow is detected.

Inferior Mesenteric Artery

Normal
❑ No plaque visualized
❑ Laminar and forward flow throughout diastole

Pressure-Reducing Stenosis (Greater Than 50% Stenosis)
❑ Plaque visualized
❑ Color Doppler evidence of focal and poststenotic turbulence
❑ Velocity ratio greater than 2

Occlusion
No flow is detected.

Proposed ultrasound criteria for the detection of severe inferior mesenteric artery stenosis are presented in Table 9-3.

PRACTICE GUIDELINES

The 2005 American College of Cardiology/American Heart Association (ACC/AHA) Practice Guidelines on Peripheral Artery Disease include indications for duplex ultrasonography of the splanchnic, mesenteric, and visceral arteries.[7]

Acute Nonocclusive Intestinal Ischemia
Etiology: Recommendations—Class I
1. Nonocclusive intestinal ischemia should be suspected in patients with low flow states or shock, especially cardiogenic shock, who develop abdominal pain. *(Level of Evidence: B)*
2. Nonocclusive intestinal ischemia should be suspected in patients receiving vasoconstrictor substances and medications (e.g., cocaine, ergots, vasopressin, or norepinephrine) who develop abdominal pain. *(Level of Evidence: B)*
3. Nonocclusive intestinal ischemia should be suspected in patients who develop abdominal pain after coarctation repair or after surgical revascularization for intestinal ischemia caused by arterial obstruction. *(Level of Evidence: B)*

Diagnosis: Recommendations—Class I
1. Chronic intestinal ischemia should be suspected in patients with abdominal pain and weight loss without other explanation, especially those with cardiovascular disease. *(Level of Evidence: B)*
2. Duplex ultrasound, computed tomography angiography, and gadolinium-enhanced magnetic resonance angiography are useful initial tests for supporting the clinical diagnosis of chronic intestinal ischemia. *(Level of Evidence: B)*
3. Diagnostic angiography, including lateral aortography, should be obtained in patients suspected of having chronic intestinal ischemia for whom noninvasive imaging is unavailable or indeterminate. *(Level of Evidence: B)*
4. Arteriography is indicated in patients suspected of having nonocclusive intestinal ischemia whose condition does not improve rapidly with treatment of their underlying disease. *(Level of Evidence: B)*

Interventional Treatment: Recommendation—Class I
Percutaneous endovascular treatment of intestinal arterial stenosis is indicated in patients with chronic intestinal ischemia. *(Level of Evidence: B)*

Surgical Treatment: Recommendations

Class I
Surgical treatment of chronic intestinal ischemia is indicated in patients with chronic intestinal ischemia. *(Level of Evidence: B)*

Class IIb
Revascularization of asymptomatic intestinal arterial obstructions may be considered for patients undergoing aortic/renal artery surgery for other indications. *(Level of Evidence: B)*

Class III

Surgical revascularization is not indicated for patients with asymptomatic intestinal arterial obstructions, except in patients undergoing aortic/renal artery surgery for other indications. *(Level of Evidence: B)*

Visceral Artery Aneurysms: Recommendations

Class I

Open repair or catheter-based intervention is indicated for visceral aneurysms measuring 2.0 cm in diameter or larger in women of childbearing age who are not pregnant and in patients of either gender undergoing liver transplantation. *(Level of Evidence: B)*

Class IIa

Open repair or catheter-based intervention is probably indicated for visceral aneurysms 2.0 cm in diameter or larger in women beyond childbearing age and in men. *(Level of Evidence: B)*

ACCREDITATION

The 2007 Intersocietal Commission for Accreditation of Vascular Laboratories (ICAVL) Standards for accreditation in visceral vascular testing are summarized below[8]:

- ❐ The entire course of the accessible portions of each visceral vessel should be examined.
- ❐ Limited examinations may occur for an appropriate or recurring indication. The reason for a limited examination must be documented.
- ❐ Visceral vascular examinations must include standard components that provide sufficient documentation for interpretation.
- ❐ A written protocol must be in place that defines the extent of the study, the components and documentation of the complete examination. The protocol should also describe how color-coded Doppler is utilized to supplement grayscale imaging and spectral Doppler. If other flow imaging modes (e.g., power Doppler) are used, the protocol should describe how they are utilized.
- ❐ The entire course of the accessible portions of each visceral vessel should be examined. Representative grayscale, spectral Doppler, and/or color Doppler images from the following vessel groups must be documented as required by the protocol. Abnormalities require additional images that demonstrate the type and severity of the abnormality present. In the mesenteric arterial system, it is necessary to image the:
  - Adjacent aorta
  - Celiac artery
  - Superior mesenteric artery
  - Inferior mesenteric artery
- ❐ Abnormalities require additional images that demonstrate the type and severity of the abnormality

present. Documentation of areas of suspected stenosis must include representative waveforms recorded at and distal to the stenosis.

- ❐ Interpretation of the visceral vascular duplex examination must use validated diagnostic criteria to assess the presence of disease, and to document its location, etiology, extent, and severity.
- ❐ Diagnostic criteria must be laboratory specific and documented.
- ❐ There must be criteria for interpretation of grayscale images; spectral Doppler; and when utilized, plaque morphology and color-coded Doppler images specific for each examination performed.
- ❐ The findings generate an interpretation and report that indicates the absence or presence of abnormalities in the vessels that were investigated. Disease, if present, must be characterized according to its location, etiology, extent, and severity.
- ❐ In general, a laboratory should perform a minimum of 100 complete splanchnic examinations annually.
- ❐ Results of visceral vascular duplex examinations must be regularly correlated with angiographic or surgical findings.
- ❐ The laboratory must have a written procedure for regular correlation of visceral vascular examinations with angiographic findings produced by digital subtraction arteriography, contrast-enhanced computed tomography, or magnetic resonance angiography. The correlation must be reported using the categories of stenosis and/or disease defined by the diagnostic criteria utilized by the laboratory. Surgical correlations may be used when angiographic correlation is not available.
- ❐ A minimum of 15 patient examinations are to be correlated. These correlations must reflect a mix of all vessel groups performed by the laboratory and have been completed within the three years preceding submission of the application.
- ❐ The correlation matrix should demonstrate greater than 70% agreement.

REFERENCES

1. Horton KM, Talamini MA, Fishman EK. Median arcuate ligament syndrome: evaluation with CT angiography. *RadioGraphics.* 2005;25:1177-1182.
2. Moneta GL, Yeager RA, Dalman R, Antonovic R, Hall LD, Porter JM. Duplex ultrasound criteria for diagnosis of splanchnic artery stenosis or occlusion. *J Vasc Surg.* 1991;14(4):511-518.
3. Moneta GL. Screening for mesenteric vascular insufficiency and follow-up of mesenteric artery bypass procedures. *Semin Vasc Surg.* 2001;14(3):186-192.
4. Zwolak RM, Fillinger MF, Walsh DB, et al. Mesenteric and celiac duplex scanning: a validation study. *J Vasc Surg.* 1998;27(6):1078-1087.
5. Mitchell EL, Moneta GL. Mesenteric duplex scanning. *Perspect Vasc Surg Endovasc Ther.* 2006;18(2):175-183.

6. Gentile AT, Moneta GL, Lee RW, Masser PA, Taylor Jr LM, Porter JM. Usefulness of fasting and postprandial duplex ultrasound examinations for predicting high-grade superior mesenteric artery stenosis. *Am J Surg.* 1995;169(5):476-479.

7. Hirsch AT, Haskal ZJ, Hertzer NR, et al. ACC/AHA 2005 practice guidelines for the management of patients with peripheral arterial disease (lower extremity, renal, mesenteric, and abdominal aortic): executive summary. *Circulation.* 2006:1474-1547.

8. Intersocietal Commission for Accreditation of Vascular Laboratories (ICAVL). ICAVL Standards. <http://www.icavl.org/icavl/main/standards.htm>: Accessed March 26, 2009.

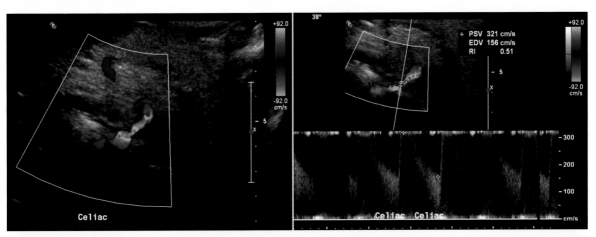

Figure 9-1. Significant stenosis of the ostium of the celiac artery localized by the color Doppler flow mapping and demonstrated by the severely elevated velocities, of which the systolic velocity exceeds the selected scale. Note, as the pulse repetition frequency is reduced to decrease the color aliasing, the aorta is rendered invisible.

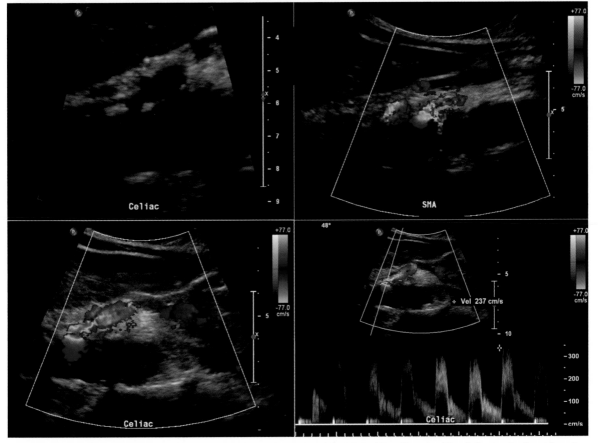

Figure 9-2. Grayscale imaging establishes the presence of plaque and narrowing of the ostium of the celiac artery. There is flow acceleration at the ostium of the superior mesenteric and celiac arteries. The flow velocity is significantly elevated, consistent with a hemodynamically relevant stenosis.

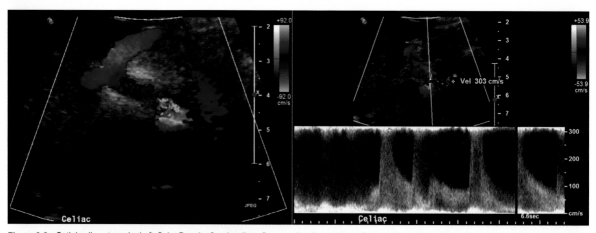

Figure 9-3. Ostial celiac stenosis. *Left,* Color Doppler flow localizes flow acceleration and turbulence at the ostium of the celiac artery and depicts the typical ("seagull") branching pattern of the celiac axis (common hepatic) and splenic artery. *Right,* The spectral display establishes significant increase of the systolic flow velocity consistent with hemodynamically significant stenosis. The true peak of the systolic velocity is unknown, given the selected scale.

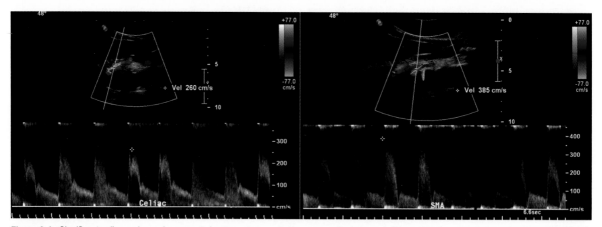

Figure 9-4. Significant celiac and superior mesenteric artery stenoses in the same patient shown in Figure 9-3. Concurrent visceral artery ostial stenosis is common.

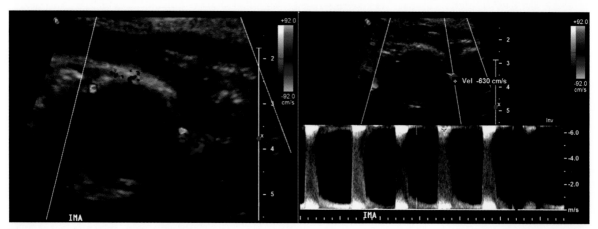

Figure 9-5. Significant stenosis of the ostium of the inferior mesenteric artery (IMA). Color Doppler flow mapping localizes turbulence at the ostium of the IMA, and the spectral Doppler sampling establishes the presence of significant flow acceleration consistent with stenosis.

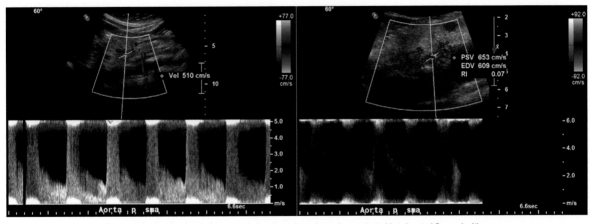

Figure 9-6. Proximal superior mesenteric artery stenosis as demonstrated by elevated flow velocities.

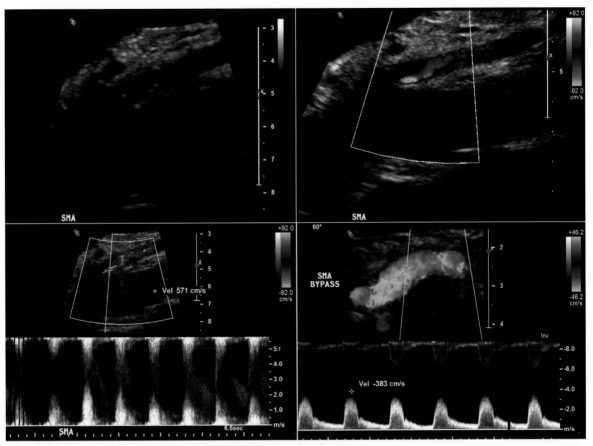

Figure 9-7. Superior mesenteric artery (SMA) stenosis and bypass graft. *Top left,* Plaque at the origin of the celiac and the superior mesenteric arteries. *Top right,* Turbulent flow at the proximal SMA within a narrowed channel of flow. *Bottom left,* Spectral display of markedly elevated flow velocities in the proximal SMA. *Bottom right,* Color flow mapping and spectral display of flow within an SMA bypass graft.

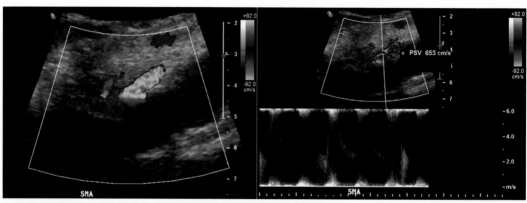

Figure 9-8. Color Doppler flow mapping depicts flow acceleration and turbulence at the ostium of the superior mesenteric artery, and the spectral display of the flow velocity establishes severely elevated velocities consistent with significant stenosis.

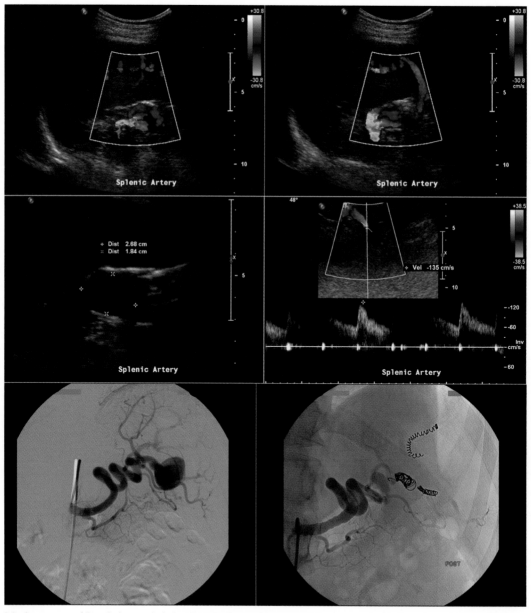

Figure 9-9. An aneurysm of the splenic artery is depicted by color Doppler flow mapping and seen on the grayscale imaging (*top left and right, middle left and right*). The flow velocities through the arteries are normal. Selective angiography confirming the aneurysm before (*bottom left*) and after coil embolization (*bottom right*).

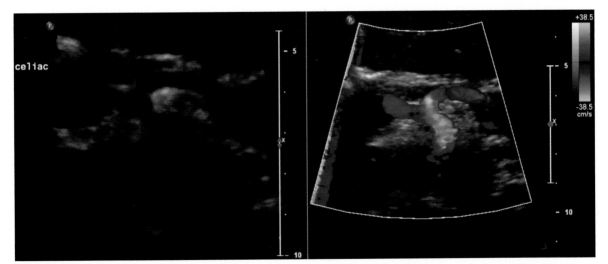

Figure 9-10. Color Doppler flow mapping depicts flow and turbulence, although imperfectly seen, in the proximal superior mesenteric artery. The spectral display of the flow velocity establishes severely elevated velocities consistent with significant stenosis. The spectral recording is clearer than the grayscale and color Doppler images.

Figure 9-11. Grayscale (*left*) and color Doppler flow mapping (*right*) of the distinctive "seagull" shape of the celiac artery trunk branching.

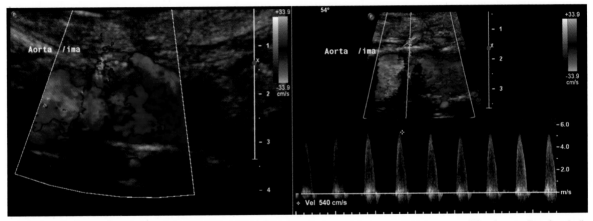

Figure 9-12. Inferior mesenteric artery ostial stenosis suggested by color Doppler flow mapping and confirmed by spectral Doppler recording of markedly elevated systolic flow velocities.

10 Venous Disease of the Upper Extremity

Key Points

- Knowledge of normal and variant anatomy of the upper extremity venous vasculature is critical.
- A standardized and comprehensive duplex examination protocol is critical.
- Knowledge of possible diseases/lesions potentially within the upper extremity venous vasculature, and how to maximize their recognition, is critical.

VENOUS ANATOMY OF THE UPPER EXTREMITY

The veins of the neck, which drain blood from the face and head, consist of the anterior jugular vein, the posterior external jugular vein, and the external jugular and internal jugular veins. However, only the internal and the external jugular veins are clearly seen on a typical duplex scan of the neck.

The external jugular vein drains blood primarily from the scalp and face. It contains two valves in the lower portion and runs superficially in the neck parallel to the posterior border of the sternomastoid muscle to terminate in the subclavian vein. No artery accompanies the external jugular vein. The external jugular vein's size (in the absence of disease) varies inversely in size with that of its internal jugular vein.

The internal jugular vein receives blood from the deep structures of the neck and the brain. It contains two valves, which may or may not prevent regurgitation, 2.5 cm above its terminus. The internal jugular vein runs down in the neck lateral, first to the internal carotid and then the common carotid artery. On the right side, the internal jugular vein crosses the first segment of the subclavian artery and joins the subclavian vein to form the right innominate vein.

The left internal jugular vein, which is usually smaller in caliber than the right internal jugular vein, crosses the common carotid artery before joining the left subclavian vein to form the left innominate vein, which then crosses the innominate artery to form, together with the right innominate vein, the superior vena cava.

The left and right vertebral veins drain blood from the muscles of the neck.

Several veins from the chest wall (the thoracodorsal vein, lateral thoracic vein, pectoral branch of the thoracoacromial vein, and subscapular vein) join the axillary vein between receiving the brachial and cephalic veins. All these veins may play an important role in supplying collateral flow in the presence of subclavian and axillary vein thrombosis.

A study of 127 arm venograms revealed that as a result of the ability of these chest wall veins to reverse flow if required, axillary vein thrombosis was commonly associated with chest wall collateral pathways. The study has demonstrated that subclavian thrombosis was most often bypassed by neck veins, especially by venous arches that connect the left and right external jugular veins.[1]

There are both deep and superficial dorsal and volar veins of the hand. The superficial veins connect via a network of interlacing branches to eventually form the dorsal venous network on the back of the hand. Digital veins extend from a venous plexus on the volar aspect of the hand. The deep and superficial arterial arches of the hand are flanked by the venae comitantes, which form the superficial and deep venous volar arches.

The cephalic vein, a long superficial vein, runs from the lateral aspect of the wrist and continues up to the shoulder to join the axillary vein just below the clavicle, where it is known as the cephalic arch. An accessory cephalic vein arises variably from segments along the main cephalic vein rejoining more proximally. A common anatomic variant is dominance of the upper arm basilic vein, with one or two diminutive cephalic veins.

The median cubital vein connects the cephalic vein just below the elbow with the basilic vein above the elbow. Occasionally, the median antebrachial vein, which drains the palmar aspect of the hand, courses along the ulnar side of the forearm and drains into the basilic vein. The median antebrachial vein may form the median cubital vein or divide and send a branch each to the cephalic and basilic veins, supplanting the median cubital.

On the medial aspect of the wrist arises the basilic vein, another superficial vessel, which courses up the posterior aspect of the ulnar side of the forearm, receives the median cubital vein slightly above the

Clinical Pearls

- During scanning of the subclavian vein, have the patient take a "sniff" breath to collapse the vein, because manual compression of the vein by the transducer is not possible due to the overlying clavicle.
- Scan the subclavian and innominate vein from the head of patient because this affords better opportunity for maximum downward angulation and maneuverability of the transducer.
- When scanning the axillary vein within the axilla, raise the patient's arm and rest it on the bed at 90 degrees to the body, so that the vein can be followed along its course into the subclavian segment.
- To establish the location of the proximal subclavian vein on either side, it is useful to scan down from the internal jugular vein and slide into the confluence with the innominate vein, on both sides.
- When vein mapping before upper extremity arteriovenous fistula creation, consider placing the patient in a steep reverse Trendelenburg (head up) to pool blood in the forearm veins and distend the veins—and in the supine position to scan the subclavian and axillary veins.
- Use sufficient gel to enable the transducer probe to be offset from the skin to avoid compression of such veins, so that their measurements are true.

elbow, and crosses the brachial artery to run along the medial border of the biceps. The basilic vein then joins one of the brachial veins (often on the medial side) to form the axillary vein.

The radial and ulnar veins are the venae comitantes of the arteries in the forearm, with the radial vein usually the smaller of the two. These are the continuation of the deep and superficial volar arches, uniting at the elbow to form the brachial veins.

The deep veins of the forearm anastomose freely with both each other and with the superficial veins.

VENOUS THROMBOSIS OF THE UPPER EXTREMITY

Venous thrombosis within the upper extremities may occur as a result of trauma, line insertion, pacemaker/implantable cardioverter defibrillator (ICD) insertion, pericardial constriction, or thrombophilia.

DUPLEX EVALUATION OF THE UPPER EXTREMITY VEINS

Purpose
- ❑ To demonstrate the presence or absence of partial or complete venous obstruction caused by either venous thrombosis or extrinsic compression
- ❑ To identify other abnormalities recognizable by ultrasound that may be related to the patient's

symptoms (e.g., enlarged and ± compressive lymph nodes, abnormal fluid collection such as a hematoma or abscess, or an abnormal ± compressive solid mass)

Common Indications and Contraindications
Indications
- ❑ Arm swelling
- ❑ Arm redness
- ❑ Palpable cord

Contraindications
- ❑ Presence of wound dressings
- ❑ Open wounds

Equipment
- ❑ Color duplex imaging system
- ❑ Higher frequency (e.g., 5- to 17-Hz) linear transducer for superficial imaging
- ❑ Medium frequency (e.g., 3- to 9-Hz) linear transducer for deeper imaging
- ❑ Lower frequency (e.g., 2- to 5-Hz) sector/curved array transducer for deep coupling gel
- ❑ Digital reporting

Procedure
- ❑ Explain procedure to the patient and answer any questions.
- ❑ Obtain and document applicable patient history on appropriate forms.
- ❑ Verify that the procedure requested correlates with the patient's symptoms.
- ❑ Obtain an appropriate history. Consider the following questions:
  - Is there a history of deep vein thrombosis (DVT)?
  - Is there a history of peripheral or central venous line insertion or of pacemaker or ICD insertion?
  - Is there a history of trauma?
  - Is there a recognized thrombophilia?
- ❑ Perform a limited physical examination of the limbs in question, looking for venous distention, swelling, or a palpable cord.
- ❑ Review any previous duplex studies available.
- ❑ Set up the duplex examination:
  - Select appropriate venous extremity menus and settings.
  - Select annotation menus that are appropriate for the examination.
- ❑ Record images.
- ❑ Complete the technologist's preliminary report when necessary.

Technique
- ❑ The patient lies supine with the head flat on a pillow.
- ❑ The scan is performed from the side and/or top of the bed.

- ❑ If the patient is symptomatic on one side, the internal jugular vein/subclavian vein on the contralateral side is included.
- ❑ The patient lies supine with the head flat on a pillow to scan the subclavian and axillary veins and in the reverse Trendelenburg (head raised 45 degrees) to scan the remainder of the arm veins.
- ❑ As with usual venous scanning technique, transverse views (the order chosen at the technologist's discretion) are used to follow the anatomy of the venous system distally, and to establish the presence or absence of intraluminal material/noncompressibility. Longitudinal views are used with color Doppler imaging and spectral display of pulsed-wave Doppler interrogation to depict flow, partial obstruction, or complete obstruction.
- ❑ The following veins are interrogated (Table 10-1):
  - Internal jugular vein
  - Subclavian vein
  - Axillary vein
  - Brachial vein
  - Basilic vein
  - Cephalic vein
  - Paired veins (radial and ulnar) if the local area is symptomatic

Additional Scanning Information

To optimally scan the internal jugular vein, the patient's head is turned slightly away from the side being examined. The vein is scanned in an anterolateral plane from the base of the neck to the angle of the mandible. It is seen to lie just superficial to the carotid artery. In the transverse plane, the internal jugular vein can be compressed with minimal probe pressure, but if compression is difficult and yet no intraluminal echoes are seen, compression may be facilitated by scanning with patient sitting up (thereby reducing venous distending pressure). The patient's arm is then supinated and abducted slightly.

The subclavian vein in its distal and mid-segments can be scanned subclavicularly via an anterior approach. The proximal subclavian vein and the innominate/brachiocephalic vein can be imaged by angling caudad toward the sternal notch.

In the presence of subclavian venous thrombosis, large collaterals may develop. It may be difficult to identify the subclavian vein by duplex scanning. Visualization of the accompanying subclavian artery may assist in locating the subclavian vein. Transverse views are used to identify the subclavian vein (and others), to follow along its length, to assess for intraluminal echoes consistent with thrombus, and to observe for compressibility.

With deep inspiration, the subclavian vein may normally collapse.

To scan the axillary vein, with the patient's arm bent 90 degrees and raised toward the head, it is necessary to scan with compression, in transverse profile, and using pulsed Doppler and color flow mapping in

TABLE 10-1	Upper Extremity Venous Duplex Protocol	
ANATOMIC SEGMENT	**TECHNIQUE**	**DUPLEX MODALITY**
Internal jugular vein	SAX sweep	Grayscale
	LAX sweep	Grayscale, color/spectral Doppler
Subclavian vein	LAX sweep Distal Mid Proximal	Grayscale, color/spectral Doppler
Axillary vein	SAX sweep With/without compression in axilla	Grayscale
	LAX sweep Distal Mid Proximal	Grayscale, color/spectral Doppler
*Basilic vein (upper arm)	SAX sweep With/without compression	Grayscale
	LAX sweep Distal Mid Proximal	Grayscale, color/spectral Doppler
Brachial veins	SAX sweep With/without compression	Grayscale
	LAX sweep Distal Mid Proximal	Grayscale, color/spectral Doppler
*Cephalic vein (upper arm)	SAX sweep With/without compression	Grayscale
	LAX sweep Distal Mid Proximal	Grayscale, color/spectral Doppler

*If symptoms involve the distal arm, the forearm basilic and cephalic veins may be scanned.
LAX, long-axis; SAX, short-axis.

the sagittal plane. The patient's arm is then lowered to its original position and rotated externally to scan the remainder of the veins in transverse and sagittal planes using flow parameters as described in the lower extremity protocol. From the axilla, the basilic and brachial veins can be imaged along the medial aspect of the upper arm.

The cephalic vein, the median cubital vein (if present), the basilic vein, and the paired veins are scanned distally. The radial and ulnar veins are interrogated only when they lie within the symptomatic area.

The left and right vertebral veins drain blood from the muscles of the neck and after being joined by the deep cervical and anterior vertebral vein, drain into the brachiocephalic vein. Major collateral pathways in the neck involve anterior, posterior, and internal venous plexuses, but flow reversal can be seen in the vertebral vein when intrathoracic pressure increases (e.g., during a Valsalva maneuver).

Signs of Deep Vein Thrombosis
Noncompressibility
The venous system is normally distended under low pressure and therefore, veins can be compressed easily with very little pressure from the transducer. With venous thrombosis, the presence of intraluminal thrombus material renders the vein incompletely compressible or noncompressible. Compression maneuvers are best performed in transverse imaging because it can be assured that the plane of imaging is not moving off to the side of the vessel, giving a false impression of compressibility as may happen with imaging along the longitudinal plane of the vessel. Generally, soft tissue material within the vessel is seen at sites of noncompressibility. Compression maneuvers should be performed at the following sites:

- Internal jugular vein
- Subclavian vein
- Axillary vein
- Brachial vein
- Cephalic vein
- Basilic vein

Flow Obstruction
Normally, flow velocity in the veins exhibits spontaneous variation according to the phase of the respiratory cycle and in proportion to respiratory effort. As well, normally, abrupt compression of a muscle bed distally to a site of sampling results in a surge of blood through the vein. With complete obstruction to flow by DVT, the signs of spontaneity, phasicity, and augmentation are lost. With partial obstruction, these signs are attenuated. Therefore, flow signs corroborate some cases of DVT; however, from a diagnostic and therapeutic standpoint, there is no difference between occlusive and nonocclusive DVT.

ACCREDITATION

The Intersocietal Commission for Accreditation of Vascular Laboratories (ICAVL) summary points for upper extremity venous testing are:[2]
- Grayscale imaging in long-axis and short-axis views to assess anatomy and lesions and color Doppler and spectral Doppler to assess physiology are to be used.
- Written disease-specific protocols are required.
- Examinations are to be in accordance with protocols.
- Indications are to be recorded.
- Examinations are to be comprehensive and documented comprehensively.
- Representative grayscale, grayscale color Doppler, and spectral Doppler waveforms to show respiratory variation/manual augmentation of the following are to be obtained:
  - Internal jugular vein
  - Subclavian vein
  - Axillary vein
  - Brachial veins
  - Basilic vein
  - Cephalic vein
- If a unilateral study is performed, a contralateral subclavian vein spectral waveform must be documented.
- When appropriate or as required by the laboratory's written protocol, further examination and recording is to be performed.
- Diagnostic criteria must be laboratory specific and documented.
- In general, a laboratory should perform a minimum of 100 complete (upper and lower) examinations annually.
- Records must be maintained that permit evaluation of annual procedure volumes. These records must include information on the indication, test(s) performed, and the findings.
- The laboratory must have a written procedure for regular correlation of venous duplex examinations. These correlations must reflect a mix of upper and lower extremities as performed by the laboratory.
- Documentation of correlation must be maintained.

REFERENCES

1. Richard HM, Selby JB, Gay SB, Tegtmeyer CJ. Normal venous anatomy and collateral pathways in upper extremity venous thrombosis. *RadioGraphics*. 1992;12: 527-534.
2. Intersocietal Commission for the Accreditation of Vascular Laboratories (ICAVL). ICAVL standards. <http://www.icavl.org/icavl/main/standards.htm>; Accessed March 26, 2009.

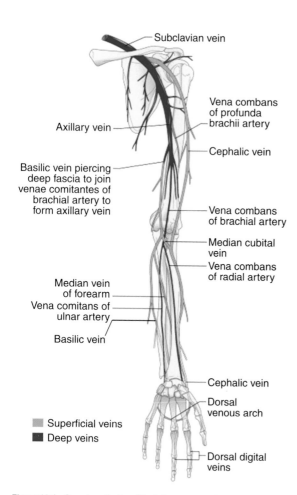

Subclavian vein

Axillary vein

Vena combans of profunda brachii artery

Cephalic vein

Basilic vein piercing deep fascia to join venae comitantes of brachial artery to form axillary vein

Vena combans of brachial artery

Median cubital vein

Vena combans of radial artery

Median vein of forearm

Vena comitans of ulnar artery

Basilic vein

Cephalic vein

Dorsal venous arch

Superficial veins
Deep veins

Dorsal digital veins

Figure 10-1. Overview of veins of the left upper extremity. (From Standring S. *Gray's Anatomy*. 40th ed. Philadelphia: Elsevier; 2009; Fig. 45-5; used with permission.)

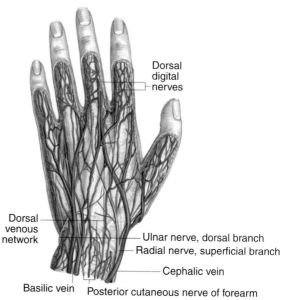

Dorsal digital nerves

Dorsal venous network

Ulnar nerve, dorsal branch

Radial nerve, superficial branch

Cephalic vein

Basilic vein

Posterior cutaneous nerve of forearm

Figure 10-2. The veins of the dorsum of the hand. (From Standring S. *Gray's Anatomy*. 40th ed. Philadelphia: Elsevier; 2009; Fig. 50-44; used with permission.)

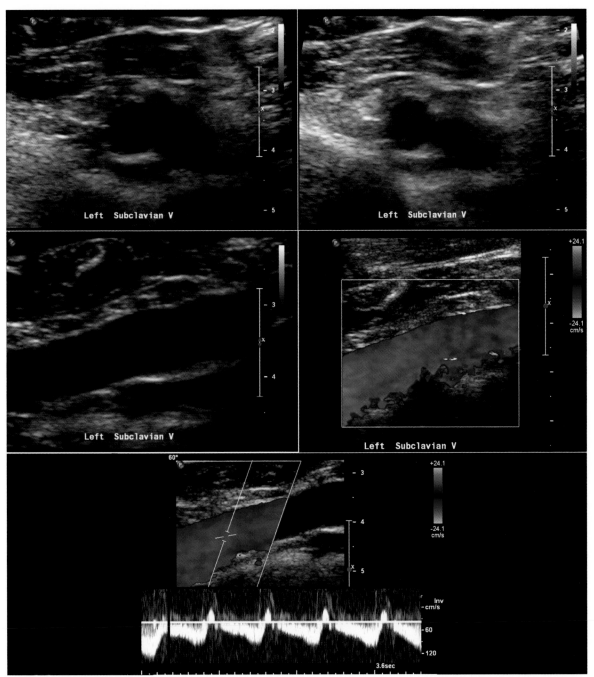

Figure 10-3. Duplex examination of the subclavian vein. *Top,* The images depict the subclavian vein in cross-section, with the top right image demonstrating partial compressibility of the subclavian vein (compressibility of the subclavian vein is variable). *Middle left and right,* Subclavian vein in its long axis. No echogenic material is seen within the lumen of the subclavian vein, and color Doppler flow mapping depicts flow filling the lumen. The color Doppler gain settings have resulted in blooming of the color Doppler signal into the adjacent subtissue. *Bottom,* The spectral display of pulse Doppler recording from within the subclavian vein. Typically, there is a phasic pattern to the venous flow due to the effects of the cardiac cycle and some respiratory variation. No respiration has taken place during the period of this recording because there is no inspiratory augmentation of flow velocities. Subclavian flow patterns are variable depending on cardiac and respiratory function and dysfunction. There is a superimposed faint Doppler signal from the adjacent subclavian artery of oppositely directed flow.

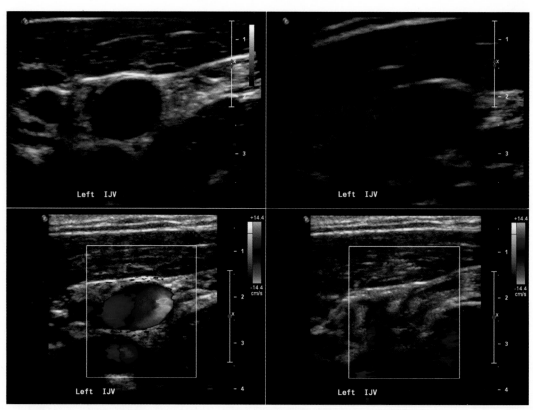

Figure 10-4. Duplex interrogation of the internal jugular vein in cross-section. *Top left and right,* Internal jugular vein in cross-section overlying the deeper carotid artery, with the top right image depicting uncertain compressibility of the internal jugular vein. In general, there is little need to compress the internal jugular vein because its imageability is good. *Bottom left and right,* Color Doppler flow mapping, which corroborates the compressibility of the vein. With compression (*bottom right*), neither lumen nor flow are depicted. No intraluminal echogenic material is present.

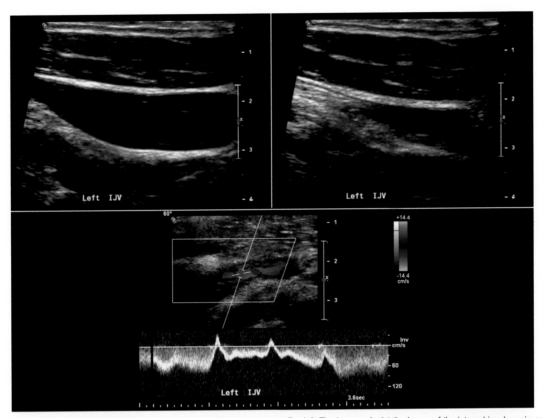

Figure 10-5. Duplex interrogation of the internal jugular vein in long-axis view. *Top left,* The images depict the lumen of the internal jugular vein and the absence of the echogenic material within the lumen. However, there are reverberation artefacts, which mildly contaminate the appearance of the lumen. *Top right,*The image reveals compressibility of the internal jugular vein, although transverse imaging depiction of compression is more reliable. *Bottom,* The image depicts the spectral Doppler flow display from within the internal jugular vein. There is phasicity due to the effect of the cardiac cycle and also augmentation due to inspiration.

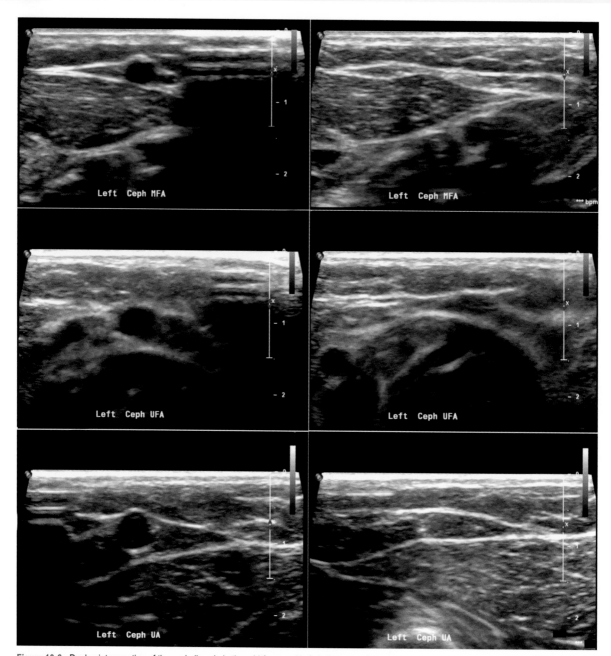

Figure 10-6. Duplex interrogation of the cephalic vein in the mid-forearm (*top*), in the upper forearm (*middle*), and in the upper arm (*lower*). The vessel is imaged in its transverse plane without compression (*left*) and with compression (*right*). Many upper extremity venous studies to detect thrombosis stop at the elbow; this study was performed for venous mapping.

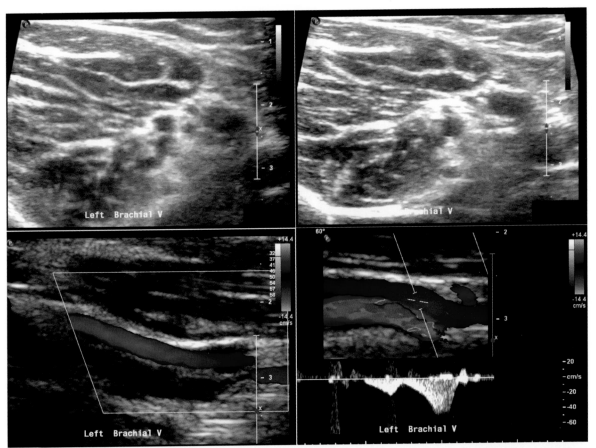

Figure 10-7. Duplex interrogation of the brachial veins. *Top left,* The images depict the brachial artery and adjacent brachial veins in cross-section. *Top right,* The image reveals compressibility of the brachial veins. *Bottom left,* The image depicts flow filling the lumen of one of the brachial veins. *Bottom right,* The image depicts the spectral display of pulsed-wave interrogation. There is phasicity to the flow and augmentation due to squeezing the forearm of the side being sampled. Note that the basilic vein on the right side of the image is not compressed, which would probably require a different compression plane.

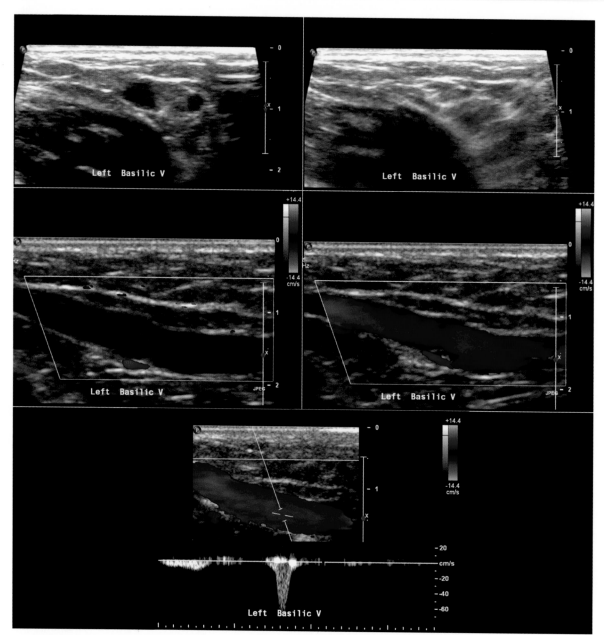

Figure 10-8. *Top,* Duplex interrogation of the basilic vein in transverse axis without (*left*) and with compression (*right*). There is full compressibility of the basilic vein. *Middle,* The images depict the basilic vein in its longitudinal access. No intraluminal soft tissue is seen, and flow is depicted by color Doppler flow mapping throughout entire lumen. *Bottom,* The image depicts the spectral display from pulsed Doppler sampling. Augmentation has been achieved by compression of the forearm. The basilic vein drains into the brachial vein at variable level in the upper arm.

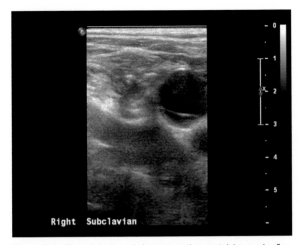

Figure 10-9. The subclavian vein in cross-section, containing a valve flap.

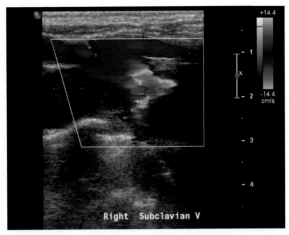

Figure 10-10. Thrombosis of the subclavian vein. Intraluminal soft tissue material consistent with thrombus is seen filling the subclavian vein across the left side of the image. Color Doppler flow mapping corroborates the absence of flow, coinciding with the observed thrombus.

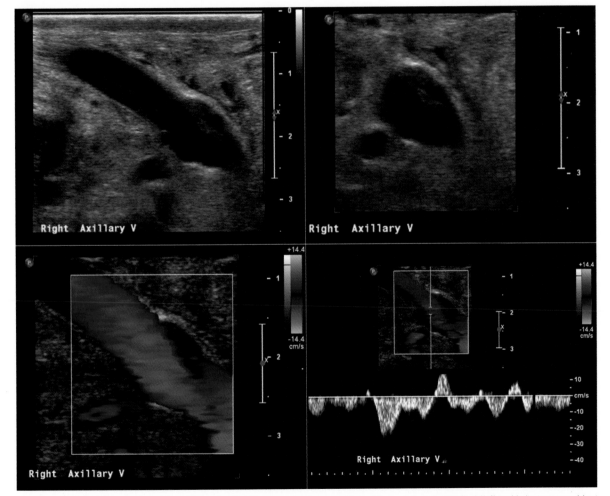

Figure 10-11. Duplex interrogation of the axillary vein. *Top,* The upper images reveal the axillary vein in its longitudinal (*left*) and in its transverse/short axis (*right*). Intraluminal echogenic material is seen involving part of the lumen. As well, there is a long linear structure along the length of the vessel, with a nonocclusive residual thrombus, and a cast from a prior central line. *Bottom left,* The image reveals flow within the lumen except at the site of the observed soft tissue as seen in the corresponding image above. *Bottom right,* Spectral display of pulse Doppler sampling reveals phasicity to the flow and inspiratory augmentation, consistent with the small burden of thrombus being nonocclusive.

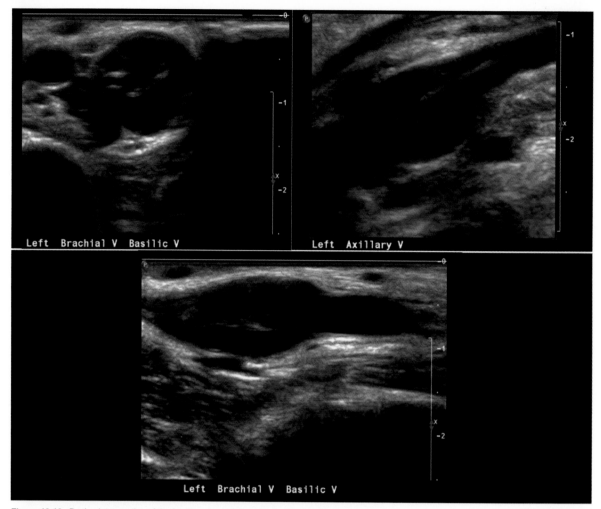

Figure 10-12. Duplex interrogation of the basilic vein, with thrombosis. *Top left,* The image depicts the brachial vein in cross-section. It can be seen to contain soft tissue filling approximately half the lumen. *Top right,* The image depicts the axillary vein (long axis [LAX]), which again contains the soft tissue and the cast of a peripherally inserted catheter. *Bottom,* The basilic vein in LAX is again seen to be containing soft tissue filling approximately half the lumen.

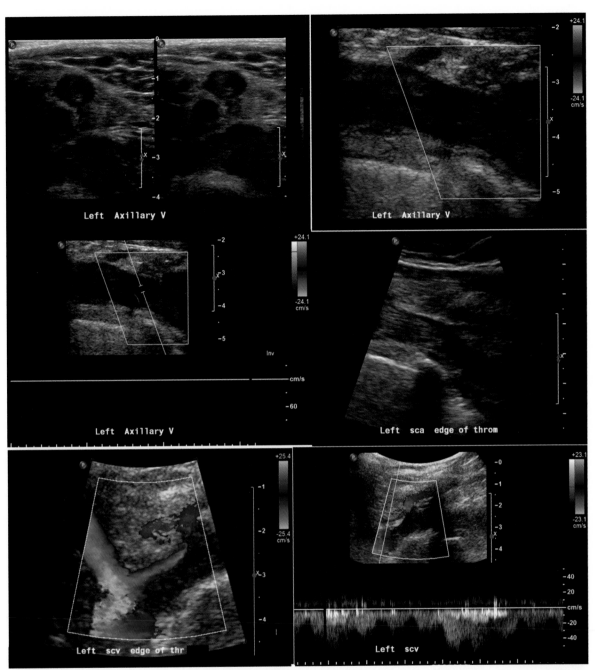

Figure 10-13. Duplex interrogation of the axillary vein thrombosis. *Top left,* The image depicts the axillary vein in cross-section without compression. No compressibility of the vein has been achieved. There is soft tissue seen throughout the lumen of the axillary vein, which is distended. *Top right,* The image depicts the axillary vein in long axis, with compression, with color Doppler flow mapping. Soft tissue is seen throughout the lumen of the axillary vein, and there is an absence of flow signal within the axillary vein lumen consistent with occlusive thrombus. *Middle left,* The pulsed-wave Doppler recording again demonstrates absence of flow. *Middle right,* Grayscale image of the junction of the axillary vein and the subclavian vein. Thrombus extends to the beginning of the subclavian vein. *Bottom left,* Color Doppler flow mapping of the junction of the internal jugular and subclavian veins. The internal jugular vein has flow throughout its lumen, and there is flow along the edge of the thrombus in the subclavian vein. There is collateral flow returning blood to the thrombus in the proximal subclavian vein alongside the distal margin of the thrombus. *Bottom right,* Spectral display of pulsed Doppler flow recording within the subclavian vein depicting a phasic pattern that exhibits inspiratory augmentation. Upper extremity deep venous thrombosis is associated with bronchogenic carcinoma.

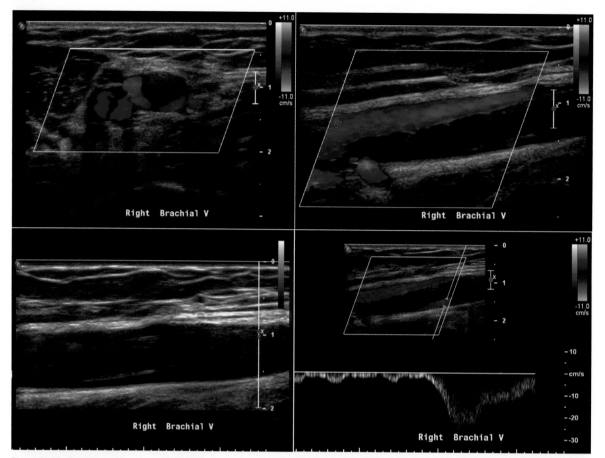

Figure 10-14. Brachial vein thrombosis. *Top left,* The brachial artery and vein in cross-section, with color Doppler flow mapping. *Top right,* Long-axis view of the brachial vein, also with color Doppler flow mapping. There is a large amount of intraluminal echogenic material, and part of the lumen remains, with flow evident by flow mapping. *Bottom left,* Grayscale imaging alone of the large amount of intraluminal echogenic material consistent with thrombus. *Bottom right,* Spectral Doppler display of flow within the residual lumen, revealing augmentation due to the nonocclusive nature of the thrombus.

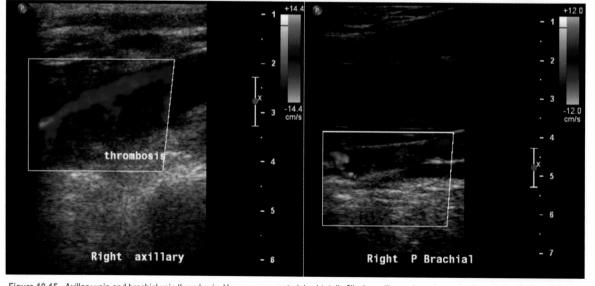

Figure 10-15. Axillary vein and brachial vein thrombosis. Homogenous material subtotally fills the axillary vein and completely occludes the brachial vein.

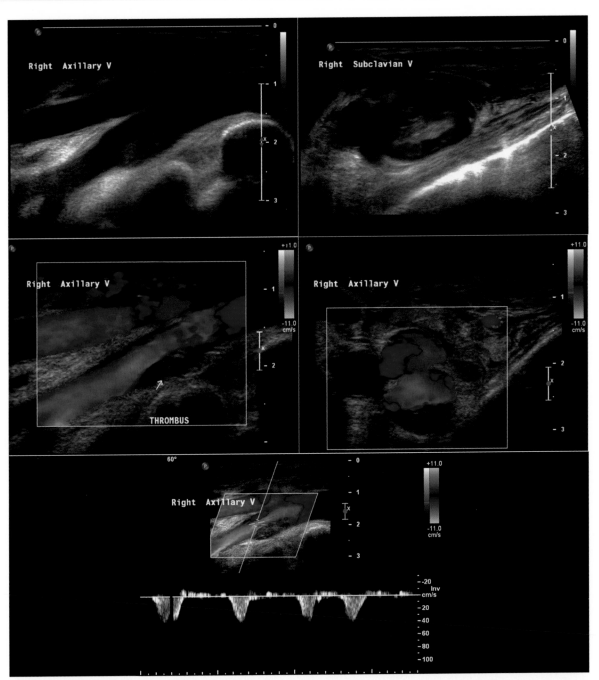

Figure 10-16. *Top left,* Nonocclusive subclavian and axillary vein thrombosis shown in grayscale long-axis imaging. *Top right,* Short-axis grayscale compression view of the partly incompressible subclavian portion of the thrombus. *Middle left and right,* The images that reveal that the axillary vein is bifid with thrombus within the deeper vein. *Bottom,* Color and spectral Doppler images outline the extent of the thrombus in the axillary vein and an essentially normal venous flow pattern.

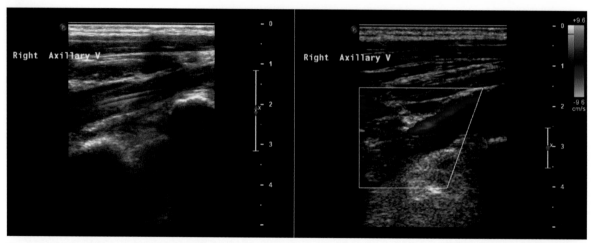

Figure 10-17. Thrombosis around the axillary vein portion of a peripherally inserted central catheter (PICC) line, revealed by grayscale imaging (*left*) and the resultant narrowed stream of venous flow (*right*).

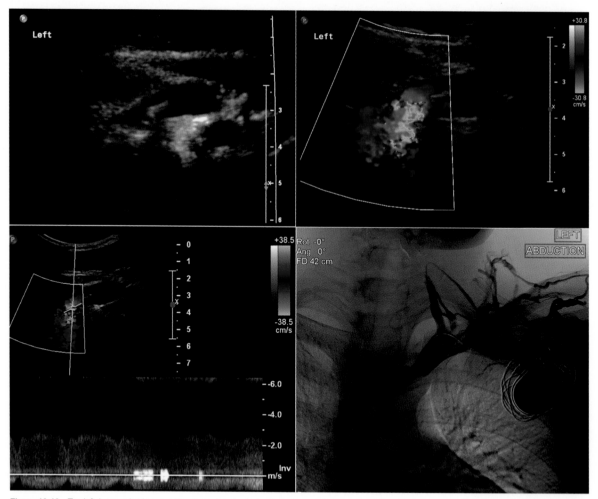

Figure 10-18. *Top left,* Long-axis view reveals a linear intraluminal echo in the subclavian vein arising from a segment of pacemaker wire. *Top right,* Color Doppler long-axis view depicts obvious color Doppler flow aliasing, suggesting narrowing of the subclavian vein at the site of the wire. *Bottom left,* The Doppler spectral sampling confirms elevated flow velocity with minimal respiratory influence. *Bottom right,* The venogram corroborates the duplex findings.

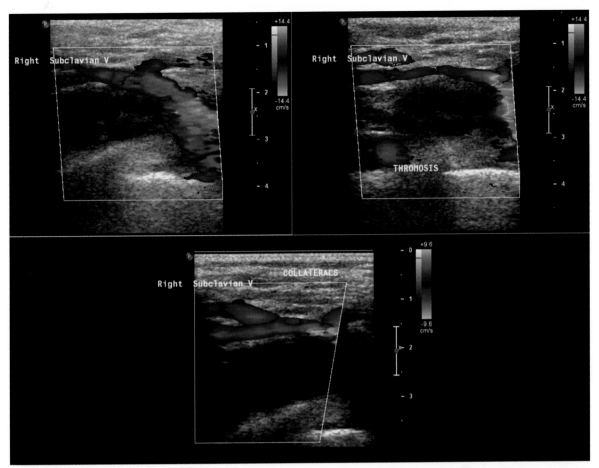

Figure 10-19. A large thrombus is present obstructing the subclavian vein (*top left*) and numerous branching collaterals circumventing the blockage (*top right and bottom*).

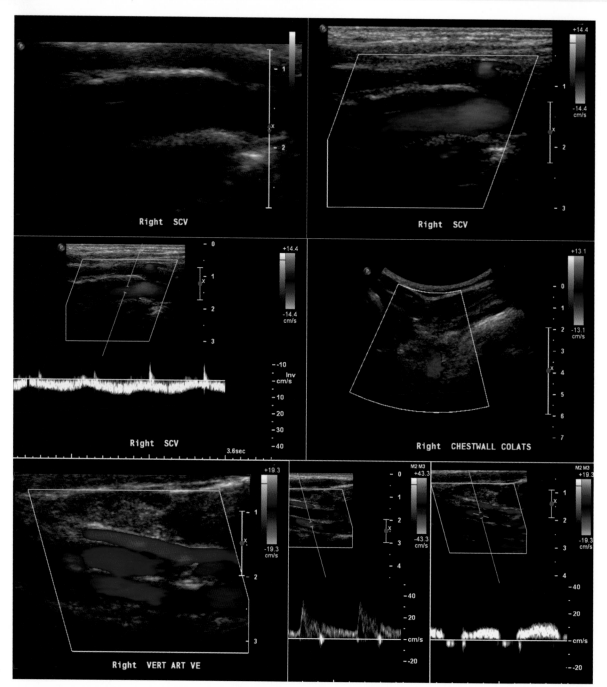

Figure 10-20. Thrombus involving the anterior wall of the subclavian vein (*top left and right*), with relatively normal flow patterns (*middle left*). Deep chest wall collaterals are quite large and prominently displayed (*middle right*). Reversal of flow in the vertebral vein (artery [*bottom left*] and vein [*bottom right*]) is depicted, suggesting extensive collateralization.

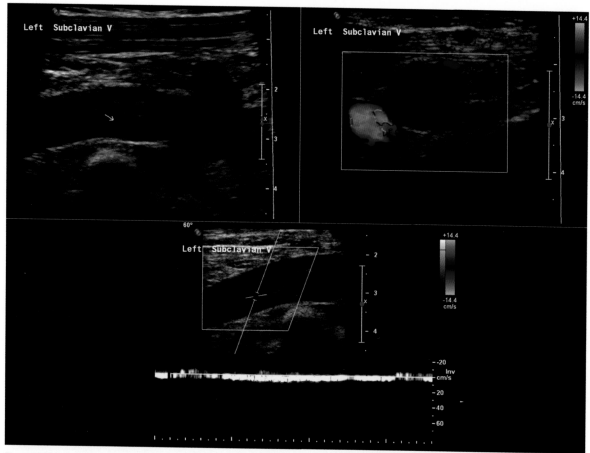

Figure 10-21. *Top left and right,* Views show a long fibrous band, suggesting chronic recanalized thrombosis of the subclavian vein. *Bottom,* Reduced pulse repetition frequency is insufficient to detect the low flow present, suggesting a more occlusive process further proximally.

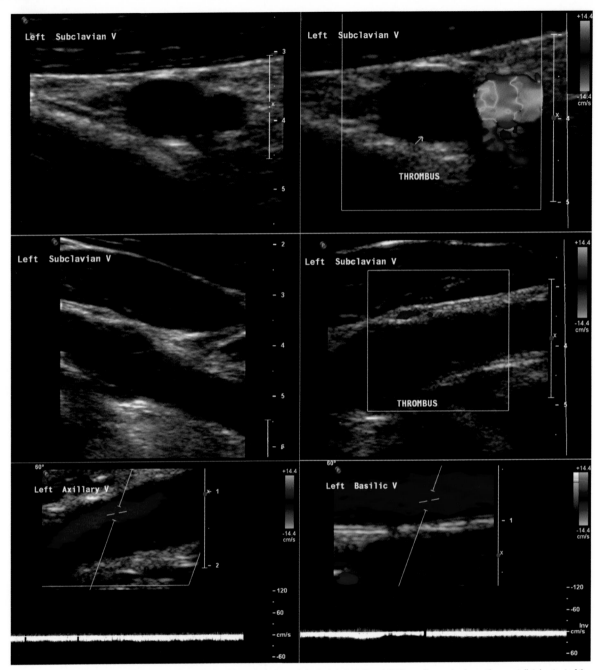

Figure 10-22. *Top and middle left and right,* Thrombosis of the subclavian vein is depicted. *Bottom left,* The axillary vein shows the most distal extent of the thrombus. *Bottom right,* This view shows a completely patent basilic vein.

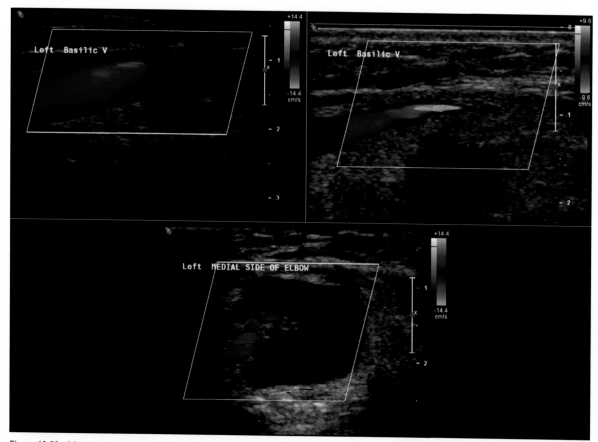

Figure 10-23. A large complex mass on the medial side of the upper arm is depicted (*bottom*), compressing the basilic vein as depicted (*top left and right*). The image of the mass taken in a slightly different plane reveals that there is only partial compression (*bottom*).

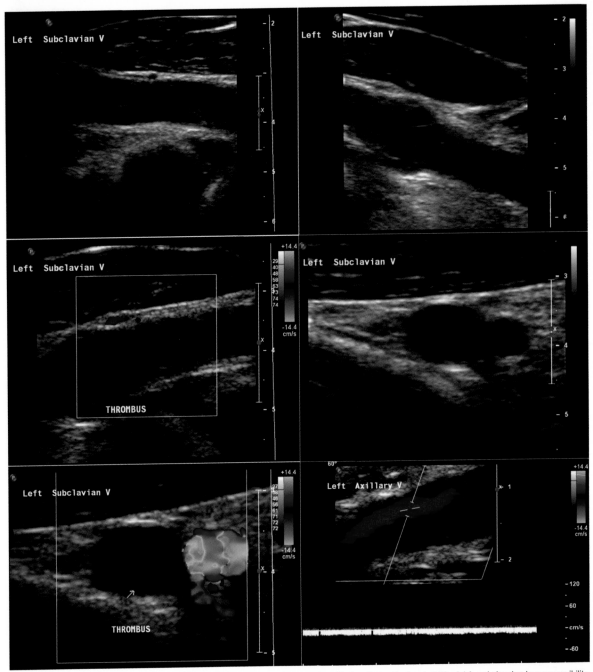

Figure 10-24. Subclavian thrombosis in the two long-axis views (*top left and right*) and in the short-axis view (*middle right*) and showing incompressibility. Color Doppler views (*middle left and bottom left*) confirm an absence of flow. There is partial involvement of the axillary vein (*bottom right*).

11 Venous Disease of the Lower Extremity

Key Points

- Knowledge of normal and variant anatomy of the lower extremity venous vasculature is critical.
- A standardized and comprehensive duplex examination protocol is critical.
- Knowledge of possible diseases/lesions potentially within the lower extremity venous vasculature, and how to maximize their recognition, is critical.

VENOUS ANATOMY OF THE LOWER EXTREMITY

The venous system of the lower extremity consists of three components:

1. Thick-walled superficial veins
2. Thin-walled deep veins
3. Perforating veins, which cross the fascia and drain blood from the superficial to the deep system

Approximately 85% of the venous return is accomplished by the deep venous system and 15% by the superficial system.[1]

All of the vein components mentioned previously contain one-way bicuspid valves, preventing reflux, and they are embedded in an area referred to as a venous sinus, an enlargement of the vein wall that allows unimpeded movement of the valve. There are fewer valves in the superficial venous system compared with the deep venous system, where, for example, in the posterior and peroneal veins of the calf, there may be one valve per inch. In approximately 20% of people, there are no valves between the groin and the heart; in approximately 20% of people, there is one valve in the external iliac vein; and in 60% of people, there is one valve in the common femoral vein.[2]

The Superficial Venous System

The main veins of the superficial system are the:

❑ Greater or long saphenous vein
❑ Lesser or short saphenous vein

The long saphenous vein, which contains up to 20 valves (mostly within the calf), runs from the medial marginal vein of the foot and along the medial aspect of the calf and thigh. This vein terminates in the common femoral vein at the level of the groin, at what is known as the saphenofemoral junction.

Large accessory saphenous veins, which run parallel with the main vein but anterior to the saphenous fascia (either anterior-laterally or posteriorly), are said to be present in 50% to 70% of people, and are thinner walled and considerably less muscular than the main vein.[3] They can appear as duplicated veins, may enter the main vein at variable levels, and drain parts of the thigh and lower abdominal wall.

Several other superficial veins drain into the greater saphenous vein before it enters into the common femoral vein: the superficial external pudendal vein, the superficial circumflex iliac vein, and the superficial epigastric veins, which drain the parts of the hip, genital, and pubic areas.

The lesser or short saphenous vein is a continuation of the lateral marginal vein. This vein runs along the line that at one time was known as the "stocking" line, referring to the nylon stockings worn by women after World War II where the seam was supposed to run straight down the middle of the back of the leg. The terminus is variable; it could drain into the deep system anywhere from the popliteal to the distal superficial femoral vein and might also join the popliteal vein via the gastrocnemius vein.

The long saphenous vein is often duplicated in the thigh, but the short saphenous vein is less frequently duplicated in the calf.

The vein of Giacomini, named after the anatomist who first identified this vein in 1837, is another superficial vein, present in approximately 70% of limbs. It connects the proximal short saphenous and proximal long saphenous veins.[4]

The Perforating Veins

Perforating veins are so-named because they pierce (traverse) the fascia. They are also referred to as "communicating veins" because they carry blood from one venous system to another. Some perforating veins carry blood from the superficial to the deep venous system and are short, straight vessels that can become dilated and tortuous when the valves are congenitally either absent or become damaged, and others connect the gastrocnemius and soleal veins with the superficial veins.

The Deep Venous System

The deep veins begin in the foot, where the plantar and dorsal digital veins communicate via a network of interlacing branches with the plantar cutaneous venous part of the deep venous system. The soleal veins drain blood from the flat soleal muscle, which lies anterior to the gastrocnemius muscle, and in turn drain into the paired peroneal and posterior tibial veins.

At the level of the popliteal fossa, three components of the venous system—the subcutaneous, intermuscular, and intramuscular veins—run in three superimposed planes.

The mostly paired and occasionally triplicate deep veins of the calf consist of the posterior tibial, anterior tibial, and peroneal veins, and they accompany a single artery in each case. The peroneal and posterior tibial veins join to become the tibioperoneal trunk.

The popliteal vein is formed by the confluence of anterior tibial and tibioperoneal trunks and begins at various levels—below, above, or at the level of the knee joint. It is duplicated in approximately 5% of limbs[5] and becomes the superficial femoral vein at approximately the level of the adductor hiatus, then running in parallel with its accompanying artery to the saphenofemoral junction.

The superficial femoral vein is duplicated in as many as 33% of patients. It may have a complicated course in 1% to 2% of cases, such as being triplicated in a segment (usually in the distal third).[5]

The deep femoral or profunda femoris vein receives flow from numerous branches along its course and invariably communicates distally with the popliteal vein and proximally with the inferior gluteal vein, an arrangement that supplies collateral flow when the superficial femoral vein is thrombosed. It joins the common femoral vein approximately 4 cm below the inguinal ligament.

The lateral and medial circumflex veins, draining blood from the muscles of the hip, thigh, knee, and iliopsoas, also drain into the deep femoral vein.

The common femoral vein becomes the external iliac vein as it passes under the inguinal ligament and in turn becomes the common iliac vein at the level of the pelvic brim, anterior to the sacroiliac joint, where it is joined by the internal iliac vein.

The pubic, inferior epigastric, and deep iliac circumflex veins all drain into the external iliac vein.

Pelvic wall, viscera, reproductive organ, and buttock venous drainage almost completely parallels the arterial supply and with a few exceptions is performed entirely by branches of the internal iliac vein, which in turn drains into the common iliac vein. Exceptions to this include various segments of the bowel, which are drained by the portal vein via branches of the inferior mesenteric, and the ovaries, which drain into the renal vein or in some cases, the IVC via the ovarian veins.

On the left side, the common iliac vein runs medial to the artery but then as it courses proximally, its position rotates and stays behind the artery. It is at this point that the vein is sometimes compressed by the artery against the fifth vertebra in May-Thurner syndrome. Interestingly, this compressive syndrome has been found to exist in healthy asymptomatic individuals.[6] The right common iliac vein runs straight up

arch to form the dorsal venous arch. The medial and lateral plantar veins leave the plantar cutaneous venous arch on either side of the foot to form the posterior tibial veins. The deep plantar venous arch, which is considered to be the venous reservoir of the foot, communicates via perforating branches with the anterior and posterior tibial veins of the deep venous system.

The gastrocnemius veins, each with its accompanying artery, are the most superficial in the calf and form a small plexus in the gastrocnemius muscle of the calf, which drains into the popliteal vein at about the same level as the short saphenous vein. They, together with the soleal veins that travel within the deep fascia, are sometimes called sural veins and are considered to be proximally and medially to a position on the right side and anterior to the fifth lumbar vertebra, where it is joined by the left common iliac vein. An iliolumbar vein drains into each common iliac vein.

The IVC, the largest vein in the body, begins at the confluence of the right and left common iliac veins on the right side of the aorta at the level of the fifth lumbar vertebra and continues proximally. There it enters the porta hepatis, a large groove, in the posterior aspect of the right lobe of the liver, then pierces through the diaphragm and enters the right atrium of the heart. Uncommon variants of the IVC include a left-sided IVC in 0.2% to 0.5% of cases, where the IVC runs to the left of the aorta, terminates in the left renal vein, and crosses over the aorta into the right renal vein, and then follows its usual course. Another uncommon variant is the double IVC, which is present in 0.2% to 0.3% of people, where typically there is a right-sided IVC running from the right common iliac vein and a left-sided IVC extending from the left common iliac vein and terminating in the left renal vein.[7]

Azygos continuation of the IVC is present in 0.6% of people, where the inferior vena cava becomes the azygos vein proximal to the diaphragm and then joins the superior vena cava draining all lower extremity blood. In the case of azygous continuation, the hepatic vein often drains directly into the right atrium.

The inferior vena cava receives six pairs of veins:

❐ Four lumbar veins, which drain the abdominal wall, skin, and muscles of the vertebral column and the spinal cord. An ascending lumbar vein connects the lumbar veins and the common iliac vein with the azygos vein on each side.

❐ Two spermatic or ovarian veins from the testes and ovaries, both containing valves. As with the uterine veins, the ovarian veins become considerably enlarged during pregnancy.

❐ Four to six hepatic veins begin in the parenchyma of the liver where they are divided into upper and lower groups. The upper group consists of three large veins that join the IVC when it is in the porta hepatis groove of the liver. The lower group consists of smaller veins and comes from the right and caudate lobes of the liver.

❐ Two renal veins (per kidney) (normally). The left renal vein receives the left testicular or ovarian vein. Renal venous anomalies include:
  • Circumaortic left renal veins (8.7%), where there are two left renal veins, the superior running across the aorta anteriorly and the inferior branch running posteriorly
  • Retroaortic left renal vein (2.7%), where the left renal vein runs behind the aorta
  • Renal and IVC anomalies, which may coexist

❐ Left and right inferior phrenic veins, which drain the diaphragm. These are thought to be a major source of collateral flow in the presence of portal hypertension.

❐ The right suprarenal vein draining the adrenal glands, which enters the IVC, and the left, which enters into either the left renal or inferior phrenic vein

The venous supply of the organs of the digestive tract drains first into the liver via the portal vein and then into the IVC via the hepatic veins. The portal veins form behind the neck of the pancreas at the level of the second lumbar vertebra, are approximately 8 cm long, and are created by the union of the splenic vein, which drains the lower duodenum and splenic flexure of the bowel, and of the superior mesenteric vein, which drains parts of the small and large intestine. The right gastric vein, which receives flow from the lesser curvature of the stomach, and the left gastric vein, which drains the lower end of the esophagus, flow into the portal vein.

The cystic vein drains blood from the gallbladder into the portal vein, and the paraumbilical vein also drains into the portal vein. The most typical pattern of the portal vein is division into right and left branches at the porta hepatis, which in turn subdivide further in the lobes of the liver. Variants are said to occur in 20% of people; the most common variant is trifurcation of the main portal vein, but there are numerous other branching variants and those associated with malposition of the gallbladder.[8]

The three most common reasons to perform a venous duplex examination of the lower extremity are for the assessment of suspected venous thrombotic disease, for the mapping of venous conduits for arterial bypass surgery, and for the evaluation of venous incompetence.

VENOUS THROMBOEMBOLISM

Approximately 0.1% of the population annually develop recognized venous thromboembolism; more develop it and die from it than are recognized. The mortality from thromboembolism is approximately 10%. Only half of fatal thromboembolic episodes are recognized and likely, far fewer nonfatal episodes. The diagnosis of deep vein thrombosis (DVT) and pulmonary embolism (PE) has shifted from invasive venography and pulmonary angiography to serum testing for D-dimer, nuclear ventilation-perfusion testing, duplex DVT scanning, and computed tomography (CT) pulmonary angiography and proximal venography. Although there are potentially benefits to the current diagnostic approach, the reality is that noninvasive testing, if not assiduously performed, is unlikely to be as accurate as what it replaced. Furthermore, inconsistencies and assumptions plague the noninvasive evaluation of venous thrombotic disease.

Although most (90%) venous thrombosis occurs within the deep lower extremity veins, venous thrombosis may be present at any level of veins in the lower and upper extremities, as well as in the visceral veins, the head and neck veins, and the superior and inferior vena cava. Again, although most pulmonary thrombo-embolism originates from the deep lower extremity veins, not all does.

USE OF DUPLEX ULTRASOUND FOR THE EVALUATION OF SUSPECTED VENOUS THROMBOSIS

Comprehensive scanning of the lower extremity veins—from the iliac veins down to the feet (including calf veins)—is the preferred duplex method to assess for suspected lower extremity DVT. Such a scan does take more time, but evaluation of the calf veins is relevant. Abridged duplex scanning protocols (scanning of only the femoral and popliteal veins to rule out DVT) are popular simply because of their brevity and ease. However, calf DVT is relevant because it may be symptomatic, may incite post–phlebitic syndrome, and may progress to proximal DVT and may result in PE. The rate of calf to proximal DVT progression is poorly characterized and is likely influenced by the clinical context but may be as high as approximately 5%. Hence, abridged scanning for suspected DVT should be used with discretion, and often it should be repeated at least once to enable detection of DVT progression.

The role of DVT scanning in the assessment of PE is controversial. Approximately 20% of cases of PE are without detectable DVT by venography because the entire bulk of DVT embolized and left insufficient residual bulk to detect. Approximately 70% of cases of PE are without detectable DVT by duplex scanning. CT pulmonary angiography protocols are often adjuncts to lower extremity CT venography. The actual yield of CT venography compared with duplex scanning is poorly established. It does not yet appear comparable. Although the identification of lower extremity DVT is a standard indication for anticoagulation unless contraindications are present, the duration of the course of anticoagulation is emergently different for DVT versus PE. Therefore, establishing whether PE has occurred in the context of recognition of DVT influences the duration of therapy and is useful information.

Risk Factors for Deep Vein Thrombosis
- History of deep or superficial venous thrombosis
- Prolonged bed rest or immobilization
- Recent surgery
- Familial history of DVT
- Pregnancy
- Congestive heart failure
- Cancer or history of cancer
- Local trauma
- Thrombophilia (protein C deficiency, protein S deficiency, antithrombin III deficiency, factor V Leiden, partial thromboplastin mutation)

Summary: Problems with the Use of Duplex Scanning for the Evaluation of Thromboembolic Disease
- DVT: abridged protocols often do not address calf level DVT, which is the original site of proximal DVT.
- Superficial venous thrombosis scanning
  - Superficial and deep venous disease may coexist or exist independently; therefore, exclusion of superficial thrombosis does not exclude DVT.
  - Rarely, a superficial thrombus may extend into the common femoral vein via the saphenofemoral junction.
- PE
  - Only a minority of patients with PE have duplex findings of DVT.
  - Identification of DVT establishes an indication for anticoagulation but not necessarily of the same duration as does identification of PE.

DUPLEX EXAMINATION FOR VENOUS THROMBOSIS OF THE LOWER EXTREMITY

Purpose
Venous Thrombosis Studies
- To demonstrate the presence or absence of DVT/obstruction
- To demonstrate the presence or absence of superficial venous thrombosis/obstruction
- To attempt to distinguish between acute and chronic venous thrombosis

Identification of Differential Pathologies
Possible pathologies are demonstrable by ultrasound and are related to the patient's symptoms:
- Venous valvular incompetence (deep and superficial)
- Ruptured popliteal (Baker) cyst
- Hematoma
- Fluid collections
- Enlarged lymph nodes
- Solid masses
- Extrinsic compression syndromes
- Compression from an adjacent arterial aneurysm

Common Clinical Indications
- Suspected DVT
  - Leg swelling or leg pain
  - Suspected PE
- Suspected superficial venous thrombosis
  - Palpable cord
  - Leg pain

Contraindications and Limitations
- Wound dressing
- Open wound
- Inability to move limbs to enable scanning

Equipment
❏ Duplex ultrasound system
❏ 3- to 9-MHz linear transducer for more superficial image
❏ 2- to 5-MHz sector/curved array transducer for deeper field imaging
❏ Coupling gel
❏ Digital reporting

Procedure
❏ Explain the procedure to the patient and answer any questions.
❏ Obtain and document applicable patient history on appropriate forms.
❏ Verify that the procedure requested correlates with patient's symptoms
❏ Determine if the patient has risk factors for DVT or a history of the condition.
❏ Perform a limited physical examination of the limbs in question.
❏ Review any previous duplex studies available.
❏ Select appropriate test preset values.
❏ Select appropriate annotation throughout test.
❏ Record images.
❏ Complete technologist's preliminary report when necessary.

Technique
❏ Both limbs are scanned.
❏ The patient lies supine with the upper body raised approximately 45 degrees (reverse Trendelenburg position) such that the veins are distended.
❏ The limb being examined is externally rotated and the knee is slightly bent.
❏ The technologist stands or sits beside the patient through the study.
❏ Gloves are worn by the technologist where there is a threat of contamination by infected body fluids.

Vary the scanning of the vein along its course:
❏ In the area of the distal thigh, scan the distal superior femoral vein from a posterior approach. The vein is closer to the transducer at this level.
❏ In the mid- and proximal thigh, apply pressure with the probe from the medial aspect while applying pressure from the free (briefly) hand on the lateral aspect, giving more heft to the maneuver.

As with usual venous scanning technique, use transverse views (the order chosen at the technologist's discretion) to follow the anatomy of the venous system distally and to establish the presence of intraluminal material/noncompressibility. Use longitudinal views with color Doppler imaging and spectral display of pulsed-wave Doppler interrogation to depict flow/partial obstruction/complete obstruction. The following veins are interrogated:
❏ External iliac vein (may be necessary to change to a lower frequency transducer)
❏ Common femoral vein
❏ Profunda femoris vein (origin)
❏ Saphenofemoral junction
❏ Femoral vein (also known as the superficial femoral vein)
❏ Popliteal vein
❏ Posterior tibial vein
❏ Peroneal/anterior tibial veins (scanned only when there is local tenderness, because normally these veins are incompressible in places because of surrounding bones)
❏ Greater saphenous origin
❏ Lesser saphenous origin
❏ Gastrocnemius vein
❏ Soleal sinus vein

The **external iliac vein** is scanned from the level of the inguinal ligament along a diagonal course toward the umbilicus. Scanning in a transverse plane, it might be possible to compress the vessel somewhat, but more reliance should be placed on grayscale visualization of intraluminal echoes, color filling, and Doppler signals in the sagittal plane.

The **common iliac vein** and **IVC** are scanned with grayscale imaging as well as color and spectral Doppler if thrombus is identified in the external iliac vein.

The **common femoral vein** in the groin is scanned with grayscale imaging to the level of the femoral bifurcation. Pressure is applied with the transducer every 1 to 2 cm (i.e., enough pressure is applied to collapse the vein completely).

The **profunda femoris vein** dives deeply at the bifurcation of the common femoral vein. (Color Doppler flow-mapping should be used where necessary to identify vessels.)

The **superficial femoral vein,** also known as the femoral vein, which is typically 1 to 2 cm distal to the femoral arterial bifurcation, is scanned along the medial aspect of the thigh (it may be necessary and desirable to apply pressure with the free hand to the lateral thigh at the site of compression). Color and spectral Doppler are added to further delineate flow channels around nonocclusive DVT. To scan the distal femoral vein at the level of the adductor hiatus, it may be necessary to move the transducer to a more posterior position just proximal to the popliteal fossa.

The **popliteal vein** is then scanned in the same manner from a posterior approach in the popliteal fossa to the level of the **tibioperoneal trunk.**

The **posterior tibial** and **peroneal veins** (transverse compression only) are scanned along the medial aspect of the calf to the ankle level.

The **gastrocnemius** and **soleal veins** are seen within the posterior calf muscle and are scanned using compression only in the transverse plane. These veins are usually too small to see if they are without pathology, but they become considerably enlarged when thrombosed.

The **perforating veins** are not routinely scanned but can sometimes be readily seen running between deep and superficial veins (and crossing fascial planes) along the medial aspect of the calf. Oblique scanning is required for clear visualization.

The **anterior tibial vein** is scanned by following along the anterolateral border of the calf from a point between the heads of the tibia and fibula to the ankle level in both transverse and sagittal. Compression of portions of the anterior tibial vein may be difficult or impossible due to depth and proximity to surrounding bone.

Signs of Deep Vein Thrombosis
Noncompressibility
The venous system is normally distended under low pressure, and therefore, veins can be compressed easily with very little pressure from the transducer. With venous thrombosis, the presence of intraluminal thrombus material renders the vein incompletely or noncompressible. Compression maneuvers are best performed in transverse imaging because it can be assured that the plane of imaging is not moving off to the side of the vessel, giving a false impression of compressibility as may happen with imaging along the longitudinal plane of the vessel. Generally, soft tissue material within the vessel is seen at sites of noncompressibility. Compression maneuvers should be performed at the following sites:

❒ External iliac vein
❒ Common femoral vein
❒ Proximal profunda femoris vein
❒ Femoral vein
  • Proximal segment
  • Middle segment
  • Distal segment
❒ Popliteal vein

Flow Obstruction
Normally, flow velocity in the veins exhibits spontaneous variation according to the phase of the respiratory cycle and in proportion to respiratory effort. Normally, abrupt compression of a muscle bed distally to a site of sampling results in a surge of blood through the vein. With complete obstruction to flow by DVT, the signs of spontaneity, phasicity, and augmentation are lost. With partial obstruction, these signs are attenuated. Therefore, flow signs corroborate some cases of DVT; however, from a diagnostic and therapeutic standpoint, there is no difference between occlusive and nonocclusive DVT.

Superficial Veins: The Greater Saphenous and Lesser Saphenous Veins
The greater saphenous vein is scanned in transverse along the medial aspect of the thigh and calf from the saphenofemoral junction at the level of the groin to a point anterior to medial malleolus using probe compression every 1 to 2 cm. In the sagittal plane, color and Doppler flow are used to assess valvular function and patency as described previously.

The lesser saphenous vein is scanned from its junction with the deep system, which can be anomalous but is usually found at the popliteal or distal femoral level, to the ankle level in the midline of the posterior calf in the same manner as for the greater saphenous vein.

A high-resolution/high-frequency linear transducer (e.g., 9- to 17-MHz) yields superior diagnostic images.

Extensive deep vein thrombosis can cause increased and continuous (less phasic) flow in the greater saphenous vein, because more venous return than usual is provided by the greater saphenous veins, through deep perforator vessels from the deep beds.

Thrombus Characteristics
Once the thrombus has been identified, its features should be further evaluated in an attempt to establish acuity versus chronicity of the thrombosis.

Acute Thrombus: Features
❒ Lightly echogenic
❒ Poorly attached. Typically, newly formed thrombus is poorly attached to the vein wall.
❒ Spongy texture. Acute thrombus usually appears to be gelatinous and echogenic.
❒ Dilated vein. As a newly formed thrombus grows, the vein enlarges to accommodate the blood flow. This continues until the vein reaches maximum size, at which time the thrombus completely fills the dilated vessel. Obstructive and occlusive thrombus distends the vessels by raising hydrostatic forces.
❒ Smooth borders. Sometimes, but not invariably, recently developed thrombus has smoother borders.

Chronic Thrombus: Features
❒ Brightly echogenic
❒ Well-attached thrombus. As the thrombus ages, it is subject to thrombolysis and fibrotic "organization." What remains in the chronic phase is more fibrotic than thrombotic and is attached firmly to the vein wall. Some thrombi recanalize through channels; they also are firmly attached to the vessel wall.
❒ Rigid texture. Fibrotic "organization" of thrombus renders it more dense and solid (collagenized). It may become so dense that it generates acoustical shadowing.
❒ Contracted vein. The fibrotic "organization" of thrombus involves collagenous contraction that causes tapering of the vein wall. The vein then appears much smaller than it did originally. The matching vein segment of the contralateral limb, if free of disease, often underscores the extent of distortion of the affected vein, which often becomes anechoic and disappears ultrasonographically into the musculature of the leg.
❒ Large collateral veins. When a major deep vein is obstructed, neighboring branch vessels dilate to accommodate for the needed increase for compensatory flow through them.

Venous Duplex Thrombosis Criteria

Criteria for venous duplex thrombosis are given in Table 11-1.

SAPHENOUS VEIN MAPPING PRIOR TO HARVESTING FOR ARTERIAL BYPASS SURGERY

Purpose

The objective is to assess the patency and size (outside diameter) of the greater and lesser saphenous veins prior to harvesting as venous conduits for arterial bypass surgery.

Technique

As described in the preceding section, the patient lies supine and the limb being examined is externally rotated. Views are obtained in the transverse axis because the vessel can be followed along its length far more easily in a transverse plane than in a longitudinal plane.

Greater Saphenous Vein

❏ Scan from its terminus with the deep system at the level of the groin along the medial aspect of the thigh to the level of the medial malleolus.
❏ Perform compression maneuvers every 1 to 2 cm along its length to assess patency and note the presence of any parallel saphenous system.
❏ Scan as per the deep venous protocol to determine patency.
❏ From the groin level measure the outside diameter of the vein at the following sites:
  • Saphenofemoral junction

• Proximal thigh
• Proximal to mid-thigh
• Mid-thigh
• Distal thigh
• Knee level
• Upper calf
• Mid-calf
• Distal calf at ankle level
❏ If a parallel greater saphenous system is identified, measure it as well.
❏ Note and document branch vessels.

Lesser Saphenous Vein

❏ Have the patient lie either prone or in an oblique position and scan the vein from the popliteal vein (or higher if anomalous). Follow it along the midline of the posterior calf to the lateral malleolus.
❏ Make outside diameter measurements as described above.
❏ Use color Doppler flow mapping and pulsed-wave spectral flow recording in the sagittal plane to corroborate patency of these vessels.

VENOUS INSUFFICIENCY ASSESSMENT

Chronic venous insufficiency may involve the superficial venous system or the deep venous system. The perforating veins are often classified within the superficial system. Valves are present at multiple levels of the deep venous system of the superficial venous system and within the perforating veins that join the two systems. Normal venous valvar function in the lower extremities, assisted by compression from the surrounding calf and

TABLE 11-1 Duplex Ultrasound Findings of Venous Thrombosis

CATEGORY	GRAYSCALE FINDINGS (SAX)	COLOR DOPPLER FINDINGS (LAX)	SPECTRAL DOPPLER FINDINGS
Normal	Vein walls coapt No intraluminal echoes	Complete intraluminal color filling	Phasic/augmented flow
Acute DVT	Expanded vein Homogenous intraluminal echoes Spongy appearance		
Occlusive	Incompressible	No color filling	No flow augmentation proximally
Partially occlusive	Partially compressible	Visible flow channel	May show reduced flow augmentation
Chronic DVT	Shrunken vein size Heterogeneous echoes Brightly echogenic		
Occlusive	Incompressible	No color filling	No flow augmentation proximally
Partially occlusive	Partially compressible	Visible flow channel	May show diminished flow augmentation May show reflux flow

DVT, deep vein thrombosis; LAX, long-axis imaging; SAX, short-axis imaging.

thigh muscles, returns venous blood despite the hydrostatic gradient. Insufficiency of the superficial system alone, often referred to as "primary venous insufficiency," is frequently observed as a familial condition (as often as in 75% of cases). Insufficiency of the deep venous system is generally held to be a less common cause of chronic venous insufficiency and to be the consequence of prior DVT that resulted in either obstruction of the veins or retraction of the valves such that they became distorted and insufficient.

Competence refers to the ability of the normal venous valves to prevent retrograde flow. Competent valves allow only a short burst of retrograde flow (<0.5 seconds) when a short squeeze is applied to the calf, or as in the case of the proximal femoral veins, when the patient performs a Valsalva maneuver. Venous valvular incompetence of the deep veins is usually, but not always, the consequence of chronic thrombosis and scarring and retraction of valve elements.

Purpose

The objective is to document the presence of venous insufficiency.

Technique

❑ The patient is examined in both supine and upright positions or in a steep reverse Trendelenburg position.

❑ No prolonged flow signal is observed after distal compression release.

❑ Competence of the common femoral or proximal superficial femoral valves is assessed by asking the patient to perform the Valsalva maneuver or by gently compressing the abdomen manually.

❑ For the remainder of the lower extremity venous system above the knee, a manual squeeze (or automatic cuff inflation) of the calf is applied. As well, the popliteal vein is assessed by compressing the thigh muscles.

❑ If a detailed study of the calf veins, including the numerous perforating veins, is required, foot compression is used.[9]

Interpretation and Reporting

Incompetent valves are present if retrograde flow is recorded for 0.5 seconds or more during proximal/distal compression or a Valsalva maneuver.

OTHER PATHOLOGIES AND CONDITIONS THAT INFLUENCE VENOUS FLOW

Arteriovenous Fistulas

In the presence of a medium (and larger) arteriovenous fistula, there is pulsatile flow in the vein at the site of the fistula and above it, transmitted from the fistula. Proximal to the fistula, the venous diameter is increased due to higher venous distending pressure. Pulsatility

and distention are absent in the context of smaller fistulas, which impart a lesser hemodynamic burden onto the vein.

Severe (Right-sided) Heart Failure

In the presence of severe tricuspid insufficiency, as a primary or secondary component of right-sided heart failure, pulsatility within systemic veins, even at the lower extremity level, may be seen. Bilateral sampling of lower extremity flow should yield similar (symmetrical) findings.

Pregnancy

During the late stages of pregnancy, the enlarged womb can exert pressure on the abdominal and pelvic veins, resulting in their extrinsic compression, which may result in abnormal or absent venous flow signals and poor ultrasound visualization. The findings can be altered by rotating the patient from side-to-side or placing the patient in a lateral decubitus position to relieve the pressure.

Cellulitis

In the presence of cellulitis, especially with extensive erythema (a sign of hyperemia), increased arterial and venous flow is present.

ACCREDITATION

The 2007 Intersocietal Commission for Accreditation of Vascular Laboratories (ICAVL) Standards for Accreditation for lower extremity venous testing, Summary Points, are:[10]

❑ Grayscale imaging in long-axis and short-axis views with compression to assess anatomy and lesions and Doppler (spectral with or without color) to assess physiology, are to be used.

❑ Written disease-specific protocols are required.

❑ Examinations are to be in accordance with protocols.

❑ Indications are to be recorded.

❑ Examinations are to be comprehensive and documented comprehensively.

❑ Representative grayscale and Doppler images and spectral Doppler waveforms to show respiratory variation/manual augmentation of the following are to be obtained:
  • Common femoral vein
  • Saphenofemoral junction
  • Proximal femoral vein
  • Mid-femoral vein
  • Distal femoral vein
  • Popliteal vein
  • Posterior tibial veins
  • Peroneal veins

❑ When appropriate or as required by the laboratory's written protocol: common and external iliac veins, IVC, great saphenous vein, small saphenous vein, proximal deep femoral vein, as well as gastrocnemius, soleal, anterior tibial, and perforating veins must be imaged.

- ❑ If a unilateral study is performed, a contralateral subclavian vein spectral waveform must be documented.
- ❑ When appropriate or as required by the laboratory's written protocol, further examination and recording is to be performed.
- ❑ Diagnostic criteria must be laboratory specific and documented.
- ❑ The components of an examination vary depending on the indication(s).
- ❑ The laboratory must have a written protocol to determine the anatomic extent of the study and when a unilateral or bilateral study is to be performed.
- ❑ A unique protocol must be defined for the examination to evaluate for DVT or venous obstruction.
- ❑ Documentation of areas of suspected thrombosis must include additional representative images.
- ❑ When assessing for obstruction, there must be criteria for interpretation of imaging, transverse compression, and Doppler waveforms.
- ❑ Interpretation of venous duplex examinations must use validated diagnostic criteria to assess the presence and extent of venous thrombosis, vessel patency, valvular competency, and/or calf muscle pump function.
- ❑ In general, a laboratory should perform a minimum of 100 complete (upper and lower) examinations annually.
- ❑ Records must be maintained that permit evaluation of annual procedure volumes.
- ❑ The laboratory must have a written procedure for regular correlation of venous duplex examinations. These correlations must reflect a mix of upper and lower extremities as performed by the laboratory.
- ❑ Documentation of correlation must be maintained.

REFERENCES

1. Schuenke M, Ross LM. Neurovascular systems. In: Schuenke M, Schulte E, Schumacher U, eds. *Thieme Atlas of Anatomy: General Anatomy and Musculoskeletal System.* New York: Thieme; 2006.
2. Cockett FB. Abnormalities of the deep veins of the leg. *Postgrad Med J.* 1954;30(348):512-522.
3. Cohn JD, Caggiati A, Korver KF. Accessory and great saphenous veins as coronary artery bypass conduits. *Interact Cardiovasc Thorac Surg.* 2006;5(5):550-554.
4. Delis KT, Knaggs AL, Khodabakhsh P. Prevalence, anatomic patterns, valvular competence, and clinical significance of the Giacomini vein. *J Vasc Surg.* 2004; 40(6):1174-1183.
5. Quinlan DJ, Alikhan R, Gishen P, Sidhu PS. Variations in lower limb venous anatomy: implications for US diagnosis of deep vein thrombosis. *Radiology.* 2003;228(2): 443-448.
6. Kibbe MR, Ujiki M, Goodwin AL, Eskandari M, Yao J, Matsumura J. Iliac vein compression in an asymptomatic patient population. *J Vasc Surg.* 2004;39(5): 937-943.
7. Bass JE, Redwine MD, Kramer LA, Huynh PT, Harris Jr JH. Spectrum of congenital anomalies of the inferior vena cava: cross-sectional imaging findings. *Radiographics.* 2000;20(3):639-652.
8. Gallego C, Velasco M, Marcuello P, Tejedor D, De Campo L, Friera A. Congenital and acquired anomalies of the portal venous system. *Radiographics.* 2002;22(1): 141-159.
9. Strandness DEJ. *Duplex Scanning in Vascular Disorders.* 3rd ed. Philadelphia: Lippincott Williams & Wilkins; 2002.
10. ICAVL Online: The Intersocietal Commission for the Accreditation of Vascular Laboratories. <http://www. icavl.org/icavl/Standards/2010_ICAVL_Standards. pdf>

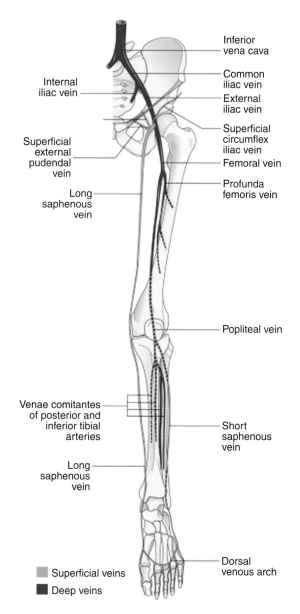

Inferior vena cava

Common iliac vein

Internal iliac vein

External iliac vein

Superficial circumflex iliac vein

Superficial external pudendal vein

Femoral vein

Profunda femoris vein

Long saphenous vein

Popliteal vein

Venae comitantes of posterior and inferior tibial arteries

Short saphenous vein

Long saphenous vein

Superficial veins

Deep veins

Dorsal venous arch

Figure 11-1. Overview of veins of the lower limb. (From Standring S. *Gray's Anatomy.* 40th ed. Philadelphia: Elsevier; 2009; Fig. 79-8; used with permission.)

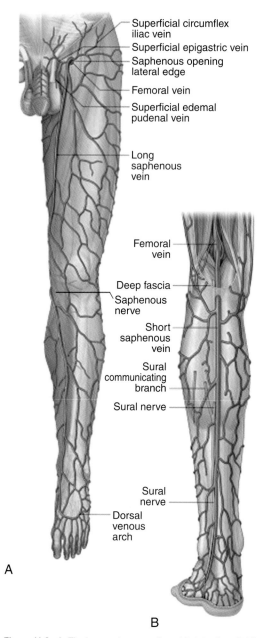

Superficial circumflex iliac vein

Superficial epigastric vein

Saphenous opening lateral edge

Femoral vein

Superficial edemal pudenal vein

Long saphenous vein

Femoral vein

Deep fascia
Saphenous nerve

Short saphenous vein

Sural communicating branch

Sural nerve

Sural nerve

Dorsal venous arch

A

B

Figure 11-2. A, The long saphenous vein and its branches. **B,** The short saphenous vein and its branches. (From Standring S. *Gray's Anatomy.* 40th ed. Philadelphia: Elsevier; 2009; Fig. 79-9; used with permission.)

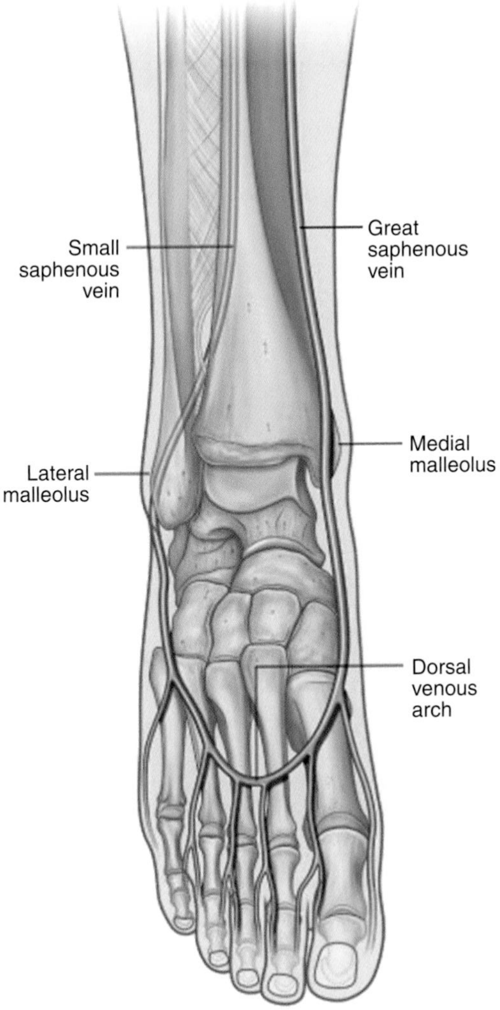

Figure 11-3. Superficial veins of the foot. (From Drake R, Vogl AW, Mitchell AWM. *Gray's Anatomy for Students.* 2nd ed. Philadelphia: Elsevier; 2010; Fig. 6-119; used with permission.)

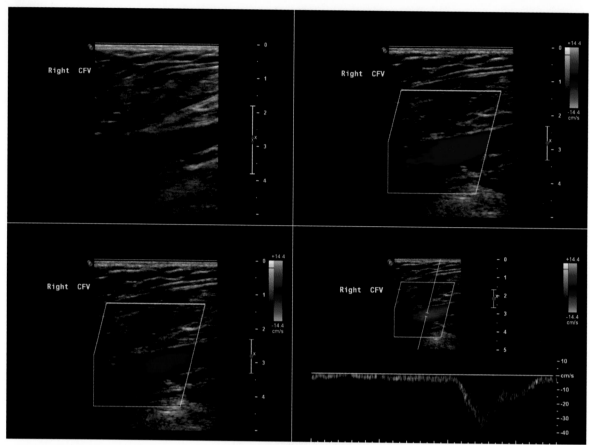

Figure 11-4. Normal venous duplex examination, common femoral vein. *Top left,* long-axis view revealing an absence of intraluminal echoes. *Top right,* Color Doppler flow mapping covers the lumen. *Bottom left,* Color flow mapping reveals respiratory variation. *Bottom right,* Pulsed-wave Doppler spectral display depicts flow velocity augmentation with distal leg compression.

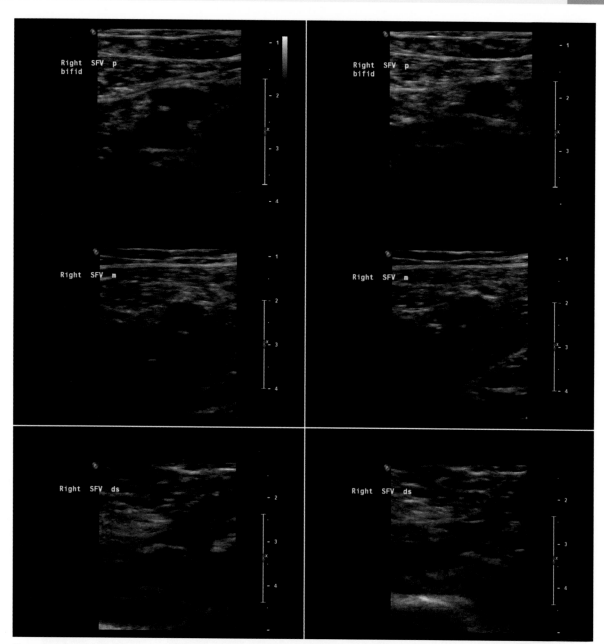

Figure 11-5. Normal venous duplex examination, superficial femoral veins (bifid system). *Top left and right* (short-axis view), proximal superior femoral artery. *Middle left and right,* middle superior femoral artery. *Bottom left and right,* superior femoral artery. The left images are without compression, and the right images are with compression. There is an absence of intraluminal echoes in each section and normal compressibility section in all segments.

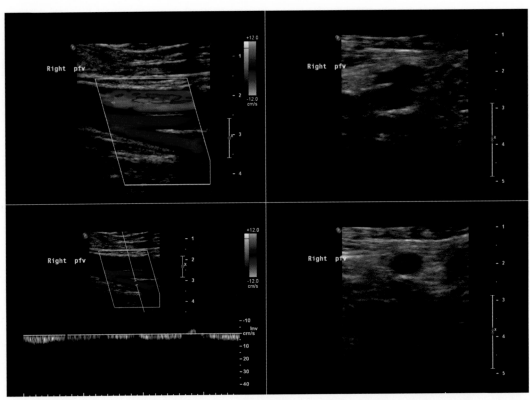

Figure 11-6. Normal venous duplex examination, profunda femoris vein. *Top left,* Color flow mapping depicts normal flow at the level of the femoral vein bifurcation, throughout the observed section of the superior femoral artery. *Top right,* Profunda femoris vein and superior femoral vein in short-axis view, without compression. *Bottom left,* Normal spectral Doppler flow pattern (respiratory variation). *Bottom right,* Profunda femoris vein and superior femoral vein in short-axis view, with compression. Absence of intraluminal echoes, normal compressibility, and normal flow pattern.

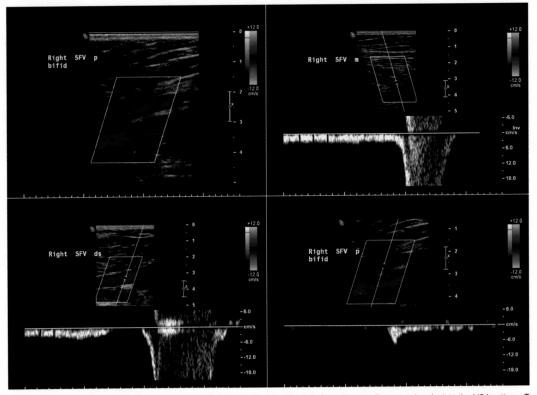

Figure 11-7. Normal venous duplex examination, bifid superficial femoral artery. *Top left,* Color Doppler flow mapping depicts the bifid pattern. *Top right, bottom left and right,* Spectral displays of augmentation within the main and the bifid superficial femoral vein vessels.

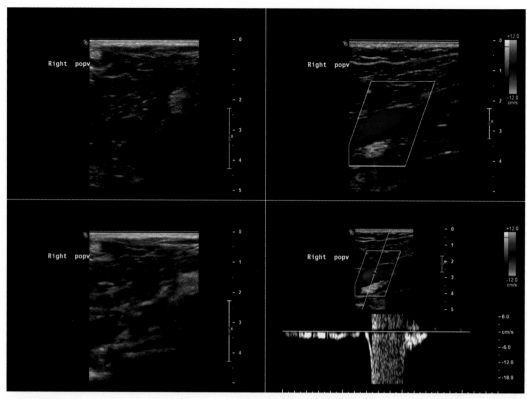

Figure 11-8. Normal venous duplex examination, popliteal veins. *Top left,* Short-axis view without compression. *Top right,* Color Doppler flow mapping revealing normal flow throughout the vein. *Bottom left,* Short-axis view with compression. *Bottom right,* Spectral Doppler display of normal augmentation with distal limb compression.

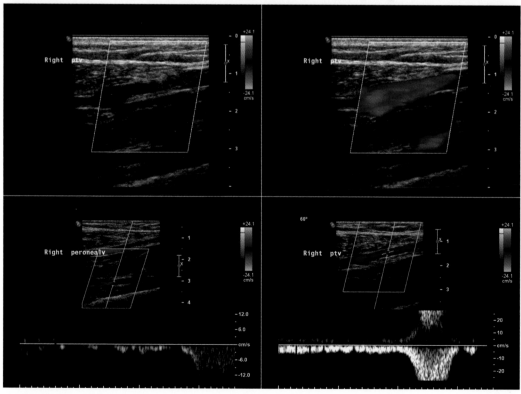

Figure 11-9. Normal venous duplex examination, veins of lower limb. *Top left,* Posterior tibial vein in long-axis view with an absence of intraluminal echoes. *Top right,* Color Doppler flow mapping during augmentation showing one of the posterior tibial and one of the peroneal veins, revealing normal flow augmentation. *Bottom right,* Posterior tibial vein spectral Doppler display revealing normal augmentation. *Bottom left,* Peroneal vein spectral Doppler display of normal augmentation.

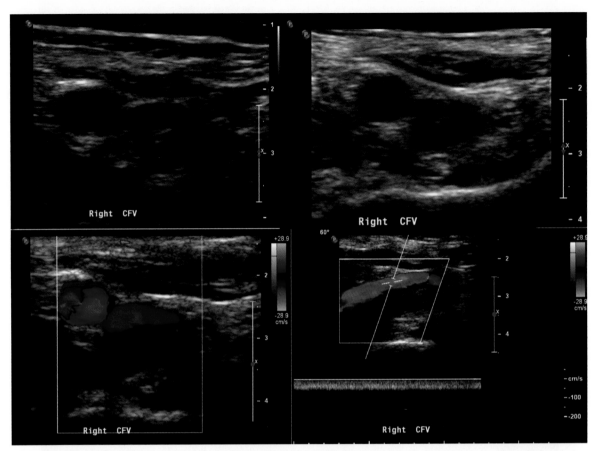

Figure 11-10. Duplex interrogation of the common femoral vein, with thrombus. *Top left,* The short-axis image depicts the common femoral vein and artery in cross-section without compression. *Top right,* Same view with compression. It can be seen that the common femoral vein, which is filled with echogenic material, is incompressible. *Bottom left,* Color Doppler flow mapping of the common femoral vein in transverse plane. In the nearfield aspect of the common femoral vein, there is still some flow within the lumen. *Bottom right,* Spectral display of pulsed-wave Doppler interrogation of the remaining lumen. Flow is again seen to be present but without respiratory variation. There is nonoccclusive deep venous thrombosis.

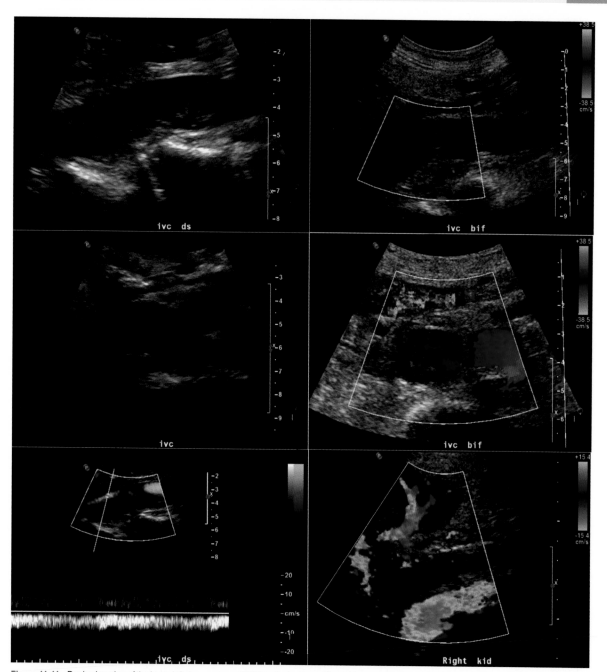

Figure 11-11. Duplex imaging of the lower inferior vena cava (IVC) in short-axis and long-axis views without and with color Doppler flow mapping. The IVC is dilated, and the lumen is largely filled with echogenic material. There is only a small amount of flow along the walls of the IVC. The *bottom left* image shows power angiography mode enhancing the depiction of color on color Doppler imaging. The flow variation seen on spectral display is minimal. The renal vein is also solidly filled with material and is not apparent in the *bottom right* image of the kidney and patent renal artery. Renal adenocarcinoma with extension through the renal vein into the IVC, then continuing into the heart. The IVC beneath the renal veins appeared to have thrombosed from the obstruction in the proximal IVC due to the tumor.

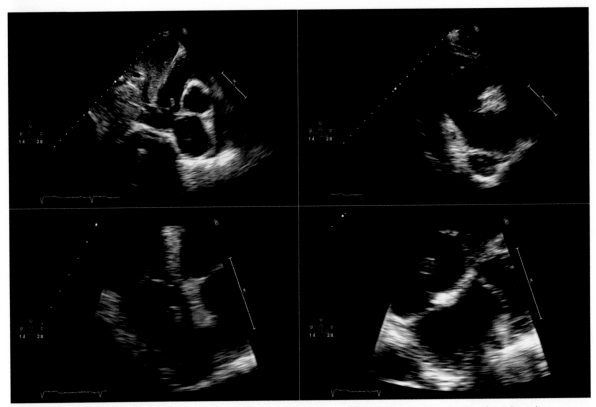

Figure 11-12. Same patient as in Figure 11-11, showing extension of tumor up the inferior vena cava into the right atrium by echocardiography.

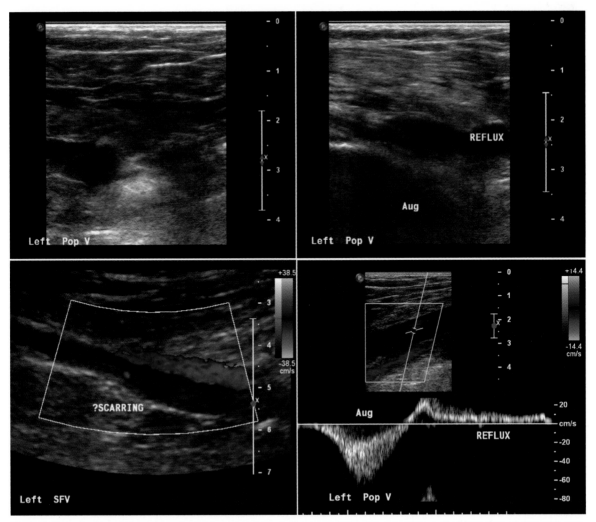

Figure 11-13. Duplex interrogation of the popliteal and superficial femoral veins demonstrating venous insufficiency. *Top left,* Popliteal vein imaged in cross-section without Valsalva maneuver. *Top right,* Same vein with Valsalva maneuver. The popliteal vein seems to distend with Valsalva maneuver—an abnormal finding. *Bottom left,* Image that depicts soft tissue occupying proximally half of the lumen at the superficial femoral vein, due to previous deep venous thrombosis. *Bottom right,* Spectral display of pulsed-Doppler sampling at the popliteal vein. With compression of the calf, there is augmentation of flow. Notably, there is reflux of flow as well following the augmentation, consistent with venous insufficiency.

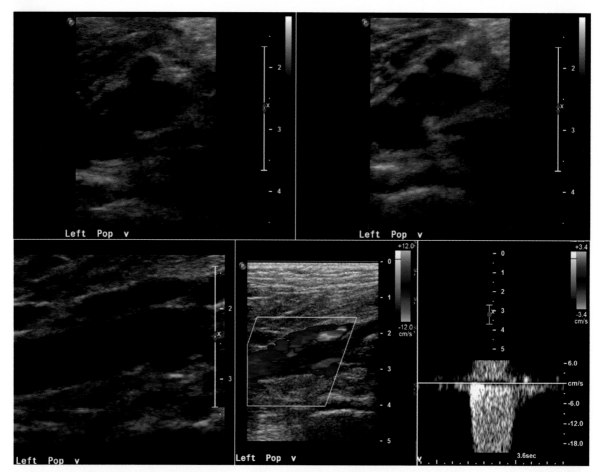

Figure 11-14. Partially occlusive popliteal vein thrombosis. *Top left,* Short-axis views of the popliteal vein and artery, without compression. *Top right,* Same view with compression. There is intraluminal echogenic material, and the vein is partially incompressible. *Bottom left,* Long-axis view of the popliteal vein with extensive intraluminal echogenic material. *Bottom middle,* Color Doppler flow mapping does not fill the lumen of the vessel where there is echogenic material. *Bottom right,* Spectral display demonstrating augmentation to calf compression, due to nonocclusiveness of the deep vein thrombosis.

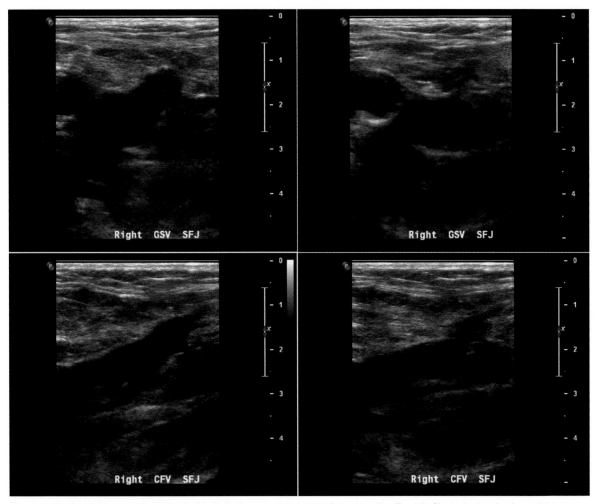

Figure 11-15. *Top left,* Short-axis views showing intraluminal echoes at the saphenofemoral junction. *Top right,* Short-axis view showing partial compressibility. *Bottom left,* Long-axis view at the same site showing thrombus extending well into the common femoral vein. *Bottom right,* Long-axis view with compression showing partial compressibility, corroborating the short-axis finding.

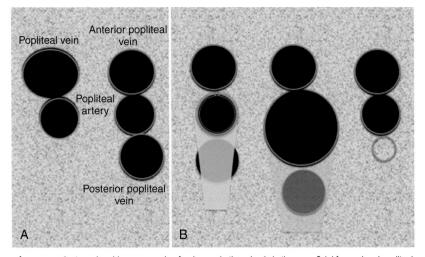

Figure 11-16. Diagram of venous variants and problems assessing for deep vein thrombosis in the superficial femoral and popliteal venous system. **A:** *Left,* The normal anatomy of a superior femoral artery or popliteal artery above and the corresponding vein below. *Right,* A bifid venous system with an accessory vein anterior to the artery as well as the main vein posterior to the artery. **B:** Problems identifying pathology in a bifid venous system. In these examples, the deep bifid vein is difficult to image as (*left*) the more interior artery is calcified and is shadowing the main vein, (*middle*) a more interior large artery/aneurysm is shadowing the main vein, and (*right*) a completely thrombosed deep bifid vein is inapparent as its appearance is indistinguishable from the surrounding tissue.

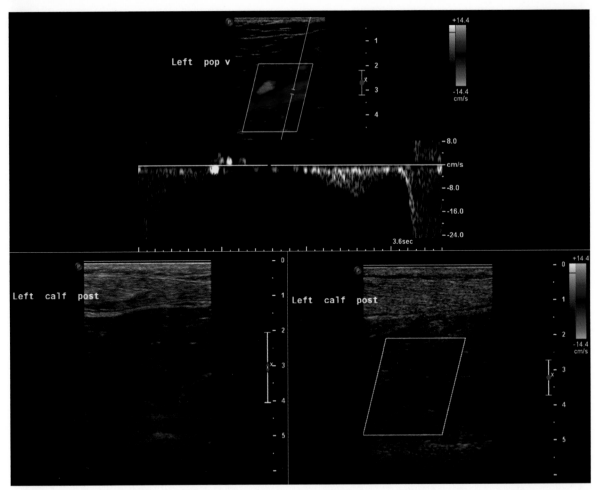

Figure 11-17. *Top,* Long-axis color and spectral Doppler depiction of the popliteal vein, showing a good response to calf compression giving the impression of calf vein patency. *Bottom left,* Short-axis grayscale view showing incompressibility of an engorged calf vein, suggesting deep vein thrombosis. *Bottom right,* Long-axis color Doppler showing no evidence of flow during compression, corroborating the finding of deep vein thrombosis in the calf. In this case, the thrombus lies in one of the calf muscle veins and the paired deep veins are patent, thus maintaining augmentation through to the popliteal vein.

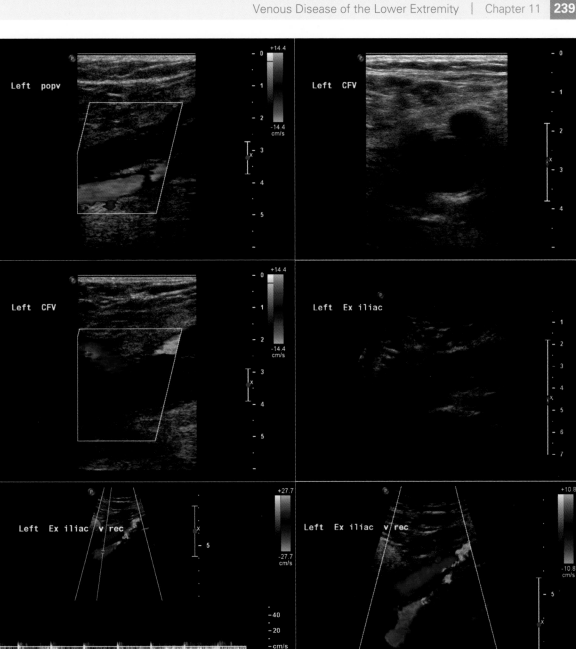

Figure 11-18. *Top left,* Long-axis view of the popliteal vein showing intraluminal echoes consistent with deep vein thrombosis. *Top right,* Short-axis view of the same. *Middle left,* The thrombus extended beyond the common femoral vein. *Middle right,* The thrombus also extended into the external iliac vein, where the fibrous cap appears to float in mid-lumen. *Bottom left,* Color and spectral Doppler of the site of reconstitution in the external iliac vein. *Bottom right,* Color Doppler shows a large collateral crossing anteriorly over the external iliac artery.

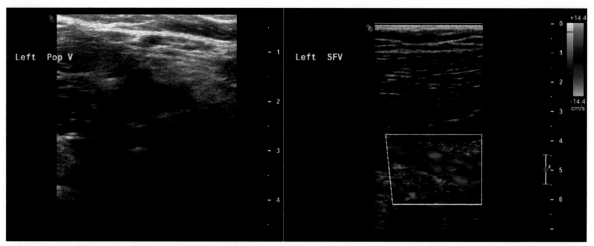

Figure 11-19. *Left,* A partially compressible popliteal vein. *Right,* Color Doppler of the popliteal and distal superficial femoral vein showing patent channels of flow consistent with chronic recanalized venous thrombosis.

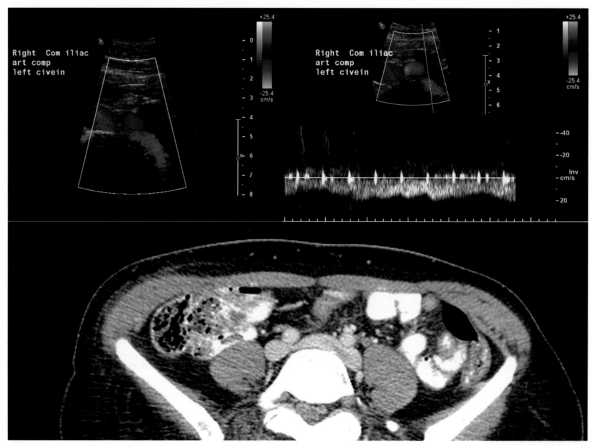

Figure 11-20. *Top left,* Color Doppler view showing the right common iliac artery in short-axis view, causing compression of the left iliac vein seen in long-axis view. *Top right,* Color and spectral Doppler depiction of transmitted arterial pulsation into the vein from the artery as a result of the compression. The Doppler sampling also picks up some of the iliac artery flow. *Bottom,* Computed tomography scan corroborating the finding.

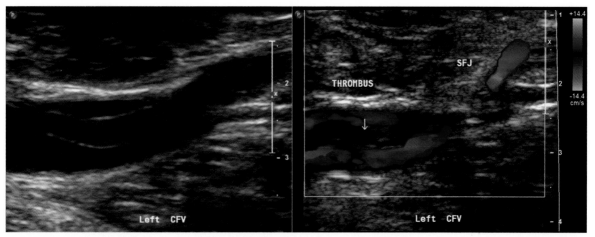

Figure 11-21. *Left,* Long-axis grayscale view of the proximal tail of a deep vein thrombus extending from the long saphenous vein at the saphenofemoral junction into the common femoral vein. *Right,* Color Doppler long-axis view showing flow around the thrombus.

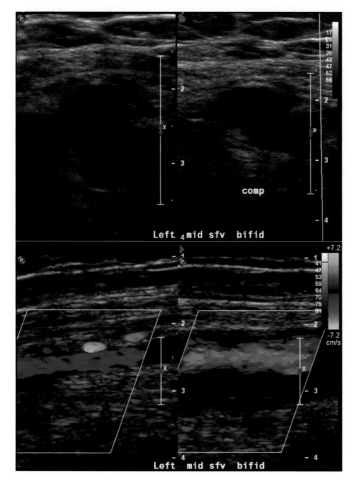

Figure 11-22. *Top left,* Grayscale short-axis view of a bifid superficial femoral vein (and the superficial femoral artery shallow to the bifid/second femoral vein). The bifid system consists of the accessory vein to the viewer's left side of the central femoral vein and the main vein deep and slightly to the right of the artery. *Top right,* With compression, only the more shallow of the superficial veins but not the deeper (nor the artery) compress. Faintly seen are intraluminal echoes in the deeper of the bifid veins. *Bottom left,* Long-axis image through the accessory vein without compression, demonstrating flow. *Bottom right,* Long-axis view through the artery and deeper main vein without compression. There is prominent flow signal in the artery and no flow depicted in the deeper main vein, also consistent with deep venous thrombosis.

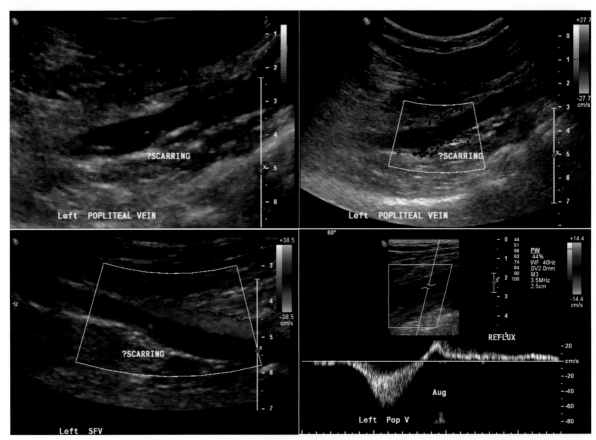

Figure 11-23. *Top left and right,* Grayscale images of the left popliteal vein revealing a peel of chronic organized thrombus—a scar. *Top right,* Color flow mapping does not depict flow among the intraluminal echoes of chronic thrombus. *Bottom left,* Grayscale/color Doppler view with chronic thrombus and flow restricted to a narrow lumen. *Bottom right,* Spectral display of flow in the popliteal vein with augmentation by calf squeeze. Initially, there is anterograde surge of flow, but following that there is reversal of flow (due to valvular insufficiency) of greater than 0.5-second duration, establishing venous incompetence due to vein scarring from prior deep venous thrombosis.

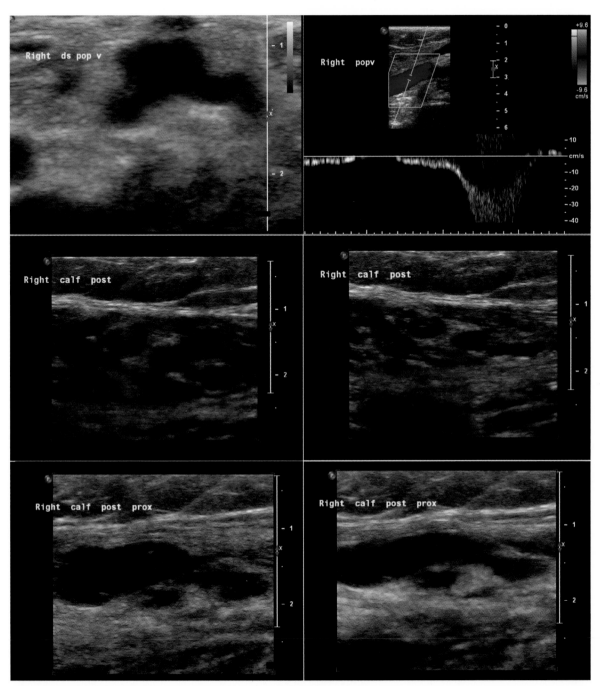

Figure 11-24. Calf deep vein thrombosis. *Top left,* The popliteal vein (center) appears to be patent; there are no intraluminal echoes, as in a branch vessel entering it from the right side. (The artery is beneath and to the left.) *Top right,* Spectral recording of flow in the popliteal vein demonstrates normal brisk flow augmentation. *Middle left,* Short-axis views of three calf veins. The one on the left has intraluminal echoes on its left side. The other two do not. *Middle right,* The artery is the smallest vessel with compression. The left vein (with intraluminal echoes) does not compress, and neither does the middle one. Both are incompressible, the sign of venous thrombosis. Only the right vein compresses. *Bottom left and right,* A large branch immediately before joining the popliteal vein contains intraluminal echoes and does not compress, due to the presence of thrombus. This case underscores the point that although there may not be thrombus within the popliteal vein, thrombus may be in close proximity to it within calf veins.

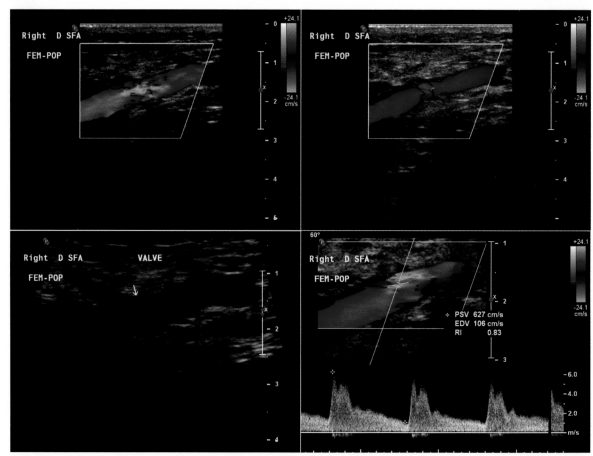

Figure 11-25. Reversed saphenous vein graft with valve stenosis. (In these images it is not possible to say whether one or both cusps are responsible.) *Top left,* Color long-axis view showing high-velocity aliased (systolic) flow in the distal thigh segment of a reversed saphenous vein graft. *Top right,* Color long-axis view showing a lower order of aliased flow in diastole. *Bottom left,* Grayscale long-axis view depicting intraluminal echoes, suggesting a single, thickened protruding venous valve at the same site. *Bottom right,* Color and spectral Doppler images clearly identifying high systolic and diastolic velocities flow through the valve site consistent with significant stenosis.

12 Intravascular Ultrasound

JUNYA AKO and KATSUHISA WASEDA

Key Points

- IVUS can be used to characterize, with high resolution, coronary artery architecture and coronary artery plaque, and other lesional architecture.
- IVUS can be used to guide coronary stent deployment by assessing the adequacy of the stent apposition to the vessel well.

INTRODUCTION

Intravascular ultrasound (IVUS) is a device used to visualize the vessel wall in a two-dimensional tomographic format. The ultrasound signal penetrates below the luminal surface, imaging the entire cross section of the vessel in real time. The current IVUS system for coronary artery imaging uses a miniaturized transducer with high-frequency ultrasound (20 to 45 MHz), achieving a resolution of 150 microns. IVUS is the first imaging modality that directly visualizes atherosclerosis and other pathologic conditions from within the vessel wall. Today, IVUS is often used in the catheterization laboratory at the time of percutaneous coronary intervention (PCI) for pre-PCI lesion assessment and post-PCI evaluation of the results.

BASIC IMAGE INTERPRETATION

The coronary arterial wall consists of three concentric layers. The layer adjacent to the arterial lumen is called the intima and is made up of a superficial lining of endothelial cells immediately exposed to the blood. The media is composed of many layers of smooth muscle cells interspersed with connective fibers embedded in a glycoprotein matrix. The external elastic lamina separates the medial layer from the adventitia. The adventitia is fibrous in nature and has the highest density of collagen. It offers the architectural support to the vessel. IVUS images of coronary arteries generally demonstrate the three major layers of the arterial wall: intima, media, and adventitia (Fig. 12-1).

PRACTICAL INTRAVASCULAR ULTRASOUND USE IN THE CATHETERIZATION LABORATORY

Typical IVUS indications in the catheterization laboratory include pre-PCI assessment of the lesions and evaluation of post-PCI results (Table 12-1). In particular, arterial stenting has become one of the most important applications for IVUS in clinical settings. On IVUS examination, stent struts are easily visualized as a collection of bright, distinct echoes. IVUS imaging can show the apposition of the stent to the vessel wall, which is essential for achieving optimal PCI results. In bare metal stents, IVUS guidance has been shown to improve stent deployment with dramatic reduction of the risk of stent thrombosis, which ultimately leads to the diminishing need for aggressive anticoagulation in most cases.

PREINTERVENTIONAL ASSESSMENT

Preinterventional IVUS has been used to assess the severity and morphology of coronary artery stenosis as well as to measure reference vessel size and lesion length, especially when angiography yields equivocal or difficult-to-interpret images. Based on physiologic approaches, including fractional flow reserve, coronary flow reserve, and stress scintigraphy, the ischemic minimal lumen area threshold has been reported to be 3 to 4 mm^2 for major epicardial coronary arteries[1,2] and 5.9 mm^2 for the left main coronary artery (LMCA).[3] The presence, location, and extent of calcium can significantly affect the results of angioplasty, atherectomy, and stent deployment. Precise measurement of lesion length, vessel size, and plaque burden can also help optimize the PCI results.

ASSESSMENT OF ANGIOGRAPHICALLY EQUIVOCAL LESIONS

Ostial Lesion
The severity of ostial lesions, especially LMCA lesions, is sometimes difficult to assess using conventional angiography alone. IVUS may help provide more accurate

TABLE 12-1   IVUS Assessment Pre- and Post-PCI

Pre-PCI Assessment

Quantitative assessment	Minimal lumen area
	Vessel size
	Lesion length
Qualitative assessment	Plaque types (fibrous, fibrofatty, calcified)
	Patterns of calcification
	Plaque eccentricity
	Plaque rupture
	Presence of thrombus
	Vascular remodeling

Post-PCI Assessment

Quantitative assessment	Minimal lumen area (minimal stent area)
Qualitative assessment	Stent apposition
	Dissection/edge tears
	In-stent protrusions

PCI, percutaneous intervention.

assessment of the severity of this lesion subset. Because of the recent increase in use of PCI with the LCMA, assessment of this artery has become an important indication for IVUS imaging. The cutoff value of significant LMCA stenosis is 5.9 mm^2 based on a previous physiologic study.[3] Deep engagement of the catheter to the LCMA prohibits the assessment of LMCA ostium, and the operator sometimes has to purposefully disengage the catheter from the orifice of the artery (Figs. 12-2 and 12-3).

Calcified Lesion

Calcified lesions are yet another lesion subset difficult to diagnose using angiography alone. With IVUS, regions of calcified plaque are characterized by bright echogenic areas that create a dense shadow more peripherally from the catheter. Shadowing is sometimes accompanied by reverberation, which causes the appearance of multiple ghost images of the leading calcium interface spaced at regular intervals radially. Because of the shadowing, the presence of calcium inhibits further evaluation of the plaque behind the calcification. The location and the severity of calcification, as well as the lumen, can be assessed with IVUS (Figs. 12-4 and 12-5).

EVALUATION OF PERCUTANEOUS INTERVENTION RESULTS

Incomplete Stent Apposition

Incomplete stent apposition (ISA) is a lack of contact between stent struts and the underlying vessel wall, which is best described by IVUS. By IVUS, ISA is

defined as one or more stent struts clearly separated from the vessel wall without involvement of side branches.[4] The etiology of ISA can be multifactorial; possible mechanisms may include stent underexpansion, artery/stent mismatch, calcification, and acute recoil. Postprocedural ISA, or ISA observed poststenting, is considered to be partly dependent on technique. Postprocedural ISA may be treatable with high-pressure postdilatation and/or use of larger sized balloons (Figs. 12-6 and 12-7).

ISA draws clinical attention because of its possible association with stent thrombosis. Although no definitive study has yet been performed, several reports show a possible association between postinterventional ISA and stent thrombosis, a catastrophic adverse event after stent implantation.[5,6] Complete stent apposition is an important factor in a classic IVUS guidance criteria.[7] Because apposition cannot be diagnosed with conventional angiography, IVUS plays an essential role in achieving adequate apposition in clinical practice.

In addition to postprocedural ISA, late-acquired ISA has been frequently reported following drug-eluting stent implantation.[4] Late-acquired ISA is an unusual form of ISA, defined as ISA observed at the time of follow-up catheterization but not at the time of stent implantation. Late-acquired ISA is also suggested as a potential risk factor for stent thrombosis[8] (Fig. 12-8).

Measurement of Minimal Stent Area

Quantitative assessment of stent expansion is an important step for achieving adequate results of stent implantation. Minimal stent area (MSA), measured as the smallest cross-sectional area within the stent, is one of the strongest predictors for angiographic and clinical restenosis following intracoronary stenting. With bare metal stents, the risk of restenosis decreases 19% for every one square millimeter increase in MSA.[9] With sirolimus-eluting stents, the prognostic value of MSA is even stronger; it is a powerful predictor of in-stent restenosis.[10] Furthermore, several studies have suggested that a smaller MSA is a predictor for stent thrombosis.[5,11] The utility of IVUS to ensure adequate stent expansion has become even more important with drug-eluting stents (Fig. 12-9).

REFERENCES

1. Abizaid AS, Mintz GS, Mehran R, et al. Long-term follow-up after percutaneous transluminal coronary angioplasty was not performed based on intravascular ultrasound findings: importance of lumen dimensions. *Circulation.* 1999;100:256-261.
2. Takagi A, Tsurumi Y, Ishii Y, et al. Clinical potential of intravascular ultrasound for physiological assessment of coronary stenosis: relationship between quantitative ultrasound tomography and pressure-derived fractional flow reserve. *Circulation.* 1999;100:250-255.

3. Jasti V, Ivan E, Yalamanchili V, et al. Correlations between fractional flow reserve and intravascular ultrasound in patients with an ambiguous left main coronary artery stenosis. *Circulation.* 2004;110:2831-2836.

4. Ako J, Morino Y, Honda Y, et al. Late incomplete stent apposition after sirolimus-eluting stent implantation: a serial intravascular ultrasound analysis. *J Am Coll Cardiol.* 2005;46:1002-1005.

5. Cheneau E, Leborgne L, Mintz GS, et al. Predictors of subacute stent thrombosis: results of a systematic intravascular ultrasound study. *Circulation.* 2003;108:43-47.

6. Uren NG, Schwarzacher SP, Metz JA, et al. Predictors and outcomes of stent thrombosis: an intravascular ultrasound registry. *Eur Heart J.* 2002;23:124-132.

7. de Jaegere P, Mudra H, Figulla H, et al. Intravascular ultrasound-guided optimized stent deployment. Immediate and 6 months clinical and angiographic results from the Multicenter Ultrasound Stenting in Coronaries Study (MUSIC Study). *Eur Heart J.* 1998;19:1214-1223.

8. Cook S, Wenaweser P, Togni M, et al. Incomplete stent apposition and very late stent thrombosis after drug-eluting stent implantation. *Circulation.* 2007;115:2426-2434.

9. Kasaoka S, Tobis JM, Akiyama T, et al. Angiographic and intravascular ultrasound predictors of in-stent restenosis. *J Am Coll Cardiol.* 1998;32:1630-1635.

10. Sonoda S, Morino Y, Ako J, et al. Impact of final stent dimensions on long-term results following sirolimus-eluting stent implantation: serial intravascular ultrasound analysis from the sirius trial. *J Am Coll Cardiol.* 2004;43:1959-1963.

11. Fujii K, Carlier SG, Mintz GS, et al. Stent underexpansion and residual reference segment stenosis are related to stent thrombosis after sirolimus-eluting stent implantation: an intravascular ultrasound study. *J Am Coll Cardiol.* 2005;45:995-998.

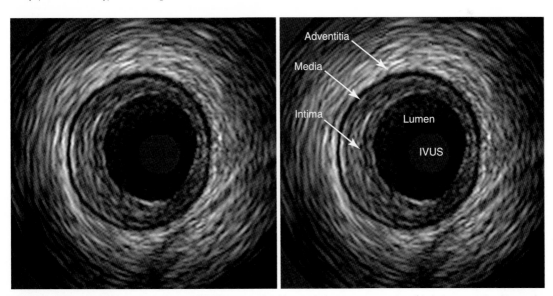

Figure 12-1. A representative intravascular ultrasound (IVUS) cross-sectional image of a human coronary artery. A typical cross-sectional image shows the lumen, intima, media, and adventitia.

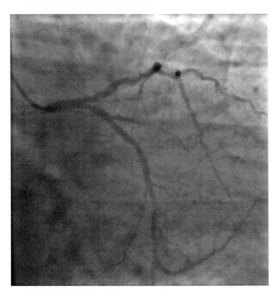

Figure 12-2. Left main ostial lesion. With this angiogram alone, it is difficult to assess the severity of the left main ostial lesion accurately.

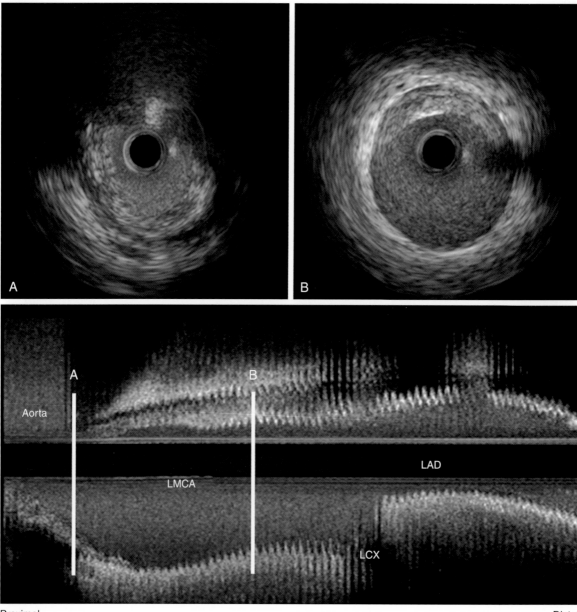

Figure 12-3. Intravascular ultrasound images (same case as Figure 12-2). **A** and **B** (*top*), Cross-sectional images corresponding to the sections of the longitudinal image (*bottom*). The cross-sectional lumen area is 4.2 mm^2 in **A,** while the cross-sectional lumen area (mid-LMCA)is 11.6 mm^2 in **B.** LAD, left anterior descending artery; LCX, left circumflex artery; LMCA, left main coronary artery.

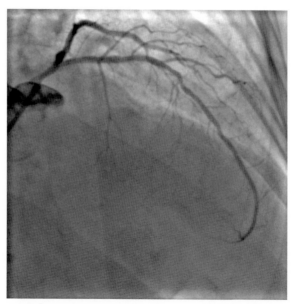

Figure 12-4. Calcified lesion. Angiography yields ambiguous results with no clear sign of focal stenosis in the left anterior descending artery.

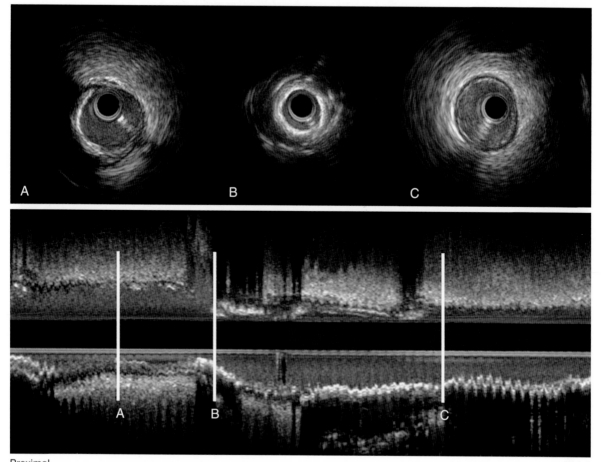

Proximal

Distal

Figure 12-5. Intravascular ultrasound (IVUS) analysis of the left anterior descending artery (same case as Figure 12-4). **A, B,** and **C** (*top*),Cross-sectional images correspond to the cross sections of the longitudinal image (*bottom*). **B,** High echoic lesion with acoustic shadow behind it, a characteristic IVUS finding of heavily calcified plaque. Lumen area at cross section B shows a significant stenosis of 2.7 mm^2.

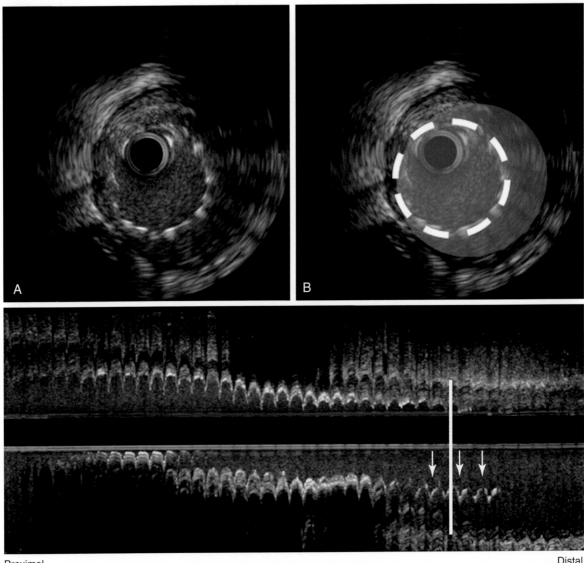

Proximal

Distal

Figure 12-6. Postprocedural incomplete stent apposition. **A** and **B,** Cross-sectional images (*top*) correspond to the vertical line in the longitudinal image (*bottom*). **B,** Stent (*dotted line*) and lumen (*gray area*). The stent is not appropriately apposed to the vessel wall. It is also shown in the longitudinal image (*arrows*).

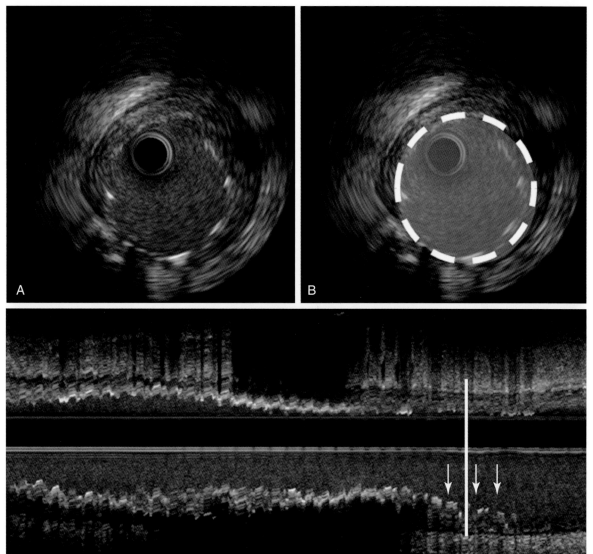

Proximal

Distal

Figure 12-7. After postdilatation with a bigger balloon with higher pressure, the stent is adequately apposed to the vessel wall (same case as in Figure 12-6). **A** and **B**, Cross-sectional images (*top*) corresponding to the vertical line in the longitudinal image (*bottom*). **B,** Complete apposition of the stent (*dashed line*) to the vessel wall. The longitudinal image (*bottom*) also confirms adequate stent apposition (*arrows*).

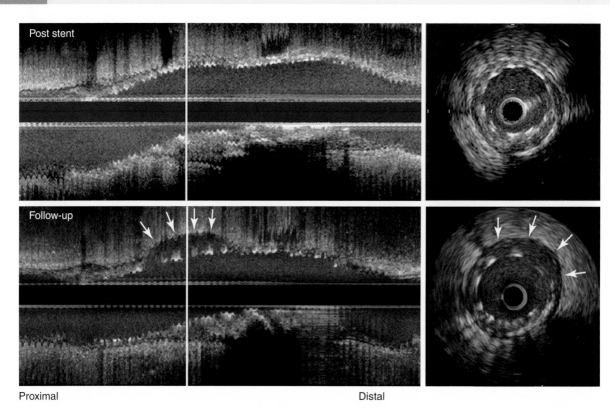

Proximal   Distal

Figure 12-8. A case of late-acquired incomplete stent apposition following drug-eluting stent implantation. *Top,* Postprocedural images (*left,* longitudinal image; *right,* cross-sectional image). *Bottom,* Eight-month follow-up images. The stent shows complete apposition at the time of stent implantation, whereas the 8-month follow-up image shows incomplete stent apposition accompanied by positive vessel remodeling (*arrows*).

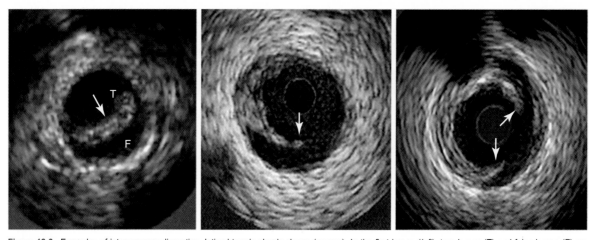

Figure 12-9. Examples of intracoronary dissection. Intimal tear is clearly shown (*arrows*). In the first image (*left*), true lumen (T) and false lumen (F) are also observed.

13

Intravascular Ultrasound Imaging of the Descending Aorta and Iliac Arteries

GEORGE E. KOPCHOK, JOE CHAUVAPUN, and RODNEY A. WHITE

Key Points

- IVUS can be used to characterize, with high resolution, the architecture of the aorta and, importantly, the architecture of its branch vessel ostia, as well as aortic plaque, thrombus, and intimal flaps.
- IVUS can be used to guide thoracic and abdominal aortic and iliac-level stent deployment.

INTRODUCTION

The continued expansion of endovascular devices and procedures has led to a major shift in the treatment of vascular disease. These procedures, which were first successful in small-caliber vessels, have quickly become quite useful in larger-caliber vessels such as the aorta and iliac arteries. The continued success and advancement of these procedures depends on the ability to image and evaluate the patient's anatomy adequately prior to the procedure, as well as during it. Accurate assessment of the patient's anatomy and disease are crucial in the selection of the appropriate device. Furthermore, during the procedure, precise imaging is needed to confirm the initial computed tomography (CT) interpretation of the anatomy, to evaluate landing zones or neck length, and to confirm that the devices are in the correct location and are fully expanded. Intravascular ultrasound (IVUS) is ideally suited to provide these real-time imaging needs. The use of IVUS can add another level of imaging accuracy to further increase the information available to the endovascular surgeon. The goals of this chapter are (1) to demonstrate the utility of IVUS imaging for thoracic and abdominal aorta and iliac artery interventions and (2) to be an atlas or guide to image interpretation of these various anatomies.

INTRAVASCULAR ULTRASOUND IMAGING

Catheters

Two types of peripheral IVUS catheters are available for use: multielement phase array catheters and mechanically rotating element type catheters. Mechanical IVUS catheters rotate a small transducer located at the tip of the catheter using a flexible, high-torque cable that extends the length of the device (Fig. 13-1). The phase array catheters incorporate a miniature integrated circuit with 64 imaging elements located on the tip of the catheter (Fig. 13-2). Both catheters can be used over a 0.035-inch guidewire and can pass through 9F sheaths. Two slight advantages of the phase array catheter are the lack of moving parts and the concentric guidewire location, which allows easy passage through tortuous anatomy and has no guidewire artifact. The key to optimizing IVUS catheter use is to not delay the procedure or add additional guidewire exchanges. IVUS should provide quick and easy assessment of the device and/or anatomy.

Rotational Orientation

On-screen image orientation, although not crucial in the diagnosis, can be helpful for image interpretation. The image can be easily electronically rotated by pushing a button on the IVUS machine. The investigator should avoid rotating the catheter, especially in tortuous anatomy. The best way to identify vessel orientation is to use known anatomical landmarks. For example, as the catheter crosses the aortic bifurcation, it is possible to rotate the IVUS display electronically such that the common iliac arteries are positioned side-by-side, in a correct anatomical location. Occasionally, this anatomical arrangement is not true, especially in tortuous, dilated vessels, and it is necessary to check the alignment against other parameters. The location of anterior visceral vessels (i.e., celiac and superior mesenteric arteries, renal vein) are also useful when imaging in the abdominal aorta. For the iliac bed, the posterior-medial position of the internal iliac artery orifices can be used to adjust for angulations.

Longitudinal Grayscale Imaging

The longitudinal grayscale image is obtained by mechanically withdrawing the catheter through the vessel at a controlled rate. The cross-sectional images are then stacked by the processing unit and rotated 90 degrees to produce a longitudinal view, very similar to an angiogram, except that detailed wall morphology and luminal dimensions are depicted. Length measurements can be made if a mechanical pull-back device is used. However, the current pull-back devices available are too slow to use for peripheral-aortic type of procedures. Therefore, length measurements cannot be obtained.

Measurements

Luminal dimensions and wall thickness determined by IVUS of normal and minimally diseased arteries (both in vitro and in vivo) are accurate to within 0.05 mm.[1–7] The luminal cross-sectional areas calculated from biplanar angiograms and measured from IVUS correlate well for normal or minimally diseased peripheral arteries in vivo. In severely diseased vessels with elliptical lumens, angiography is less accurate in calculating luminal cross-sectional area and tends to underestimate the severity of atherosclerosis in the wall compared with IVUS.[8,9] Studies have shown that IVUS is an important intraoperative tool in evaluating aortic diameters for endovascular aneurysm repair and that the technique has proven efficacy in the characterization of vessel diameter, stenosis, and morphology.[10–14]

When dealing with the aorta, angulations caused by tortuosity may also cause an elliptical image of the vessel lumen. This is especially true in the thoracic arch. When this occurs, the minimal diameter (minor axis) should be used to measure the diameter. Investigators have demonstrated that the minor axis is the most accurate measurement in angled images and/or tortuous anatomy.[15] In another study, investigators found that off-center IVUS measurements may not be as accurate as centerline CT measurements.[16] In a study comparing two-dimensional versus three-dimensional CT scans for aortic measurement, investigators found that the minor axis measurement on axial CT scans had a high correlation with the centerline three-dimensional measurements.[17] Their conclusion was that the minor axis measurement can substitute for three-dimensional centerline measurements in most situations. The authors continue to use three-dimensional centerline CT scans for preoperative evaluation and sizing but use minor axis IVUS diameter measurement, at systole, to select the appropriate endoluminal device size.

THERAPEUTIC INTERVENTIONS

Aortoiliac Disease

IVUS can provide important diagnostic information that can alter the conduct of selected endovascular procedures. It is especially useful when the procedure requires deployment of arterial stents.[18,19] Proper sizing, stent selection, and deployment are critical for improving chances of long-term patency. Researchers have shown that inadequate stent expansion can lead to early thrombosis or stent migration, whereas overexpansion can result in excessive intimal hyperplasia or vessel perforation.[5] IVUS is effective in assessing the result of the primary intervention, establishing the need for stenting, and guiding stent deployment. Studies have found that it improves long-term patency rates.[20–24] Additional studies have revealed that contrast angiography, which is thought to be the "gold standard" for assessing endovascular therapy, has limitations in the evaluation of stent-based procedures. Specifically, the monoplanar images produced with arteriography show the details only of the outer edges of the artery and stent. This limits the ability to evaluate stent-to-vessel apposition adequately. One study demonstrated that vessel size and lumen diameter were underestimated 62% of the time by arteriography and that 40% of the stents placed in the iliac arterial system were underdeployed, which might lead to related treatment failure.[21,24]

It is also possible to use IVUS to differentiate intimal versus subintimal guidewire location and to choose appropriate endovascular technique based on that data. In cases where the investigator cannot reenter the true lumen, research has demonstrated that IVUS can be used to guide a trans-septal needle from the subintimal space to the true lumen, followed by successful angioplasty and stenting.[25] Figure 13-3 illustrates the use of IVUS to determine guidewire location and assess the area of treatment for a total occlusion of the right iliac artery. Figure 13-3A shows pre-IVUS images. The patient underwent treatment with bilateral iliac stents and primary stent ballooning, followed by IVUS. After the clinician used the same balloon to further dilate the stent, the patient had a final IVUS and angiogram, which can be seen in Figure 13-3B.

IVUS can also be useful in cases where the quality of the fluoroscopic imaging is limited (due to equipment and/or size [density] of the patient) and when the investigator wishes to limit the amount of contrast. Once the clinician advances the guidewire past the lesion of interest, an IVUS catheter can completely interrogate the vessel morphology without the use of contrast or fluoroscopy. A radiopaque scale placed behind the patient can be used to identify the location of IVUS catheter at specific areas of interest. If this technique is used, the landmarks should be centered on the screen to eliminate fluoroscopic parallax or the fluoroscopic unit should be locked in place. Figure 13-4 illustrates this use of IVUS.

Endoluminal Grafts for Abdominal Aortic Aneurysm

IVUS can be an important adjuvant in the deployment and evaluation of endoluminal grafts for the treatment of abdominal aortic aneurysms. Currently, most of the preprocedural evaluations can be performed using contrast-enhanced spiral CT imaging. However, during the procedure, IVUS is useful to confirm diameters and lengths of proximal and distal fixation points as well as to ensure normal healthy arterial wall at those fixation points.[8,25–27] Cinefluoroscopy and IVUS are complementary in enabling expedient placement of endoluminal grafts. The use of IVUS can significantly reduce the fluoroscopy time and contrast usage during the procedures, minimizing the exposure of both personnel and the patient. Several investigators have reported deploying both thoracic and abdominal endoluminal grafts without the use of contrast agents.[28,29]

The authors commonly place the radiopaque scale beneath the patient, positioned parallel to the spine along the left psoas muscle, to locate the major landmarks such as the aorta just distal to the lowest renal artery, the aortic bifurcation, and the hypogastric arteries. At each given point, the IVUS catheter is centered on the fluoroscopic screen to eliminate fluoroscopic parallax, and the diameter is measured to confirm pre-CT measurements (Fig. 13-5). If the aorta is tortuous and/or the IVUS image is elliptical, the minor axis is measured to determine diameter, as described earlier. The catheter is then retracted to the next landmark and measurement repeated.

This technique allows the interventionalist to interrogate the entire aortoiliac system with minimal fluoroscopy time and no contrast. It also verifies the interpretation of the CT scan and enables the physician to further examine the fixation points. Several times, in the authors' experience, the normal aortic wall seen on the CT scan was aneurysmal or had evidence of a pseudoaneurysm on IVUS evaluation. Once the landmarks are located and measured, the investigator can verify the length from the infrarenal fixation point to the iliac bifurcation by placing the IVUS catheter at the level of the distal renal orifice and grasping the IVUS catheter as it exits the access sheath. He or she then withdraws the catheter to the level of the iliac orifice and measures the distance between the sheath and fingers. Leaving the fingers in place, it is possible to withdraw the catheter to the external iliac artery and measure the overall (shortest) length.

Once the anatomy is interrogated and mapped out, the authors routinely advance the endoluminal graft device into the approximate location. They then position an angiographic catheter alongside the device and inject a small bolus of contrast to confirm the renal orifice and infrarenal fixation point relative to the endoluminal graft. They repeat small injections until the device is in position and deployed.

For two-component abdominal aortic aneurysm endograft systems, once the ipsilateral device is deployed, it is necessary to gain access to the contralateral limb. After access is obtained, IVUS is very useful to confirm that the wire is in the device lumen and not outside of the device. Some clinicians simply rotate a pigtail catheter or inflate a small balloon. However, if the device was mis-sized or not fully expanded, enfolding can occur, which can lead to misinterpretation. Following deployment of the contralateral limb, IVUS is used to evaluate device location and to confirm good device to artery apposition and proximity to the renal orifice.

Thoracic Aorta and Thoracic Aortic Dissections

In 1994, investigators first described endovascular treatment of thoracic aortic dissections.[30,31] Since then, improvements of endoluminal graft design and delivery systems have broadened their use throughout the world.[32,33] Accurate screening and evaluation are critical to the decision-making process for treatment of the thoracic aorta. Multislice spiral CT or magnetic resonance imaging have been proven to provide detailed information of thoracic aneurysms and dissections.[33,34] However, once the decision has been made to intervene with an endovascular graft, these imaging modalities are limited during the deployment procedure.

Preliminary investigations confirm the utility of IVUS in identifying and reconfirming the important parameters required for successful endoluminal treatment of acute and chronic type B thoracic aortic dissection.[33–35] IVUS provides real-time evaluation of (1) proximal entry site and distal extent of the dissection, (2) relationship of the false lumen to major aortic branches, (3) measurement of aortic dimensions to allow selection of correct stent size, (4) confirmation that the device is being deployed in the true lumen, and (5) confirmation that blood supply to major branch vessels has not been compromised during device deployment. As with abdominal aortic aneurysm intervention, it is possible to use IVUS to identify major branch vessels of the arch as well as location of visceral vessels and to confirm that the morphology has not changed in the time between initial evaluation and treatment. IVUS can also reduce the overall fluoroscopy time and contrast usage.

Proximal and distal entry points and intimal tears can usually be visualized with IVUS examination. If the dissection propagates into the visceral vessels, IVUS can be useful in confirming that visceral blood flow is being supplied by the true and/or false lumens—a crucial factor in determining if the patient is a candidate for endoluminal repair. This is also something that can change from the time of the CT scan to the actual treatment. As shown in Figure 13-6, IVUS can confirm the pre-CT evaluation and the current relationship of major arch and visceral vessels to true and false lumens. Many times, a change in the false lumen flow is apparent immediately after device deployment (Fig. 13-7).

Thoracic Aneurysms and Ulcerations

The treatment of thoracic aneurysms and ulcerations is a little more straightforward and generally associated with more favorable primary success rates than the treatment of aortic dissections.[36] However, given the high flow of the thoracic aorta, IVUS can be very useful for identifying the extent of the aneurysm, to confirm healthy aortic wall for proximal and distal fixation, and to identify the site for endoluminal graft deployment.[37] Figure 13-8 demonstrates the use of IVUS to identify the morphology of the thoracic aneurysm, as well as the landing zones prior to deployment. Following deployment, with graft material placed over the subclavian artery, bare struts are apparent at the left carotid artery orifice. Stagnant flow is evident in the aneurysm sac outside of the endoluminal graft. Device enfolding was also apparent at the distal end of the device, requiring balloon dilation.

The importance of evaluating aortic wall integrity when evaluating proximal and distal fixation points can be demonstrated in Figure 13-9. In this case, the preoperative contrast CT scan revealed healthy aortic wall distal to the subclavian artery as an optimal landing zone. The angiogram would have confirmed the diagnosis and a thoracic endovascular aortic repair (TEVAR) would have been placed distal to the subclavian artery. However, IVUS examination revealed a circumferential intramural thrombus starting at the level of the subclavian artery and extending to the aneurysm. Based on the IVUS findings, the TEVAR was placed just distal to the left carotid artery.

It is not within the scope of this chapter to discuss techniques and procedures for deploying devices at the level of the carotid artery and covering the subclavian artery. However, when deploying devices around the arch, in tortuous anatomy and brisk blood flow, there is always a risk of the device moving forward and covering the carotid artery with graft material. If the graft material is porous, or the orifice not completely covered, flow may still be visualized into the carotid artery. IVUS has been very useful in determining the exact level of graft material relative to the carotid artery orifice. Figure 13-10 demonstrates the bare strut across the carotid orifice versus graft material, excluding flow.

All of the previously described clinical thoracic cases (including those involving thoracic dissection) were performed as part of a single-center, investigator-sponsored, Food and Drug Administration–approved study, with an investigational device exemption (IDE).

POSTPROCEDURAL ASSESSMENTS AND TROUBLESHOOTING

As noted earlier, IVUS is an invaluable tool in the assessment of endoluminal graft apposition following deployment. Although it is usually difficult to image an endoluminal graft along its length, due to the air in the porosity of the graft material, IVUS can be very useful to assess proximal and distal fixation points. Advancing and retracting the IVUS catheter over the transition area can accomplish this. Any gap between the device and arterial wall verifies poor apposition and a potential endoleak. It is also invaluable to determine lumen characteristics following deployment (Fig. 13-11).

Any time guidewire access through an endoluminal graft is compromised (guidewire is accidentally withdrawn), or if there is a reintervention in a previously deployed device, endoluminal position should be verified. IVUS is very useful to confirm access through a device and ensure that the guidewire is not positioned between the device and aorta.

CONCLUSION

With ongoing refinements, endovascular devices will continue to be an important part of the armamentarium of the endovascular specialist. The authors believe that IVUS will be an important part of that refinement and help optimize the future successes.

REFERENCES

1. Gussenhoven WJ, Essed CE, Lancee CT. Arterial wall characteristics determined by intravascular ultrasound imaging: an in-vitro study. *J Am Coll Cardiol.* 1989;14:947-952.
2. Gussenhoven WJ, Essed CE, Frietman P, et al. Intravascular echographic assessment of vessel wall characteristics: a correlation with histology. *Int J Cardiac Imaging.* 1989;4:105-116.
3. Tobis JM, Mahon D, Lehmann K, et al. The sensitivity of ultrasound imaging compared to angiography for diagnosing coronary atherosclerosis. *Circulation.* 1990;82(suppl 3):439:[abstract].
4. Kopchok GE, White RA, Guthrie C, et al. Intraluminal vascular ultrasound: preliminary report of dimensional and morphologic accuracy. *Ann Vasc Surg.* 1990;4:291-296.
5. Kopchok GE, White RA, White G. Intravascular ultrasound: a new potential modality for angioplasty guidance. *Angiology.* 1990;41:785-792.
6. Mallery JA, Tobis JM, Griffith J, et al. Assessment of normal and atherosclerotic arterial wall thickness with an intravascular ultrasound imaging catheter. *Am Heart J.* 1990;119:1392-1400.
7. Nissen SE, Grines CL, Gurley JC, et al. Application of new phased-array ultrasound imaging catheter in the assessment of vascular dimensions. *Circulation.* 1990;81:660-666.
8. Nissen SE, Gurley JC, Grines CL, et al. Intravascular ultrasound assessing of lumen size and wall morphology in normal subjects and patients with coronary artery disease. *Circulation.* 1993;84:1087-1099.

9. Tabbara MR, White RA, Cavaye DM, et al. In-vivo human comparison of intravascular ultrasound and angiography. *J Vasc Surg*. 1991;14:496-504.

10. Nolthenius RP, van den Berg LC, Moll FL. The value of intraoperative intravascular ultrasound for determining stent graft size (excluding the abdominal aortic aneurysm) with modular system. *Ann Vasc Surg*. 2000;14:311-317.

11. White RA, Donayre CE, Kopchok G, et al. Intravascular ultrasound: the ultimate tool for abdominal aortic aneurysm assessment and endovascular graft delivery. *J Endovasc Surg*. 1997;4:45-55.

12. van Sambeek MR, Gussenhoven EJ, van Overhagen H, et al. Intravascular ultrasound in endovascular stent-grafts for peripheral aneurysm: a clinical study. *J Endovasc Surg*. 1998;5:106-112.

13. Garret HE, Abdulla AH, Hodgkiss TD, et al. Intravascular ultrasound aids in the performance of endovascular repair of abdominal aortic aneurysm. *J Vasc Surg*. 2003;37:615-618.

14. van Essen JA, van der Lugt A, Gussenhoven EJ, Leertouwer TC, Zondervan P, Sambeek MR. Intravascular ultrasonography allows accurate assessment of abdominal aortic aneurysm: an in vitro validation study. *J Vasc Surg*. 1998;27(2):347-353.

15. Geselschap JH, Heilbron MJ, Hussain FM, et al. The effect of angulation on intravascular ultrasound imaging observed in vascular phantoms. *J Endovasc Surg*. 1998;5:126-133.

16. Fernandez JD, Donovan S, Garrett Jr E, Burgar S. Endovascular thoracic aorta aneurysm repair: evaluating the utility of intravascular ultrasound measurements. *J Endovasc Ther*. 2008;15(1):68-72.

17. Dillavou ED, Buck DG, Muluk SC, Makaroun MS. Two-dimensional versus three-dimensional CT scan for aortic measurement. *J Endovasc Ther*. 2003;10:531-538.

18. Busquet J. The current role of vascular stents. *Int Angiol*. 1993;12(3):206-213.

19. Arko F, McCollough R, Manning L, Buckley CJ. Use of intravascular ultrasound in the endovascular management of atherosclerotic aortoiliac occlusive disease. *Am J Vasc Surg*. 1996;172:546-550.

20. Tobis JM, Mahon DJ, Goldberg SL, et al. Lessons from intravascular ultrasonography: observations during interventional angioplasty procedures. *J Clin Ultrasound*. 1993;21:589-607.

21. Lee SD, Arko FR, Buckley CJ. Impact of intravascular ultrasonography in the endovascular management of aortoiliac occlusive disease. *J Vasc Nurs*. 1998;16(3):57-61.

22. Diethrich EB. Endovascular treatment of abdominal aortic occlusive disease: the impact of stents and intravascular ultrasound imaging. *Eur J Vasc Surg*. 1993; 7:228-236.

23. Cavaye DM, Diethrich EB, Santiago OJ, et al. Intravascular ultrasound imaging: an essential component of angioplasty assessment and vascular stent deployment. *Int Angiol*. 1993;12:212-220.

24. Arko F, Mettauer M, McCollough R, Patterson D, Manning L, Buckley CJ. Use of intravascular ultrasound improves long-term clinical outcome in the management of atherosclerotic aortoiliac occlusive disease. *J Vasc Surg*. 1998;27(4):614-623.

25. van Essen JA, Gussenhoven EJ, Blankensteijn JD, et al. Three dimensional intravascular ultrasound assessment of abdominal aortic aneurysm necks. *J Endovasc Ther*. 2000;7(5):380-388.

26. White RA, Donayre C, Kopchok GE, et al. Utility of intravascular ultrasound in peripheral interventions. *Tex Heart Inst J*. 1997;24:28-34.

27. Nishanian G, Kopchok GE, Donayre CE, White RA. The impact of intravascular ultrasound (IVUS) on endovascular interventions. *Seminars Vasc Surg*. 1999;12(4):285-299.

28. Irshad K, Reid DB, Miller PH, Velu R, Kopchok GE, White RA. Early clinical experience with color three-dimensional ultrasound in peripheral interventions. *J Endovasc Ther*. 2001;8:329-339.

29. Slovut DP, Ofstein LC, Bacharach JM. Endoluminal AAA repair using intravascular ultrasound for graft planning and deployment. *J Endovasc Ther*. 2003;10: 463-475.

30. Dake MD, Miller DC, Semba CP, et al. Transluminal placement of endovascular stent-grafts for the treatment of descending thoracic aortic aneurysms. *N Engl J Med*. 1994;331:1729.

31. Dake MD, Kato N, Mitchell RS, et al. Endovascular stent-graft placement for treatment of acute aortic dissection. *N Engl J Med*. 1999;340:1546-1554.

32. Nienaber CA, Fattori R, Lund G, et al. Nonsurgical reconstruction of thoracic aortic dissection by stent graft placement. *N Engl J Med*. 1999;340:1539-1545.

33. Greenberg RK, Haulon S, Khwaja J, Fulton G, Ouriel K. Contemporary management of acute aortic dissection. *J Endovasc Ther*. 2003;10:476-485.

34. Quint LE, Platt JF, Sonnad SS, Deep GM, Williams DM. Aortic intimal tears: detection with spiral computed tomography. *J Endovasc Ther*. 2003;10:505-510.

35. White RA, Donayre C, Walot I, Lee J, Kopchok GE. Regression of a desending thoracoabdominal aortic dissection following staged deployment of thoracic and abdominal aortic endografts. *J Endovasc Ther*. 2002; 9(suppl 2):84-92.

36. Chabbert V, Otal P, Bouchard L, et al. Midterm outcomes of thoracic aortic stent-grafts: complications and imaging techniques. *J Endovasc Ther*. 2003;10:494-504.

37. Woody JD, Walot I, Donayre CE, Eugene J, Carey JS, White RA. Endovascular exclusion of leaking thoracic aortic aneurysms. *J Endovasc Ther*. 2002;9(suppl 2): 1179-1183.

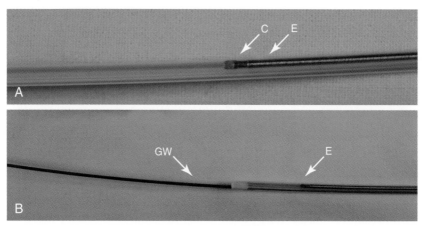

Figure 13-1. A, Mechanically rotating catheter (C), with the imaging element (E) and 0.035-inch guidewire in the catheter lumen. **B,** The catheter can be advanced past the area of interest and the guidewire (GW) removed to eliminate the artifact. When intravascular ultrasound (IVUS) imaging is completed, the guidewire is readvanced and the IVUS catheter removed (Atlantis SR Pro Imaging Catheter, Boston Scientific, Natick, MA).

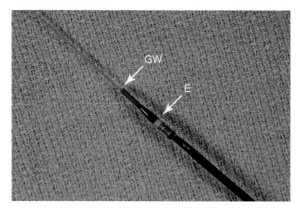

Figure 13-2. Phase array catheter (8.2F) coaxial over a 0.035-inch guidewire (GW). The gold-colored band contains 64 imaging elements (E) arranged circumferentially around the tip of the catheter (Visions PV8.2F catheter, Volcano Therapeutics, Rancho Cordova, CA).

Figure 13-3. A, Pre–intravascular ultrasound (IVUS) images of a total iliac occlusion prior to treatment. The guidewire is in the true lumen the entire length. Note the aorta (A) and right iliac orifice with a circumferential ring that is approximately 80% calcified (B). The lumen narrows along its length with a soft atheromatous-type disease (C, D, E). The external iliac artery is patent but has stagnant flow (bright speckle-type image) due to clamping of the distal artery (F), where areas of circumferential calcification are also apparent. **B,** Angiogram and IVUS evaluation following treatment with bilateral iliac stents (E-Luminexx Vascular Stent [10 mm × 10 cm], Bard Peripheral Vascular, Tempe, AZ) and balloon angioplasty (Dorado Balloon Dilatation Catheter [10 mm × 8 cm], Bard Peripheral Vascular, Tempe, AZ). On initial IVUS evaluation, the proximal and distal ends of the stent were widely patent, but the midsection remained stenotic and required further balloon dilation. The case took 42 mL of contrast and a fluoroscopy time of 15 minutes.

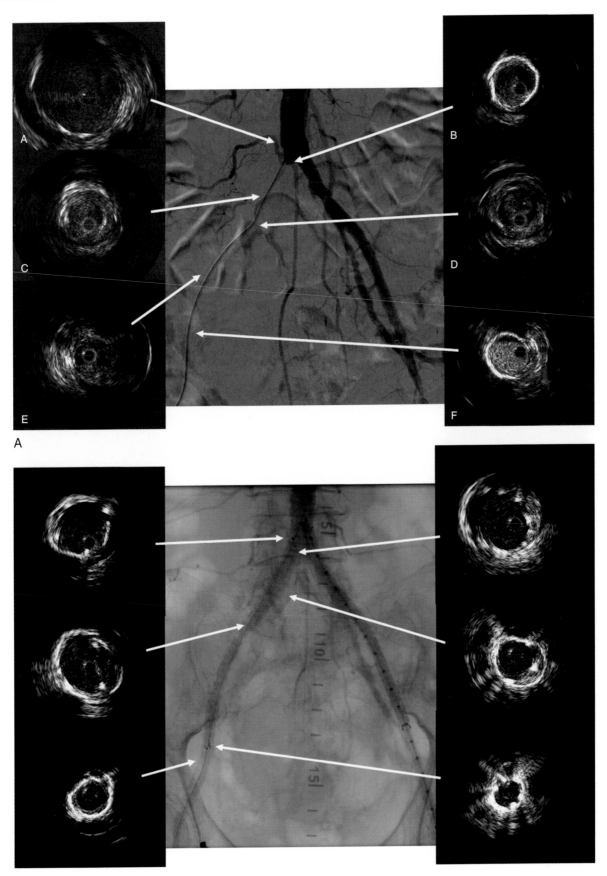

A

B

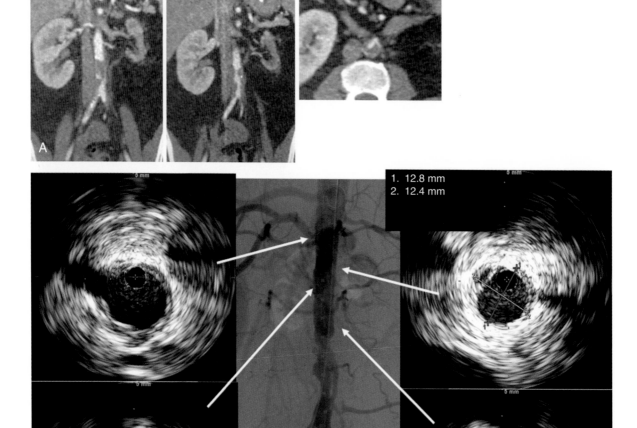

Figure 13-4. A, Computed tomography scan of a stenosis of the aorta prior to treatment. **B,** Preangiogram and intravascular ultrasound (IVUS) images along the length of the proximal aorta. Note the aortic dissection observed (*thick arrows, bottom left and right*) proximal to the stenosis at the level of the inferior mesenteric artery. The diameter of the aorta, proximal to stenosis, measured 12.8 × 12.4 mm on IVUS.

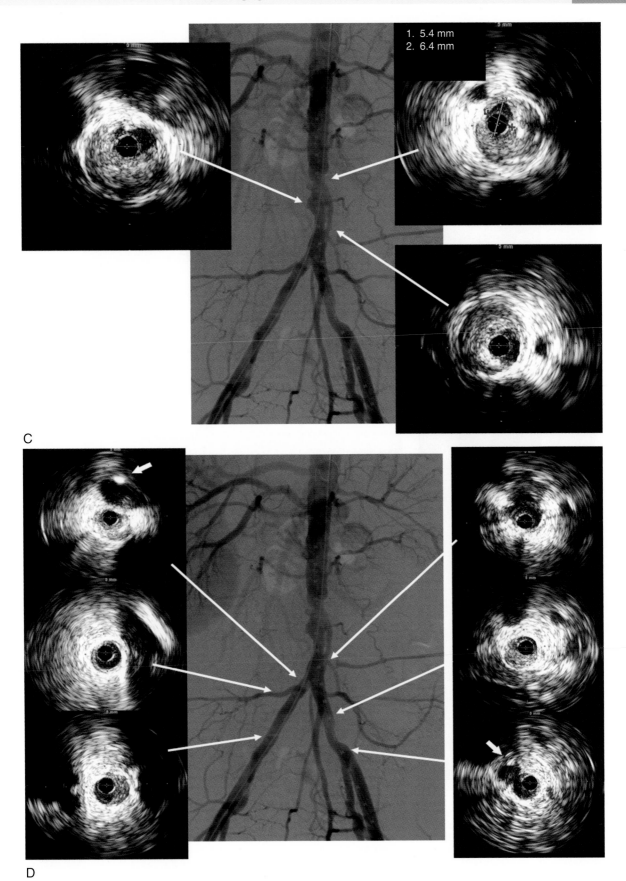

1. 5.4 mm
2. 6.4 mm

C

D

Figure 13-4, cont'd. C, An area of stenosis of the aorta, with the lumen narrowing to approximately 6 mm, is apparent. **D,** Both iliac arteries had diffuse disease to the level of the hypogastric artery (*thick arrow, right lower image*). *Continued*

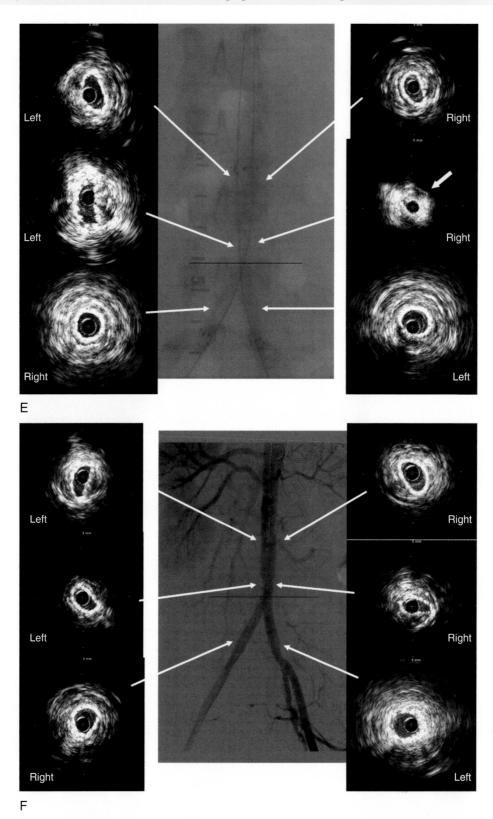

Figure 13-4, cont'd. E, Images following bilateral aortoiliac stents were deployed and primary balloon dilation was performed (two—Fluency Plus Vascular Stents [10 mm × 80 mm], C.R. Bard, Murray Hill, NJ; Dorado Balloon Dilatation Catheter [10 mm × 8 cm], Bard Peripheral Vascular, Tempe, AZ). IVUS was performed after balloon dilation, and narrowing was observed proximal to the aortic bifurcation on the device deployed from the right femoral artery. Note the luminal narrowing proximal to the aortic bifurcation on the device deployed from the right femoral artery (*thick arrow, middle right*). Based on IVUS evaluation, both stents were redilated with the same balloon. The IVUS catheter was then positioned at the level of the hypogastric artery orifice and its location marked on the fluoroscopic screen. A second iliac stent (E-Luminexx Vascular Stent [10 mm × 40 mm], Bard Peripheral Vascular, Tempe, AZ) was then deployed, with the distal end positioned at the mark signifying the hypogastric artery. The same procedure was performed for the contralateral side. **F,** The completion angiogram and selected IVUS images, demonstrating widely patent lumens. The case took of 60 mL of contrast for the preangiogram and postangiogram and a fluoroscopy time of exactly 9 minutes.

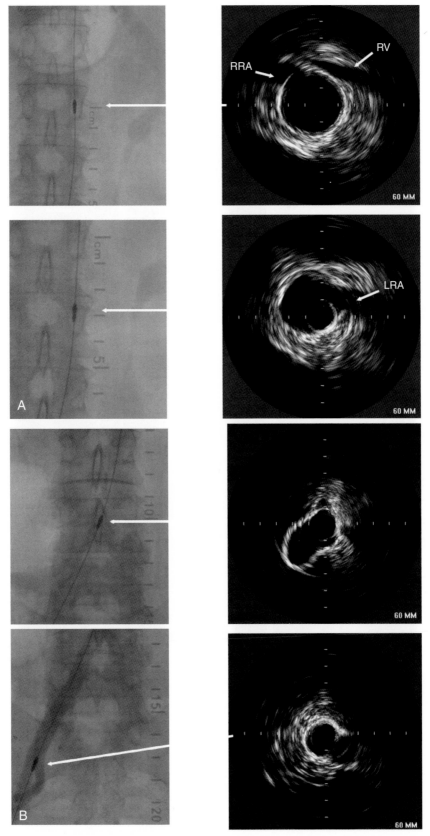

Figure 13-5. A, A radiopaque scale is placed beneath the patient and used to locate the major landmarks based on the intravascular ultrasound (IVUS) images. The widest part of the IVUS catheter tip is the imaging element's location. The right renal artery (RRA) and crossing renal vein (RV) can be observed at 0 cm on the radiopaque scale. The left renal artery (LRA) can be observed at 3 cm on the scale. **B,** The aortic bifurcation and the location of the hypogastric arteries can be identified. At each given point, the IVUS catheter is centered on the fluoroscopic screen to eliminate fluoroscopic parallax, and the diameter is measured to confirm pre–computed tomography scan measurements.

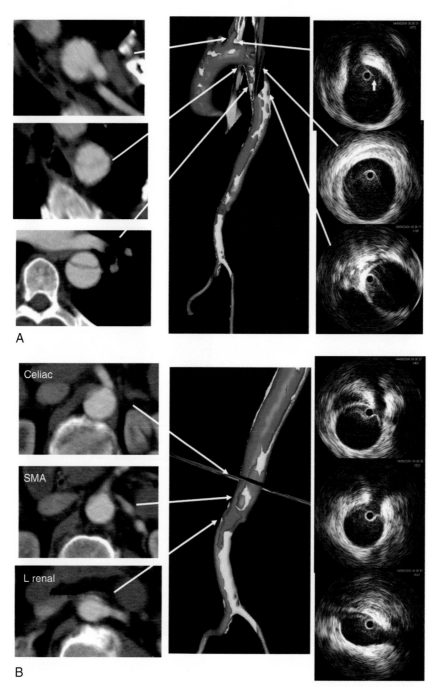

Figure 13-6. A, Pre–computed tomography (CT) evaluation and real-time intravascular ultrasound (IVUS) imaging demonstrating the relationship of the aortic branch vessels to a dissection flap. As seen on the IVUS image, the intimal tear begins just distal to the left subclavian artery (*thick arrow, top right*). **B,** Pre-intervention CT and IVUS images of the visceral vessels demonstrating true and false lumens.

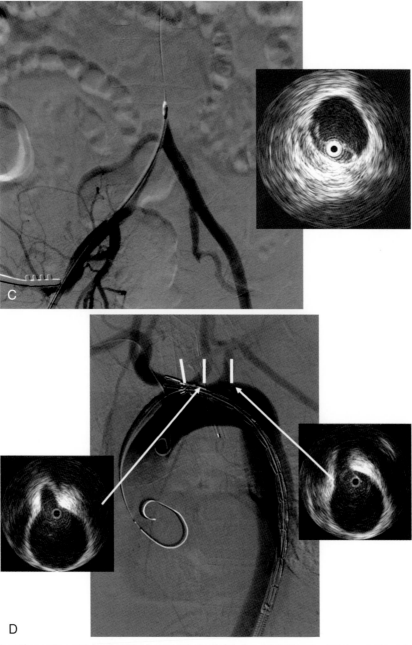

Figure 13-6, cont'd. C, IVUS can differentiate true and false lumens at the level of the iliac and distal aorta, which is crucial in gaining access and maintaining, or guiding, the guidewire through the true lumen from the femoral access site to the ascending aorta. **D,** The arch vessels are marked on fluoroscopic screen using IVUS images. The IVUS catheter is then withdrawn, the device advanced into the aortic arch, and the first angiogram is performed.

Continued

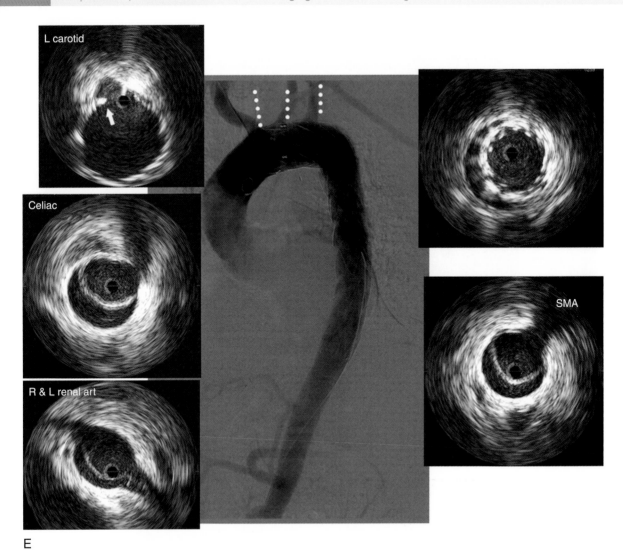

E

Figure 13-6, cont'd. E, Following deployment, IVUS is useful to evaluate changes to the true and false lumens and visceral blood flow as well as to determine if secondary devices are needed to exclude the false lumen completely. IVUS evaluation of the predeployment and postdeployment anatomy is performed with no contrast and minimal fluoroscopy. The case took 170 mL of contrast and a fluoroscopy time of 9 minutes, 31 seconds. Art, arteries, L, left; R, right; SMA, superior mesenteric artery.

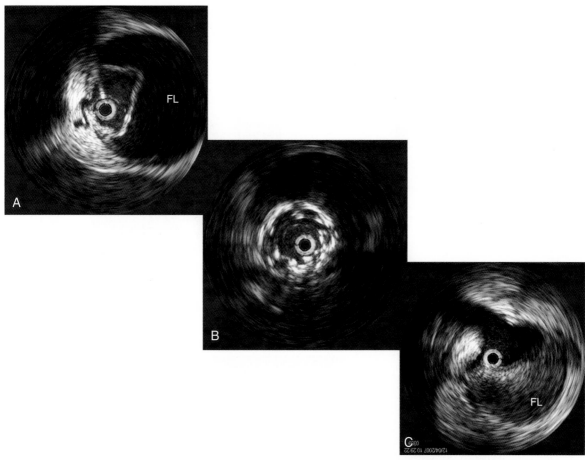

Figure 13-7. A, Intravascular ultrasound (IVUS) image of a thoracic aorta dissection proximal to the celiac artery prior to device deployment. The image demonstrates that there is blood flow in the true and false (FL) lumens. **B,** IVUS image of the distal edge of an endoluminal graft. **C,** IVUS image at the level of the celiac artery after device deployment, demonstrating good flow to the visceral vessel, and stagnant flow in the FL, immediately after device deployment.

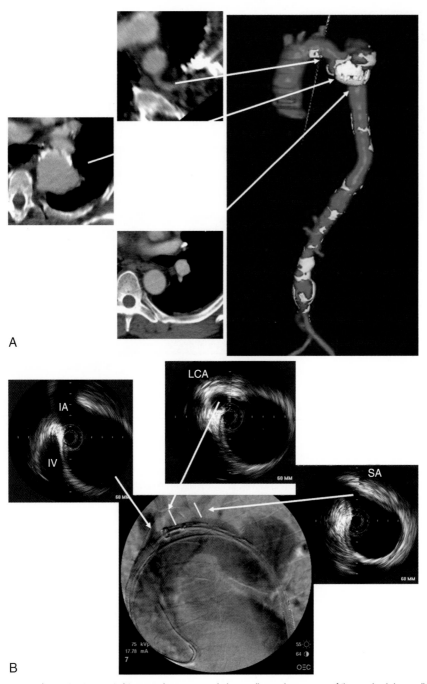

Figure 13-8. A, The preoperative contrast computed tomography scan revealed a small pseudoaneurysm of the proximal descending thoracic aorta, as seen on this M2S three-dimensional reconstruction. **B,** Intravascular ultrasound (IVUS) images of the innominate artery (IA) and innominate vein (IV), left carotid artery (LCA), and subclavian arteries (SA).

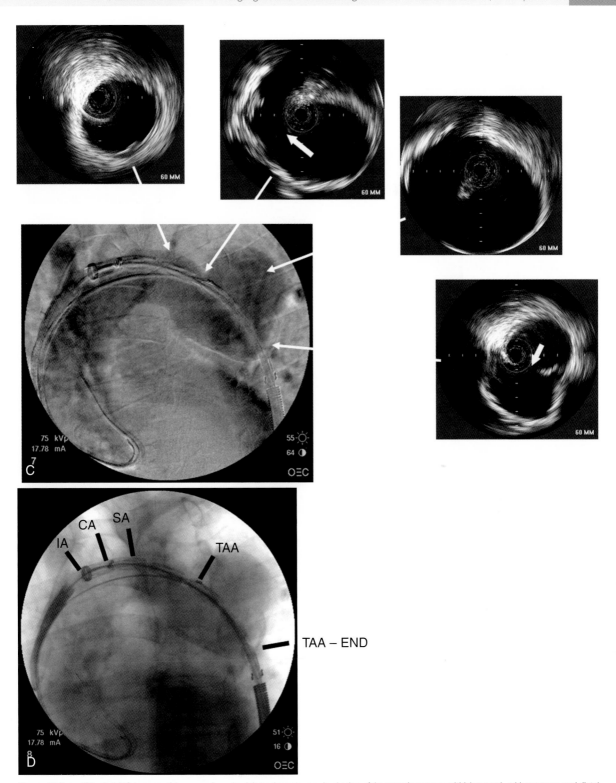

Figure 13-8, cont'd. **C,** IVUS images of the normal proximal thoracic aorta, proximal edge of the pseudoaneurysm (*thick arrows*), midaneurysm, and distal edge of the aneurysm. The *thick arrows* denote the loss of aortic wall. **D,** The IVUS images are used to locate the arch vessels and aneurysm prior to device insertion. TAA, thoracic aortic aneurysm; TAA-END, distal end of the thoracic aortic aneurysm.

Continued

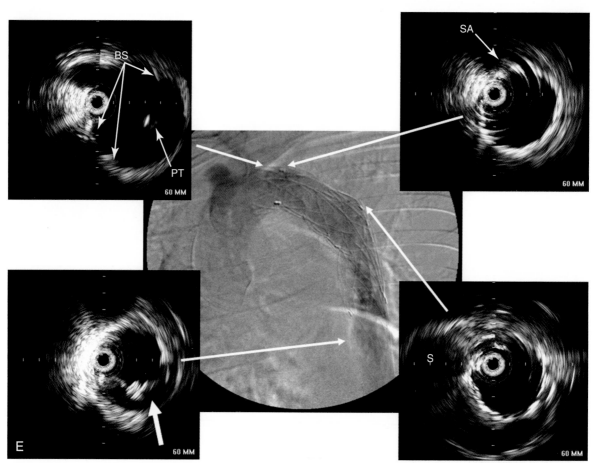

Figure 13-8, cont'd. E, Angiogram and IVUS images following device deployment. *Top left,* Note the bare stent struts (BS) and pigtail catheter (PT) at the level of the carotid artery. *Top right,* The covered subclavian artery (SA) and the bright echo of the endoluminal graft wall are apparent. *Bottom left,* Device enfolding is visible at the distal end of the endoluminal graft, which leads to balloon dilation (*thick arrow*). *Bottom right,* IVUS image demonstrates an area of stagnant blood (S) outside of the endoluminal graft in the area of the aneurysm. The case took 120 mL of contrast and a fluoroscopy time of 6 minutes, 10 seconds.

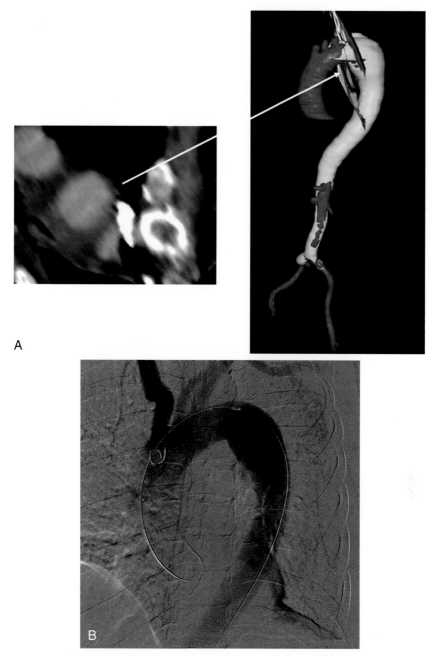

Figure 13-9. A, The preoperative contrast computed tomography scan revealed a thoracic aneurysm at the proximal descending thoracic aorta as seen on this M2S three-dimensional reconstruction. **B,** The angiogram confirmed that the proximal descending thoracic aortic wall was normal and could be used for the proximal fixation point.

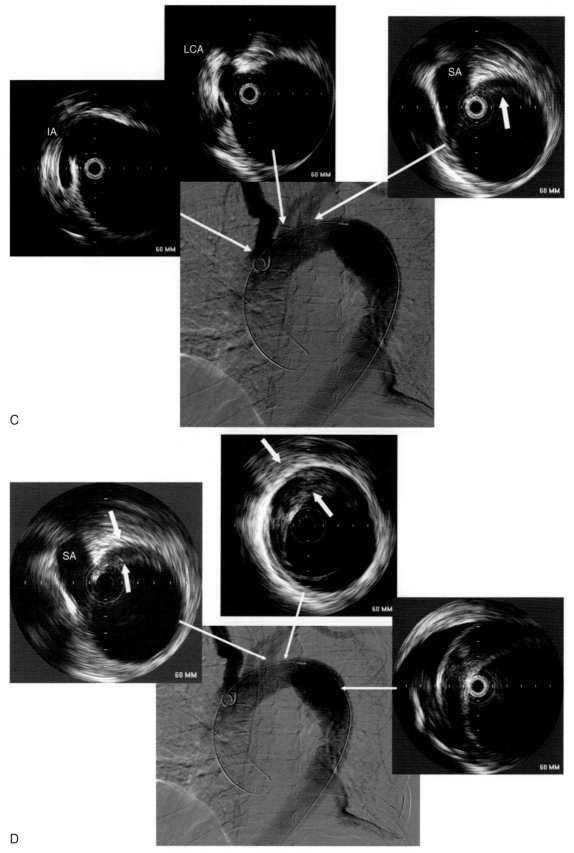

C

D

Figure 13-9, cont'd. C, Intravascular ultrasound (IVUS) evaluation revealed the innominate artery (IA) and left common carotid artery (LCA) with normal aortic wall to the level of the subclavian artery (SA). Circumferential thrombus was observed at the distal edge of the subclavian artery (*thick arrow, top right*). **D,** The thrombus continued through the aorta to the level of the aneurysm (*thick arrows, lower IVUS images*). Based on the IVUS findings, clinicians successfully deployed the device to the level of the carotid artery. The case took 180 mL of contrast and a fluoroscopy time of 20 minutes, 57 seconds.

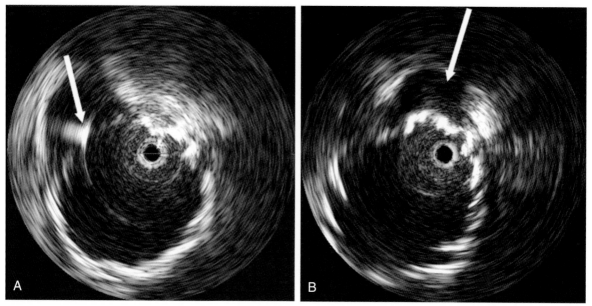

Figure 13-10. A, Intravascular ultrasound (IVUS) demonstrates the bare strut across the carotid orifice following device deployment. **B,** IVUS image of the graft material, excluding flow to the left carotid artery following graft deployment. In both cases, patients had palpable carotid pulses. In **B,** a carotid stent was deployed at the orifice to maintain the carotid lumen. *Arrows* mark left carotid artery ostium.

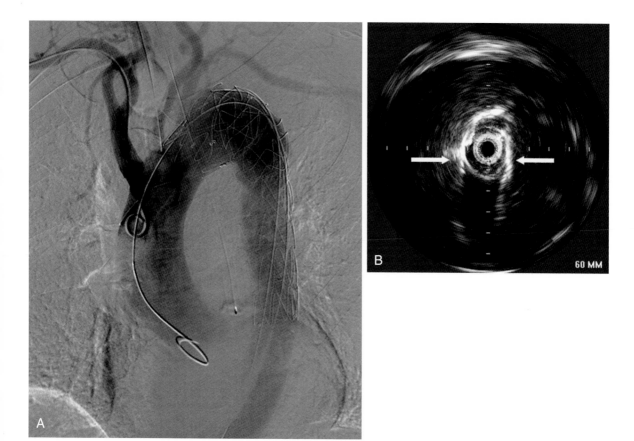

Figure 13-11. A, The completion angiogram looks very good, with a widely patent device and aorta. **B,** The intravascular ultrasound evaluation demonstrates severe narrowed lumens at the arch (*arrows*), requiring further balloon dilation and a second device.

The tables in this appendix complement Chapter 2 and are reproduced from 2011 ASA/ACCF/AHA/AANN/AANS/ACR/ASNR/CNS/SAIP/SCAI/SIR/SNIS/SVM/SVS guideline on the management of patients with extracranial carotid and vertebral artery disease. *J Am Coll Cardiol.* 2011;57:16-94.

TABLE A-1	American Heart Association/American Stroke Association Guidelines for Antithrombotic Therapy in Patients with Ischemic Stroke of Noncardioembolic Origin (Secondary Prevention)
GUIDELINE	**CLASSIFICATION OF RECOMMENDATION, LEVEL OF EVIDENCE***
Antiplatelet agents recommended over oral anticoagulants	I, A
For initial treatment, aspirin (50–325 mg/d),[†] the combination of aspirin and extended-release dipyridamole, or clopidogrel	I, A
Combination of aspirin and extended-release dipyridamole recommended over aspirin alone	I, B
Clopidogrel may be considered instead of aspirin alone	IIb, B
For patients hypersensitive to aspirin, clopidogrel is a reasonable choice	IIa, B
Addition of aspirin to clopidogrel increases risk of hemorrhage	III, A

*Recommendation: I indicates treatment is useful and effective; IIa, conflicting evidence or divergence of opinion regarding treatment usefulness and effectiveness; IIb, usefulness/efficacy of treatment is less well established; and III, treatment is not useful or effective. Level of evidence: A indicates data from randomized clinical trials; and B, data from a single randomized clinical trial or nonrandomized studies.
†Insufficient data are available to make evidence-based recommendations about antiplatelet agents other than aspirin.
Reprinted with permission from Sacco RL, Adams R, Albers G, et al. Guidelines for prevention of stroke in patients with ischemic stroke or transient ischemic attack: a statement for healthcare professionals from the American Heart Association/American Stroke Association Council on Stroke: cosponsored by the Council on Cardiovascular Radiology and Intervention. *Stroke.* 2006;37:577-617.

TABLE A-2 Event Rates in Patients with Carotid Artery Stenosis Managed without Revascularization

STUDY	NO. OF PATIENTS	SYMPTOM STATUS	STENOSIS (%)	FOLLOW-UP	MEDICATION THERAPY	ENDPOINT	EVENT RATE OVER STUDY PERIOD (%)
Observational Studies							
Hertzer et al.[1]	290	Asymptomatic	≥50	33–38 mo	Aspirin or dipyridamole (n = 104); or anticoagulation with warfarin (n = 9); or no medical treatment (n = 82)	Death TIA Stroke	22.0, or 7.33 annualized 8.21, or 2.74 annualized 9.23, or 3.1 annualized
Spence et al.[2]	168	Asymptomatic	≥60	≥12 mo	Multiple, including antiplatelet, statins, exercise, Mediterranean diet, ACE inhibitors	Stroke	3.8, or 1.3 annualized
Marquardt et al.[3]	1153	Asymptomatic	≥50	Mean 3 y	Multiple, including antiplatelet, anticoagulation, statin, antihypertensive drugs	Ipsilateral stroke	0.34 (95% CI 0.01 to 1.87) average annual event rate
Abbott et al.[4]	202	Asymptomatic	60–90	Mean 34 mo	Multiple, including antiplatelet, warfarin, antihypertensive drugs, cholesterol-lowering therapy	Ipsilateral stroke or TIA; ipsilateral carotid hemispheric stroke	Ipsilateral stroke or TIA or retinal event: 3.1 (95% CI 0.7 to 5.5) average annual rate Ipsilateral carotid hemispheric stroke: 1.0 (95% CI 0.4 to 2.4) average annual rate
Goessens et al.[5]	2684	Asymptomatic	≥50	Mean 3.6 y (SD 2.3)	Multiple, including antiplatelet, antihypertensive drugs, lipid-lowering agents, ACE inhibitors, and/or AIIA	Ischemic stroke; death	Death: 9.0 or 2.5 annualized; ischemic stroke: 2.0 or 0.54 annualized
Randomized Trial Cohorts							
ECST[6]	3024	Symptomatic	≥80	3 y	No surgery within 1 y or delay of surgery	Major stroke or death	26.5 over 3 y or annualized 8.83 for 1 y*
NASCET[7]	659	Symptomatic	≥70	2 y	Aspirin	Ipsilateral stroke	26.0 over 2 y or annualized 13.0 for 1 y†

Trial	n	Symptoms	Stenosis (%)	Treatment	Duration	Endpoint	Rate (%)
VA 309[8]	189	Symptomatic	≥50	Aspirin	1 y	Ipsilateral stroke or TIA or surgical death	19.4 over 11.9 ~12 mo
NASCET[9]	858	Symptomatic	50–69	Antiplatelet (usually aspirin)	5 y	Ipsilateral stroke	22.2 over 5 y or annualized 4.44 for 1 y[‡]
NASCET[9]	1368	Symptomatic	≤50	Antiplatelet (usually aspirin)	5 y	Ipsilateral stroke	18.7 over 5 y or annualized 3.74 for 1 y[‡]
ACAS[10]	1662	Asymptomatic	>60	Aspirin	5 y	Ipsilateral stroke, surgical death	11.0 over 5 y or annualized 2.2 for 1 y[§]
ACST[11]	3120	Asymptomatic	≥60	Indefinite deferral of any CEA	5 y	Any stroke	11.8 over 5 y or annualized 2.36 for 1 y[§]
VA[12]	444	Asymptomatic	≥50	Aspirin	4 y	Ipsilateral stroke	9.4 over 4 y or annualized 2.35 over 1 y

*Frequency based on Kaplan-Meier.

†Risk event rate based on Kaplan-Meier.

‡Failure rate based on Kaplan-Meier.

§Risk rate based on Kaplan-Meier.

AIIA, angiotensin II antagonist; ACAS, Asymptomatic Carotid Atherosclerosis Study; ACE, angiotensin-coverting enzyme; ACST, Asymptomatic Carotid Surgery Trial; CEA, carotid endarterectomy; CI, confidence interval; ECST, European Carotid Surgery Trial; n, numbers; N/A, not applicable; NASCET, North American Symptomatic Carotid Endarterectomy Trial; SD, standard deviation; TIA, transient ischemic attack; VA 309, Veterans Affairs Cooperative Studies Program 309; VA, Veterans Affairs Cooperative Study Group.

Modified from Bates ER, Babb JD, Casey DE Jr, et al. ACCF/SCAI/SVMB/SIR/ASITN 2007 clinical expert consensus document on carotid stenting: a report of the American College of Cardiology Foundation Task Force on Clinical Expert Consensus Documents (ACCF/SCAI/SVMB/SIR/ASITN Clinical Expert Consensus Document Committee on Carotid Stenting). J Am Coll Cardiol. 2007;49:126-170.

Studies cited in this table:

[1]Hertzer NR, Flanagan RA Jr, Beven EG, et al. Surgical versus nonoperative treatment of asymptomatic carotid stenosis: 290 patients documented by intravenous angiography. Ann Surg. 1986;204:163-171.

[2]Spence JD, Coates V, Li H, et al. Effects of intensive medical therapy on microemboli and cardiovascular risk in asymptomatic carotid stenosis. Arch Neurol. 2010;67:180-186.

[3]Marquardt L, Geraghty OC, Mehta Z, et al. Low risk of ipsilateral stroke in patients with asymptomatic carotid stenosis on best medical treatment: a prospective, population-based study. Stroke. 2010;41:e11-e17.

[4]Abbott AL, Chambers BR, Stork JL, et al. Embolic signals and prediction of ipsilateral stroke or transient ischemic attack in asymptomatic carotid stenosis: a multicenter prospective cohort study. Stroke. 2005;36:1128-1133.

[5]Goessens BM, Visseren FL, Kappelle LJ, et al. Asymptomatic carotid artery stenosis and the risk of new vascular events in patients with manifest arterial disease: the SMART study. Stroke. 2007;38:1470-1475.

[6]Randomised trial of endarterectomy for recently symptomatic carotid stenosis: final results of the MRC European Carotid Surgery Trial (ECST). Lancet. 1998;351:1379-1387.

[7]North American Symptomatic Carotid Endarterectomy Trial Collaborators. Beneficial effect of carotid endarterectomy in symptomatic patients with high-grade carotid stenosis. N Engl J Med. 1991;325:445-453.

[8]Mayberg MR, Wilson SE, Yatsu F, et al. Carotid endarterectomy and prevention of cerebral ischemia in symptomatic carotid stenosis. JAMA. 1991;266:3289-3294.

[9]Barnett HJ, Taylor DW, Eliasziw M, et al. North American Symptomatic Carotid Endarterectomy Trial Collaborators. Benefit of carotid endarterectomy in patients with symptomatic moderate or severe stenosis. N Engl J Med. 1998;339:1415-1425.

[10]Executive Committee for the Asymptomatic Carotid Atherosclerosis Study. Endarterectomy for asymptomatic carotid artery stenosis. JAMA. 1995;273:1421-1428.

[11]Halliday A, Mansfield A, Marro J, et al. Prevention of disabling and fatal strokes by successful carotid endarterectomy in patients without recent neurological symptoms: randomised controlled trial. Lancet. 2004;363:1491-1502.

[12]Hobson RW, Weiss DG, Fields WS, et al. Efficacy of carotid endarterectomy for asymptomatic carotid stenosis: the Veterans Affairs Cooperative Study Group. N Engl J Med. 1993;328:221-227.

TABLE A-3 Comparative Utility of Various Management Strategies for Patients with Carotid Stenosis in Clinical Trials

TRIAL (YEAR)	PATIENT POPULATION	INTER-VENTION	COMPARATOR	NO. OF PATIENTS		EVENTS (%)		EVENT USED TO CALCULATE NNT	ARR (%)	NNT*
				Treatment Group	Comparator Group	Treatment Group	Comparator Group			
Symptomatic CEA										
NASCET (1991)[1]	Symptomatic, 70% to 99% stenosis	CEA	Medical therapy	328	321	9	26	Ipsilateral stroke	17.00	12
ECST (2003)[2]	Symptomatic, 70% to 99% stenosis	CEA	Medical therapy	Not reported	Not reported	Not reported	Not reported	Ipsilateral ischemic stroke and surgical stroke or death; ARR provided in study	18.70	27
ECST (2003)[2]	Symptomatic, 70% to 99% stenosis	CEA	Medical therapy	429	850	6.80	N/A	Stroke or surgical death; ARR provided in study	21.20	24
NASCET (1998)[3]	Symptomatic, 50% to 69% stenosis	CEA	Medical therapy	430	428	15.70	22.20	Ipsilateral stroke	6.50	77
ECST (2003)[2]	Symptomatic, 50% to 69% stenosis	CEA	Medical therapy	Not reported	Not reported	Not reported	Not reported	Ipsilateral ischemic stroke and surgical stroke or death; ARR provided in study	2.90	173
ECST (2003)[2]	Symptomatic, 50% to 69% stenosis	CEA	Medical therapy	646	850	10.00	N/A	All stroke or surgical death; ARR provided in study	5.70	88
Asymptomatic CEA										
ACAS (1995)[4]	Asymptomatic	CEA	Medical therapy	825	834	5.10	11	Ipsilateral stroke and periprocedural stroke or death	6	84

Study	Status	Treatment A	Treatment B	n A	n B	% A	% B	Endpoint		
ACAS (1995)[4]	Asymptomatic	CEA	Medical therapy	825	834	13.40	13.60	Stroke or death	0.20	1351
ACST (2004)[5]	Asymptomatic	Immediate CEA	Deferred CEA	1560	1560	3.80	3.97	Ipsilateral stroke in carotid artery territory	0.17	2000
ACST (2004)[5]	Asymptomatic	Immediate CEA	Deferred CEA	1560	1560	3.80	11.00	Stroke risks	7.20	70
Symptomatic										
SPACE 2-y data (2008)[6]	Symptomatic	CEA	CAS	589	607	8.80	9.50	All periprocedural strokes or deaths and ipsilateral ischemic strokes up to 2 y after the procedure	0.70	286
SPACE 2-y data (2008)[6]	Symptomatic	CEA	CAS	589	607	1.90	2.20	Ipsilateral ischemic stroke within 31 d and 2 y	0.30	667
SPACE 2-y data (2008)[6]	Symptomatic	CEA	CAS	589	607	10.10	10.90	All stroke	0.80	250
EVA-3S 4-y data (2008)[7]	Symptomatic	CEA	CAS	262	265	1.50	1.50	Ipsilateral stroke	0	—
EVA-3S 4-y data (2008)[7]	Symptomatic	CEA	CAS	262	265	6.20	11.10	Composite of periprocedural stroke, death, and nonprocedural ipsilateral stroke during 4 y of follow-up	4.90	82
EVA-3S 4-y data (2008)[7]	Symptomatic	CEA	CAS	262	265	3.40	9.10	All strokes	5.70	71

Continued

TABLE A-3 Comparative Utility of Various Management Strategies for Patients with Carotid Stenosis in Clinical Trials—cont'd

TRIAL (YEAR)	PATIENT POPULATION	INTER-VENTION	COMPARATOR*	NO. OF PATIENTS		EVENTS (%)		EVENT USED TO CALCULATE NNT	ARR (%)	NNT*
				Treatment Group	Comparator Group	Treatment Group	Comparator Group			
Mixed Patient Populations										
SAPPHIRE 1-y data (2004)[8]	Mixed population: Symptomatic, ≥50% stenosis; Asymptomatic, ≥80% stenosis	CEA	CAS	167	167	7.90	6.20	Stroke	1.70	58
SAPPHIRE 1-y data (2004)[8]	Mixed population: Symptomatic, ≥50% stenosis; Asymptomatic, ≥80% stenosis	CEA	CAS	167	167	4.80	4.20	Ipsilateral stroke	0.60	167
SAPPHIRE 1-y data (2004)[†,8]	Mixed population: Symptomatic, ≥50% stenosis; Asymptomatic, ≥80% stenosis	CEA	CAS	167	167	20.10	12.20	Cumulative incidence of death, stroke, or MI within 30 d after the procedure or death or ipsilateral stroke between 31 d and 1 y	7.90	13

Study	Population							Outcome		
SAPPHIRE 3-y data (2008)[9]	Mixed population: Symptomatic, ≥50% stenosis; Asymptomatic, ≥80% stenosis	CEA	CAS	167	167	26.90	24.60	Composite of death, stroke, or MI within 30 d after the procedure; death or ipsilateral stroke between 31 d and 1080 d; 1080 d was converted to 3 y for normalization and NNT calculation	2.30	130
SAPPHIRE 3-y data (2008)[9]	Mixed population: Symptomatic, ≥50% stenosis; Asymptomatic, ≥80% stenosis	CEA	CAS	167	167	9.00	9.00	Stroke	0	~
SAPPHIRE 3-y data (2008)[9]	Mixed population: Symptomatic, ≥50% stenosis; Asymptomatic, ≥80% stenosis	CEA	CAS	167	167	5.40	6.60	Ipsilateral stroke	1.20	250
Symptomatic										
ICSS (2010)[10]	Symptomatic	CEA	CAS	858	855	4.10	7.70	All strokes within 120 d after randomization‡	3.60	7
ICSS (2010)[10]	Symptomatic	CEA	CAS	858	855	3.30	7.00	All strokes within 30 d after randomization‡	3.70	2

Continued

TABLE A-3 Comparative Utility of Various Management Strategies for Patients with Carotid Stenosis in Clinical Trials—cont'd

TRIAL (YEAR)	PATIENT POPULATION	INTER-VENTION	COMPARATOR	NO. OF PATIENTS		EVENTS (%)		EVENT USED TO CALCULATE NNT	ARR (%)	NNT*
				Treatment Group	Comparator Group	Treatment Group	Comparator Group			
CREST Symptomatic										
CREST 4-y data (2010)[11]	Symptomatic	CEA	CAS	653	668	8.40	8.20	All strokes, MIs, or deaths within periprocedural period and postproce-dural ipsilateral strokes	0.20	2000
CREST 4-y data (2010)[11]	Symptomatic	CEA	CAS	653	668	6.40	8.00	All periproce-dural strokes or deaths or postproce-dural ipsilateral strokes	1.60	250
CREST 4-y data (2010)[11]	Symptomatic	CEA	CAS	653	668	6.40	7.60	All periproce-dural strokes or postproce-dural ipsilateral strokes	1.20	333
CREST Asymptomatic										
CREST 4-y data (2010)[11]	Asymptomatic	CEA	CAS	587	594	4.90	5.60	All strokes, MIs, or deaths within periprocedural period and postproce-dural ipsilateral strokes	0.70	571
CREST 4-y data (2010)[11]	Asymptomatic	CEA	CAS	587	594	2.70	4.50	All periproce-dural strokes or postproce-dural ipsilateral strokes	1.80	223

CREST 4-y data (2010)[11]	Asymptomatic	CEA	CAS	587	594	2.70	4.50	All periprocedural strokes or deaths or postprocedural ipsilateral strokes	1.80	223
CREST Mixed Population										
CREST 4-y data (2010)[11]	Patient population not separated in table; mixed patient population	CEA	CAS	1240	1262	7.90	10.20	All stroke	2.30	174

*NNT indicates number of patients needed to treat over the course of 1 year with the indicated therapy as opposed to the comparator to prevent the specified event(s). All NNT calculations have been annualized.
†The 1-year data from the SAPPHIRE trial included the primary endpoint; long-term data were used to calculate rates of the major secondary endpoint.
‡Annualized data.
~Cannot be calculated because ARR is 0.

ACAS, Asymptomatic Carotid Atherosclerosis Study; ACST, Asymptomatic Carotid Surgery Trial; ARR, absolute risk reduction; CAS, carotid artery stenting; CEA, carotid endarterectomy; CREST, Carotid Revascularization Endarterectomy versus Stenting Trial; ECST, European Carotid Surgery Trial; EVA-3S, Endarterectomy Versus Angioplasty in Patients with Symptomatic Severe Carotid Stenosis; ICSS, International Carotid Stenting Study; NASCET, North American Symptomatic Carotid Endarterectomy Trial; NNT, number needed to treat; N/A, not applicable; SAPPHIRE, Stenting and Angioplasty with Protection in Patients at High Risk for Endarterectomy; SPACE, Stent-Protected Angioplasty versus Carotid Endarterectomy.

Studies cited in this table:

1North American Symptomatic Carotid Endarterectomy Trial Collaborators. Beneficial effect of carotid endarterectomy in symptomatic patients with high-grade carotid stenosis. N Engl J Med. 1991;325:445-453.
2Rothwell PM, Gutnikov SA, Warlow CP. Reanalysis of the final results of the European Carotid Surgery Trial. Stroke. 2003;34:514-523.
3Barnett HJ, Taylor DW, Eliasziw M, et al. North American Symptomatic Carotid Endarterectomy Trial Collaborators. Benefit of carotid endarterectomy in patients with symptomatic moderate or severe stenosis. N Engl J Med. 1998;339:1415-1425.
4Executive Committee for the Asymptomatic Carotid Atherosclerosis Study. Endarterectomy for asymptomatic carotid artery stenosis. JAMA. 1995;273:1421-1428.
5Halliday A, Mansfield A, Marro J, et al. Prevention of disabling and fatal strokes by successful carotid endarterectomy in patients without recent neurological symptoms: randomised controlled trial. Lancet. 2004;363:1491-1502.
6Eckstein HH, Ringleb P, Allenberg JR, et al. Results of the Stent-Protected Angioplasty versus Carotid Endarterectomy (SPACE) study to treat symptomatic stenoses at 2 years: a multinational, prospective, randomised trial. Lancet Neurol. 2008;7:893-902.
7Mas JL, Trinquart L, Leys D, et al. Endarterectomy Versus Angioplasty in Patients with Symptomatic Severe Carotid Stenosis (EVA-3S) trial: results up to 4 years from a randomised, multicentre trial. Lancet Neurol. 2008;7:885-892.
8Yadav JS, Wholey MH, Kuntz RE, et al. Protected carotid-artery stenting versus endarterectomy in high-risk patients. N Engl J Med. 2004;351:1493-1501.
9Gurm HS, Yadav JS, Fayad P, et al. Long-term results of carotid stenting versus endarterectomy in high-risk patients. N Engl J Med. 2008;358:1572-1579.
10Bonati LH, Jongen LM, Haller S, et al. New ischaemic brain lesions on MRI after stenting or endarterectomy for symptomatic carotid stenosis: a substudy of the International Carotid Stenting Study (ICSS). Lancet Neurol. 2010;9:353-362.
11Brott TG, Hobson RW, Howard G, et al. Stenting versus Endarterectomy for Treatment of Carotid-Artery Stenosis. N Engl J Med. 2010;363:11-23.

TABLE A-4 Randomized Trials Comparing Endarterectomy with Stenting in Symptomatic Patients with Carotid Stenosis

TRIAL (YEAR)	NO. OF PATIENTS	KEY FEATURES	DEATH OR ANY STROKE	OR (95% CI)	COMMENTS
Leicester (1998)[1]	17 had received their allocated treatment before trial suspension	Single center; patients with symptomatic carotid stenosis >70%.	CEA: 0/10 (0%)* CAS: 5/7 (71.4%)*	p = 0.0034; OR not reported	Terminated prematurely because of safety concerns.
CAVATAS-CEA (2001)[2]	504	Multicenter; patients of any age with symptomatic or asymptomatic carotid stenosis suitable for CEA or CAS.	CEA: 25/253 (9.9%) CAS: 25/251 (10.0%)	p = NS in original article; OR not reported	Follow-up to 3 y; relatively low stent use (26%) in CAS group.
Kentucky (2001)[3]	104	Single center; patients with symptomatic carotid stenosis >70% (events within 3 mo of evaluation).	CEA: 1/51 (2.0%) CAS: 0/53 (0%)	0.31 (0.01 to 7.90)	
SAPPHIRE (2004)[4]	334	Multicenter randomized trial of patients with ≥80% asymptomatic carotid stenosis (70%) and ≥50% symptomatic carotid stenosis (30%).	CEA: 9.3% symptomatic patients*,‡ CAS: 2.1% symptomatic patients‡	p = 0.18†	Terminated prematurely because of a drop in randomization.
EVA-3S (2006)[5]	527	Multicenter; patients with symptomatic carotid stenosis >60% within 120 d before enrollment suitable for CEA or CAS.	CEA: 10/259 (3.9%) CAS: 25/261 (9.6%)	RR 2.5 (1.2 to 5.1), p = 0.01	Study terminated prematurely because of safety and futility issues; concerns about operator inexperience in the CAS arm and nonuniform use of embolism protection devices.
SPACE (2006)[6]	1183	Multicenter; patients >50 y old with symptomatic carotid stenosis >70% in the 180 d before enrollment.	Primary endpoint of ipsilateral ischemic stroke or death from time of randomization to 300 d after the procedure: CEA: 37/584 (6.3%) CAS: 41/599 (6.8%)	1.19 (0.75 to 1.92)	Study terminated prematurely after futility analysis; concerns about operator inexperience in the CAS arm and nonuniform use of embolism protection devices.

Continued

EVA-3S 4-y follow-up (2008)[7]	527	Multicenter, randomized, open, assessor-blinded, noninferiority trial. Compared outcome after CEA with outcome after CAS in 527 patients who had carotid stenosis of at least 60% that had recently become symptomatic.	Major outcome events up to 4 y for any periprocedural stroke or death: CEA: 6.2% CAS: 11.1%	HR for any stroke or periprocedural death 1.77 (1.03 to 3.02); p = 0.04 HR for any stroke or death 1.39 (0.96 to 2.00); p = 0.08 HR for CAS versus CEA 1.97 (1.06 to 3.67); p = 0.03	A hazard function analysis showed 4-y differences in cumulative probabilities of outcomes between CAS and CEA were largely accounted for by the higher periprocedural (within 30 d of the procedure) risk of stenting compared with endarterectomy. After the periprocedural period, the risk of ipsilateral stroke was low and similar in the 2 treatment groups.
SPACE 2-y follow-up (2008)[8]	1214	Patients with symptomatic, severe (≥70%) carotid artery stenosis were recruited to this noninferiority trial and randomly assigned with a block randomization design to undergo CAS or CEA.	Intention-to-treat population: Ipsilateral ischemic strokes within 2 y, including any periprocedural strokes or deaths: CAS: 56 (9.5%) CEA: 50 (8.8%) Any deaths between randomization and 2 y: CAS: 32 (6.3%) CEA: 28 (5.0%) Any strokes between randomization and 2 y: CAS: 64 (10.9%) CEA: 57 (10.1%) Ipsilateral ischemic stroke within 31 d and 2 y: CAS: 12 (2.2%) CEA: 10 (1.9%) Per-protocol population: Ipsilateral ischemic strokes within 2 y, including any periprocedural strokes or deaths: CAS: 53 (9.4%) CEA: 43 (7.8%) Any deaths between randomization and 2 y: CAS: 29 (6.2%) CEA: 25 (4.9%) Any strokes between randomization and 2 y: CAS: 61 (11.5%) CEA: 51 (9.8%) Ipsilateral ischemic stroke within 31 d and 2 y: CAS: 12 (2.3%) CEA: 10 (2.0%)	Intention-to-treat population: Ipsilateral ischemic strokes within 2 y, including any periprocedural strokes or deaths: HR 1.10 (0.75 to 1.61) Any deaths between randomization and 2 y: HR 1.11 (0.67 to 1.85) Any strokes between randomization and 2 y: HR 1.10 (0.77 to 1.57) Ipsilateral ischemic stroke within 31 d and 2 y: HR 1.17 (0.51 to 2.70) Per-protocol population: Ipsilateral ischemic strokes within 2 y, including any periprocedural strokes or deaths: HR 1.23 (0.82 to 1.83) Any deaths between randomization and 2 y: HR 1.14 (0.67 to 1.94) Any strokes between randomization and 2 y: HR 1.19 (0.83 to 1.73) Ipsilateral ischemic stroke within 31 d and 2 y: HR 1.18 (0.51 to 2.73)	In both the intention-to-treat and per-protocol populations, recurrent stenosis of ≥70% was significantly more frequent in the CAS group than the CEA group, with a life-table estimate of 10.7% versus 4.6% (p = 0.0009) and 11.1% versus 4.6% (p = 0.0007), respectively.

TABLE A-4 Randomized Trials Comparing Endarterectomy with Stenting in Symptomatic Patients with Carotid Stenosis—cont'd

TRIAL (YEAR)	NO. OF PATIENTS	KEY FEATURES	DEATH OR ANY STROKE	OR (95% CI)	COMMENTS
SAPPHIRE 3-y follow-up (2008)[9]	260	Long-term data were collected for 260 individuals; included symptomatic carotid artery stenosis of at least 50% of the luminal diameter or an asymptomatic stenosis of at least 80%.	Stroke: CAS: 15 (9.0%) CEA: 15 (9.0%) Ipsilateral stroke: CAS: 11 (7.0%) CEA: 9 (5.4%) Death: CAS: 31 (18.6%) CEA: 35 (21%) Note: data were calculated using $n = 167$ for both groups because breakdowns of CAS and CEA for $N = 260$ were not given.	Stroke: $p = 0.99$ (−6.1 to 6.1) Death: $p = 0.68$ (−10.9 to 6.1)	
Wallstent (2005)[10]	219	Included symptomatic angiographic carotid stenosis >70%.	CAS: 13 (12.2%) CEA: 5 (4.5%)	N/A	Premature termination based on futility analysis.
SAPPHIRE (symptomatic data) (2008)[11]	96	Included patients with ≥50% carotid stenosis.	CEA: 3 (6.5%) CAS: 0	N/A	Premature termination secondary to declining enrollment.
ICSS (2010)[12]	1713	Multicenter study. In the study, the degree of carotid stenosis was 70% to 99% in 89% of stent patients and in 91% of endarterectomy patients. Study patients had >50% carotid artery stenosis measured by the NASCET criteria.	120-d follow-up data available only: CAS: 72/853 (8.5%) CEA: 40/857 (4.7%)	OR not available; HR 1.86 (1.26 to 2.74) $p = 0.001$	Primary outcome was 3-y rate of fatal or disabling stroke in any territory; interim results have been provided for 120-d rate of stroke, death, or procedural MI.

CREST (2010)[13]	2502	The study included 1321 symptomatic patients and 1181 asymptomatic patients. Symptomatic patients in the study had ≥50% carotid stenosis by angiography, ≥70% by ultrasound or ≥70% by CTA or MRA. Asymptomatic patients had carotid stenosis (patients with symptoms beyond 180 d were considered asymptomatic) ≥60% by angiography, ≥70% by ultrasound, or ≥80% by CTA or MRA.	Any periprocedural stroke or postprocedural ipsilateral stroke: Symptomatic: CAS: 37 (5.5±0.9 SE) CEA: 21 (3.2±0.7 SE) Any periprocedural stroke or death or postprocedural ipsilateral stroke: Symptomatic: CAS: 40 (6.0±0.9 SE) CEA: 21 (3.2±0.7 SE)	Any periprocedural stroke or postprocedural ipsilateral stroke: Symptomatic: $p = 0.04$ Any periprocedural stroke or death or postprocedural ipsilateral stroke: Symptomatic: $p = 0.02$	The risk of composite primary outcome of stroke, MI, or death did not differ significantly among symptomatic and asymptomatic patients between CAS and CEA.

*Death and ipsilateral stroke.

†Combined asymptomatic and symptomatic patients for death, any stroke.

‡Death, stroke, and MI.

CAS, carotid artery stent; CAVATAS, Carotid And Vertebral Artery Transluminal Angioplasty Study; CEA, carotid endarterectomy; CI, confidence interval; CREST, Carotid Revascularization Endarterectomy versus Stenting Trial; CTA, computed tomography angiography; EVA-3S, Endarterectomy Versus Angioplasty in patients with Symptomatic Severe carotid Stenosis; HR, hazard ratio; ICSS, International Carotid Stenting Study; MI, myocardial infarction; MRA, magnetic resonance angiography; N/A, not available; NASCET, North American Symptomatic Carotid Endarterectomy Trial; NS, not significant; OR, odds ratio; RR, risk reduction; SAPPHIRE, Stenting and Angioplasty with Protection in Patients at High Risk for Endarterectomy; SE, standard error; SPACE, Stent-Protected Angioplasty versus Carotid Endarterectomy.

Modified from Ederle J, Featherstone RL, Brown MM. Percutaneous transluminal angioplasty and stenting for carotid artery stenosis. *Cochrane Database Syst Rev.* 2007;CD000515.

Studies cited in this table:

1Naylor AR, Bolia A, Abbott RJ, et al. Randomized study of carotid angioplasty and stenting versus carotid endarterectomy: a stopped trial. *J Vasc Surg.* 1998;28:326-334.

2Endovascular versus surgical treatment in patients with carotid stenosis in the Carotid and Vertebral Artery Transluminal Angioplasty Study (CAVATAS): a randomised trial. *Lancet.* 2001;357:1729-1737.

3Brooks WH, McClure RR, Jones MR, et al. Carotid angioplasty and stenting versus carotid endarterectomy: randomized trial in a community hospital. *J Am Coll Cardiol.* 2001;38:1589-1595.

4Yadav JS, Wholey MH, Kuntz RE, et al. Protected carotid-artery stenting versus endarterectomy in high-risk patients. *N Engl J Med.* 2004;351:1493-1501.

5Mas JL, Chatellier G, Beyssen B, et al. Endarterectomy versus stenting in patients with symptomatic severe carotid stenosis. *N Engl J Med.* 2006;355:1660-1671.

6Ringleb PA, Allenberg J, Bruckmann H, et al. 30 day results from the SPACE trial of stent-protected angioplasty versus carotid endarterectomy in symptomatic patients: a randomised non-inferiority trial [published correction appears in *Lancet.* 2006;368:1238]. *Lancet.* 2006;368:1239-1247.

7Mas JL, Trinquart L, Leys D, et al. Endarterectomy Versus Angioplasty in Patients with Symptomatic Severe Carotid Stenosis (EVA-3S) trial: results up to 4 years from a randomised, multicentre trial. *Lancet Neurol.* 2008;7:885-892.

8Eckstein HH, Ringleb P, Allenberg JR, et al. Results of the Stent-Protected Angioplasty versus Carotid Endarterectomy (SPACE) study to treat symptomatic stenoses at 2 years: a multinational, prospective, randomised trial. *Lancet Neurol.* 2008;7:893-902.

9Gurm HS, Yadav JS, Fayad P, et al. Long-term results of carotid stenting versus endarterectomy in high-risk patients. *N Engl J Med.* 2008;358:1572-1579.

10Coward LJ, Featherstone RL, Brown MM. Safety and efficacy of endovascular treatment of carotid artery stenosis compared with carotid endarterectomy: a Cochrane systematic review of the randomized evidence. *Stroke.* 2005;36:905-911.

11Gurm HS, Nallamothu BK, Yadav J. Safety of carotid artery stenting for symptomatic carotid artery disease: a meta-analysis. *Eur Heart J.* 2008;29:113-119.

12Ederle J, Dobson J, Featherstone RL, et al. Carotid artery stenting compared with endarterectomy in patients with symptomatic carotid stenosis (International Carotid Stenting Study): an interim analysis of a randomised controlled trial. *Lancet.* 2010;375:985-997.

13Brott TG, Hobson RW, Howard G, et al. Stenting versus Endarterectomy for Treatment of Carotid-Artery Stenosis. *N Engl J Med.* 2010;363:11-23.

TABLE A-5 Trials Comparing Endarterectomy with Stenting in Asymptomatic Patients with Carotid Stenosis

TRIAL (YEAR)	NO. OF PATIENTS	KEY FEATURES	DEATH OR ANY STROKE	P	COMMENTS
SAPPHIRE (2004)[1]	334	Multicenter randomized trial of patients with >50% symptomatic carotid stenosis (58%) or >80% asymptomatic carotid stenosis (42%) with 1 or more comorbidity criteria* (high-surgical-risk group).	Asymptomatic: CEA: 10.2%† CAS: 5.4%† Combined: CEA: 9.8%† CAS: 4.8%†	0.20 0.09	Terminated prematurely because of a drop in randomization.
SAPPHIRE (2008)[2]	334	Multicenter randomized trial of patients with >80% asymptomatic carotid stenosis (70%) and ≥50% symptomatic carotid stenosis (30%).	SAPPHIRE 3-y data, Stroke: CEA: 15/167 CAS: 15/197 Death: CEA: 35/167 CAS: 31/167	Stroke: 0.99 Death: 0.68 (OR not reported)	No significant difference could be shown in long-term outcomes between patients who underwent CAS with an EPD and those who underwent CEA.
CREST (2010)[3]	2502	The study included 1321 symptomatic patients and 1181 asymptomatic patients. Symptomatic patients in the study had ≥50% carotid stenosis by angiography, ≥70% by ultrasound, or ≥70% by CTA or MRA. Asymptomatic patients in the study had carotid stenosis (patients with symptoms beyond 180 d were considered asymptomatic) ≥60% by angiography, ≥70% by ultrasound, or ≥80% by CTA or MRA.	Any periprocedural stroke or postprocedural ipsilateral stroke: Asymptomatic: CAS: 15 (2.5±0.6 SE) CEA: 8 (1.4±0.5 SE) Any periprocedural stroke or death or postprocedural ipsilateral stroke: Asymptomatic: CAS: 15 (2.5±0.6 SE) CEA: 8 (1.4±0.5 SE)	Any periprocedural stroke or postprocedural ipsilateral stroke: Asymptomatic: 0.15 Any periprocedural stroke or death or postprocedural ipsilateral stroke: Asymptomatic: 0.15	The risk of the composite primary outcome of stroke, MI, or death did not differ significantly among symptomatic and asymptomatic patients between CAS and CEA.

*Criteria for high risk (at least 1 factor required): clinically significant cardiac disease (congestive heart failure, abnormal stress test, or need for open heart surgery); severe pulmonary disease; contralateral carotid occlusion; contralateral laryngeal nerve palsy; previous radical neck surgery or radiation therapy to the neck; recurrent stenosis after endarterectomy; and age >80 years. High risk is defined by age ≥80 years, New York Heart Association class III/IV heart failure, chronic obstructive pulmonary disease, contralateral carotid stenosis 50% or more, prior CEA or CAS, or prior coronary artery bypass graft surgery.

†Death, stroke, and MI.

CAS, carotid artery stent; CEA, carotid endarterectomy; CREST, Carotid Revascularization Endarterectomy versus Stent Trial; CTA, computed tomography angiography; EPD, embolic protection device; MI, myocardial infarction; MRA, magnetic resonance angiography; OR, odds ratio; SAPPHIRE, Stenting and Angioplasty with Protection in Patients at High Risk for Endarterectomy; SE, standard error.

Studies cited in this table:

[1]Yadav JS, Wholey MH, Kuntz RE, et al. Protected carotid-artery stenting versus endarterectomy in high-risk patients. N Engl J Med. 2004;351:1493-1501.

[2]Gurm HS, Yadav JS, Fayad P, et al. Long-term results of carotid stenting versus endarterectomy in high-risk patients. N Engl J Med. 2008;358:1572-1579.

[3]Brott TG, Hobson RW, Howard G, et al. Stenting versus Endarterectomy for Treatment of Carotid-Artery Stenosis. N Engl J Med. 2010;363:11-23.

TABLE A-6   Kaplan-Meier Estimates of Event Rates in the CaRESS Trial

EVENT	≤30 DAYS (%)		≤365 DAYS (%)	
	CEA	CAS	CEA	CAS
Death	0.40	0.00	6.60	6.30
Stroke	3.60	2.10	9.80	5.50
MI	0.80	0.00	2.40	1.70
Death/stroke	3.60	2.10	13.60	10.00
Death/stroke/MI	4.40	2.10	14.30	10.90
Restenosis	N/A	N/A	3.60	6.30
Carotid revascularization	N/A	N/A	1.00	1.80

CaRESS, Carotid Revascularization Using Endarterectomy or Stenting Systems; CAS, carotid artery stenting; CEA, carotid endarterectomy; MI, myocardial infarction; N/A, not available.
Modified from CARESS Steering Committee. Carotid Revascularization Using Endarterectomy or Stenting Systems (CaRESS) phase I clinical trial: 1-year results. *J Vasc Surg.* 2005;42:213-219.

TABLE A-7   Summary of Recommendations Regarding the Selection of Revascularization Techniques for Patients with Carotid Artery Stenosis

	SYMPTOMATIC PATIENTS		ASYMPTOMATIC PATIENTS 70% TO 99% STENOSIS
	50% to 69% Stenosis	70% to 99% Stenosis	
Endarterectomy	Class I LOE: B	Class I LOE: A	Class IIa LOE: A
Stenting	Class I LOE: B	Class I LOE: B	Class IIb LOE: B

The severity of stenosis is defined according to angiographic criteria by the method used in NASCET[1] but generally corresponds as well to assessment by sonography[2] and other accepted methods of measurement.
LOE, level of evidence.
Studies cited in this table:
[1]North American Symptomatic Carotid Endarterectomy Trial (NASCET) Investigators. Clinical alert: benefit of carotid endarterectomy for patients with high-grade stenosis of the internal carotid artery. National Institute of Neurological Disorders and Stroke Stroke and Trauma Division. *Stroke.* 1991;22:816-817.
[2]Grant EG, Benson CB, Moneta GL, et al. Carotid artery stenosis: gray-scale and Doppler US diagnosis–Society of Radiologists in Ultrasound Consensus Conference. *Radiology.* 2003;229:340-346.

TABLE A-8 Sensitivity and Specificity of Duplex Ultrasonography as a Function of Degree of Carotid Stenosis

STUDY (YEAR)	DEGREE OF STENOSIS	CAROTIDS (*n*)	SENSITIVITY (%)	SPECIFICITY (%)
Serfaty et al. (2000)[1]	Occlusion	46	100	90
Hood et al. (1996)[2]	Occlusion	457	100	99
White et al. (1994)[3]	Occlusion	120	80	100
Turnipseed et al. (1993)[4]	Occlusion	34	100	100
Riles et al. (1992)[5]	Occlusion	75	100	100
Riles et al. (1992)[5]	Stenosis ≥ 80%	75	85	80
Johnson et al. (2000)[6]	Stenosis ≥ 70%	76	65	95
Serfaty et al. (2000)[1]	Stenosis ≥ 70%	46	64	97
Huston et al. (1998)[7]	Stenosis ≥ 70%	100	97	75
Link et al. (1997)[8]	Stenosis ≥ 70%	56	87	98
Hood et al. (1996)[2]	Stenosis ≥ 70%	457	86	97
Bray et al. (1995)[9]	Stenosis ≥ 70%	128	85	96–97
Patel et al. (1995)[10]	Stenosis ≥ 70%	171	94	83
Turnipseed et al. (1993)[4]	Stenosis ≥ 70%	34	94	89
Bluth et al. (2000)[11]	Stenosis ≥ 60%	40	62	100
Jackson et al. (1998)[12]	Stenosis ≥ 60%	99	89	92
White et al. (1994)[3]	Stenosis ≥ 60%	120	73	88
Walters et al. (1993)[13]	Stenosis ≥ 60%	102	88	88
Serfaty et al. (2000)[1]	Stenosis ≥ 50%	46	94	83
Hood et al. (1996)[2]	Stenosis ≥ 50%	457	99.5	89
Bray et al. (1995)[9]	Stenosis ≥ 50%	128	87–95	96
Riles et al. (1992)[5]	Stenosis ≥ 50%	75	98	69

Modified from Long A, Lepoutre A, Corbillon E, et al. Critical review of non- or minimally invasive methods (duplex ultrasonography, MR- and CT-angiography) for evaluating stenosis of the proximal internal carotid artery. *Eur J Vasc Endovasc Surg.* 2002;24:43-52.
Studies cited in this table:

[1]Serfaty JM, Chirossel P, Chevallier JM, et al. Accuracy of threedimensional gadolinium-enhanced MR angiography in the assessment of extracranial carotid artery disease. *AJR Am J Roentgenol.* 2000;175:455-463.

[2]Hood DB, Mattos MA, Mansour A, et al. Prospective evaluation of new duplex criteria to identify 70% internal carotid artery stenosis. *J Vasc Surg.* 1996;23:254-261.

[3]White JE, Russell WL, Greer MS, et al. Efficacy of screening MR angiography and Doppler ultrasonography in the evaluation of carotid artery stenosis. *Am Surg.* 1994;60:340-348.

[4]Turnipseed WD, Kennell TW, Turski PA, et al. Combined use of duplex imaging and magnetic resonance angiography for evaluation of patients with symptomatic ipsilateral high-grade carotid stenosis. *J Vasc Surg.* 1993;17:832-839.

[5]Riles TS, Eidelman EM, Litt AW, et al. Comparison of magnetic resonance angiography, conventional angiography, and duplex scanning. *Stroke.* 1992;23:341-346.

[6]Johnson MB, Wilkinson ID, Wattam J, et al. Comparison of Doppler ultrasound, magnetic resonance angiographic techniques and catheter angiography in evaluation of carotid stenosis. *Clin Radiol.* 2000;55:912-920.

[7]Huston J, Nichols DA, Luetmer PH, et al. MR angiographic and sonographic indications for endarterectomy. *AJNR Am J Neuroradiol.* 1998;19:309-315.

[8]Link J, Brossmann J, Penselin V, et al. Common carotid artery bifurcation: preliminary results of CT angiography and color-coded duplex sonography compared with digital subtraction angiography. *AJR Am J Roentgenol.* 1997;168:361-365.

[9]Bray JM, Galland F, Lhoste P, et al. Colour Doppler and duplex sonography and angiography of the carotid artery bifurcations: prospective, double-blind study. *Neuroradiology.* 1995;37:219-224.

[10]Patel MR, Kuntz KM, Klufas RA, et al. Preoperative assessment of the carotid bifurcation. Can magnetic resonance angiography and duplex ultrasonography replace contrast arteriography? 1995;26:1753-1758.

[11]Bluth EI, Sunshine JH, Lyons JB, et al. Power Doppler imaging: initial evaluation as a screening examination for carotid artery stenosis. *Radiology.* 2000;215:791-800.

[12]Jackson MR, Chang AS, Robles HA, et al. Determination of 60% or greater carotid stenosis: a prospective comparison of magnetic resonance angiography and duplex ultrasound with conventional angiography. *Ann Vasc Surg.* 1998;12:236-243.

[13]Walters GK, Jones CE, Meyd CJ, et al. The role of carotid duplex ultrasonography in the therapeutic algorithm of extracranial carotid disease. *J Vasc Technol.* 1993;17:177-182.

TABLE A-9   Sensitivity and Specificity of Computed Tomographic Angiography as a Function of Degree of Carotid Stenosis

STUDY (YEAR)	DEGREE OF STENOSIS	CAROTIDS (*n*)	SENSITIVITY (%)	SPECIFICITY (%)
Anderson et al. (2000)[1]	Occlusion	80	69–100	98
Leclerc et al. (1999)[2]	Occlusion	44	100	100
Marcus et al. (1999)[3]	Occlusion	46	100	100
Verhoek et al. (1999)[4]	Occlusion	38	66–75	87–100
Magarelli et al. (1998)[5]	Occlusion	40	100	100
Link et al. (1997)[6]	Occlusion	56	100	100
Leclerc et al. (1995)[7]	Occlusion	39	100	100
Dillon et al. (1993)[8]	Occlusion	50	81–87.5	97–100
Schwartz et al. (1992)[9]	Occlusion	40	100	100
	Stenosis ≥ 80%	NA	NA	NA
Anderson et al. (2000)[1]	Stenosis ≥ 70%	80	67–77	84–92
Leclerc et al. (1999)[2]	Stenosis ≥ 70%	44	67–100	94–97
Marcus et al. (1999)[3]	Stenosis ≥ 70%	46	85–93	93–97
Verhoek et al. (1999)[4]	Stenosis ≥ 70%	38	80–100	95–100
Magarelli et al. (1998)[5]	Stenosis ≥ 70%	40	92	98.5
Link et al. (1997)[6]	Stenosis ≥ 70%	56	100	100
Leclerc et al. (1995)[7]	Stenosis ≥70%	39	87.5–100	96–100
Dillon et al. (1993)[8]	Stenosis ≥ 70%	50	81–82	94–95
Schwartz et al. (1992)[9]	Stenosis ≥ 70%	40	100	100
	Stenosis ≥ 60%	NA	NA	NA
Anderson et al. (2000)[1]	Stenosis ≥ 50%	80	85–90	82–91

NA, not available.

Modified from Long A, Lepoutre A, Corbillon E, et al. Critical review of non- or minimally invasive methods (duplex ultrasonography, MR- and CT-angiography) for evaluating stenosis of the proximal internal carotid artery. *Eur J Vasc Endovasc Surg.* 2002;24:43-52.

Studies cited in this table:

[1]Anderson GB, Ashforth R, Steinke DE, et al. CT angiography for the detection and characterization of carotid artery bifurcation disease. *Stroke.* 2000;31:2168-2174.

[2]Leclerc X, Godefroy O, Lucas C, et al. Internal carotid arterial stenosis: CT angiography with volume rendering. *Radiology.* 1999;210:673-682.

[3]Marcus CD, Ladam-Marcus VJ, Bigot JL, et al. Carotid arterial stenosis: evaluation at CT angiography with the volume-rendering technique. *Radiology.* 1999;211:775-780.

[4]Verhoek G, Costello P, Khoo EW, et al. Carotid bifurcation CT angiography: assessment of interactive volume rendering. *J Comput Assist Tomogr.* 1999;23:590-596.

[5]Magarelli N, Scarabino T, Simeone AL, et al. Carotid stenosis: a comparison between MR and spiral CT angiography. *Neuroradiology.* 1998;40:367-373.

[6]Link J, Brossmann J, Penselin V, et al. Common carotid artery bifurcation: preliminary results of CT angiography and color-coded duplex sonography compared with digital subtraction angiography. *AJR Am J Roentgenol.* 1997;168:361-365.

[7]Leclerc X, Godefroy O, Pruvo JP, et al. Computed tomographic angiography for the evaluation of carotid artery stenosis. *Stroke.* 1995;26:1577-1581.

[8]Dillon EH, van Leeuwen MS, Fernandez MA, et al. CT angiography: application to the evaluation of carotid artery stenosis. *Radiology.* 1993;189:211-219.

[9]Schwartz RB, Jones KM, LeClercq GT, et al. The value of cerebral angiography in predicting cerebral ischemia during carotid endarterectomy. *AJR Am J Roentgenol.* 1992;159:1057-1061.

INDEX

Page numbers followed by *f* indicate figures; *t*, tables; *b*, boxes.